CONTROVERSIES

in the

MENTAL HEALTH

PROFESSIONS

Edwin L. Herr, Ed.D.
Professor and Head
Division of Counseling and
 Educational Psychology and
 Career Studies
The Pennsylvania State University

Stanley H. Cramer, Ed.D.
Professor and Chair
Department of Counseling and
 Educational Psychology
University at Buffalo
State University of New York

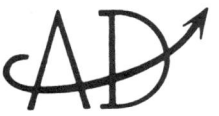 ACCELERATED DEVELOPMENT INC.
Publishers
Muncie, Indiana

CONTROVERSIES

In The Mental Health Professions

Library of Congress Number: 87-70347

International Standard Book Number: 0-915202-67-0

©Copyright 1987 by Accelerated Development Inc., Publishers

All rights reserved. No part of this book may be reproduced or transmitted in any form or by any means, electronic or mechanical, including photocopying, recording, or by an information storage and retrieval system, without permission in writing from Accelerated Development Inc.

Technical Development: Tanya Dalton
　　　　　　　　　　　　Judy McWilliams
　　　　　　　　　　　　Sheila Sheward

Cover Design: Tanya Dalton

ACCELERATED DEVELOPMENT Inc., PUBLISHERS
3400 Kilgore Avenue, Muncie, IN 47304
(317) 284-7511

DEDICATION

To Ruth McGonigal Herr (1907-) whose Irish legacy of love, resoluteness of spirit and high expectations has been a source of pride to her son for many decades. And to Pat, Amber, Chris, and Alicia whose love and support make writing possible.

To Mark, Naomi, Joel, and Marcia whose encouragement, caring and availability continue to make a crucial and happy difference to their brother and brother-in-law, Stan, through the years.

ACKNOWLEDGEMENTS

Although both the established and the emerging members of the mental health professions are young in total history, they have made major contributions to the quality of life, the productivity, and the personal dignity of many Americans. We appreciate the points of view of the authors and professional organizations reflected in these pages as well as the sincerity and the perspectives they represent. We hope our syntheses of such perspectives advances the understanding of the mental health professions of each other, demonstrates the importance of increased collaboration among them, and reaffirms their pride in being called "the helping professions."

We also acknowledge that the original idea for this book came from Dr. Joe Hollis and his late wife, Pat. We appreciate the patience and good will which was extended by Joe as we completed this effort.

Finally, we acknowledge the continuing clerical support in this project and others of three excellent "word processors": Marsha Bierly, Karen Homan, and Judy Kauffman. Thanks much.

PREFACE

Controversy *is* a basic factor in the helping professions. To a major extent the content of the helping professions *is* individual controversy, real or imagined. Persons come to mental health professionals because of conflicts with others, intrapsychic confusion, or controversies between possible behavioral options under consideration. However important those forms of controversy are to the individuals concerned and to the helping professionals who assist them, this is not the theme of this book.

The controversies which are at issue here are those which occur between different types of "helping professionals." Such controversies tend to divide or separate one group of mental health professionals from another group. They tend to create presumed status hierarchies, and territoriality, and have direct effects upon which helping professionals can help which type of client or consumer with what type of problem. The foci of these controversies, among other concerns, are theories espoused, language systems, treatments used, preparation, credentialling, and reimbursement. These classes of controversy will be treated in six major themes in this book. These include Theme One—"Identity for the Mental Health Professions" which will be covered in Chapters 1 through 4; Theme Two—"The Education and Training of Persons in the Helping Professions," Chapter 5; Theme Three—"Credentialing of Helpers," Chapter 6; Theme Four—"Ethical and Legal Standards in the Mental Health Professions," Chapter 7; Theme Five—"Controversies in the Techniques, Strategies, and Procedures of the Mental Health Professions," Chapter 8; and Theme Six,—"The Economics of the Helping Professions," Chapter 9. Within these themes major topical areas necessary to an understanding of the major controversies will be identified and examined from different points of view.

The rationale for discussing controversies among the mental health professions is not necessarily to resolve them. Rather it is to facilitate understanding by "helping professionals" of the central elements of some of the major issues which describe their field. Probably most of these controversies are not resolvable. Rather, they are realities which, if understood, can be accepted and worked around rather than being allowed to create tensions between mental health professionals without being understood. By definition, issues are controversies in which solutions are not easily found. Whether one speaks of controversies or issues they are ordinarily characterized by the presence of multiple factors which interrelate.

Without attempting to be exhaustive, in this book will be discussed elements of six major areas of controversy. In doing so, various lenses—historical, scientific, political, economic—will be used to demystify each controversy, to convert it from an abstract source of conflict among helping professionals to a dynamic whole comprised of parts which can be attributed differently to each of the separate occupations comprising the "helping professions." When appropriate, possible resolutions of the controversies addressed will be suggested; in other instances, where resolution is less a matter of some systematic action and more a matter of perceptual clarity, we will settle for a description of the elements of the controversy.

In conclusion, no historical period has been as complex or as demanding of mental health services and practitioners as is currently true. Yet, the realities of the mental health professions frequently fall short of their promise because of the competition and obstacles which tend to reduce the effectiveness of individual groups of practitioners and, as a result, the aggregate impact of the helping professions as a whole.

Edwin L. Herr

Stanley H. Cramer

CONTENTS

Dedication iii

Acknowledgements iv

Preface v

THEME ONE: IDENTITY FOR MENTAL HEALTH PROFESSIONS 1

1 THE MENTAL HEALTH PROFESSIONS—ISSUES OF IDENTITY 3

Who Are The Mental Health Professionals? 5

Psychiatrists 8
    Enter Freud 9
    Psychiatric Identity Crises 12
    Interprofessional Relationships 15

Clinical Psychologists 17
    Strangers in a Medical Culture 19
    The Provision of Psychotherapy 19
    Effectiveness of Clinical Psychologists 21
    Parity of Clinical Psychologists 21
    Perspectives on Competence 24

Counseling Psychologists 25
    Distinctions in Counseling and Clinical Psychology 26
    Blurring of the Uniqueness of Counseling Psychology 29

Clinical Social Workers 34
    Social Work 35
    Controversies in Definition 35
    Social Conditions and Human Behavior 37
    The Evolution of Social Work 37
    Current Trends 39
    Professional Controversies 40

Psychiatric Nurses 43
    Psychiatric Nurse Standards 45
    Seeds of Controversy 46
    Nurse-Physician Relationships 47
    Community Mental Health 49

Summary 51

2 NON-CORE MENTAL HEALTH PROVIDERS 53

Professional Counselors 53
    Efforts to Become Core Providers 55
    Certification of Professional Counselors and Their Training 56
    Some Historical Perspectives 58
    Current Controversies 60
    Emergence of Professional Validation 61

Family Therapists 62
    Controversies with Other Groups 63

Summary 66

3 ARE THE HELPING PROFESSIONS, PROFESSIONS? 67

Criteria of a Profession 68
    Knowledge Base 68
    Community Interests versus Self-Interests 69
    Authority or Regulation of Practitioner Behavior 70
    Community Sanction 72
    A Culture 72
    System of Rewards Symbolic of Work Achievement 73

Conclusion 74

4 THE ULTIMATE QUESTION OF PROFESSIONAL IDENTITY: WHAT IS MENTAL HEALTH AND WHO SHOULD PROVIDE IT? 75

Nature of Mental Illness 76
Perspectives of DSM-III 77
Opponents of Mental Illness 79
Health and Wellness 84

Professional Identity: A Reprise 86

THEME TWO: EDUCATION AND TRAINING 89

5 THE EDUCATION AND TRAINING OF PERSONS IN THE MENTAL HEALTH PROFESSIONS 91

Medical Model and Education of Mental Health Workers 93

Scientist-Practitioner Versus Practitioner 94

Clinical Versus Counseling Psychology 98

Differences In Training 100
    One Orientation or Multi-Orientation 100
    Tools of the Trade 100

Specialization 102
    Gerontology 103
    Cross-Cultural Counseling 103
    Sexual Orientation, Sexuality, and Gender 104
    Substance Abuse 105
    Fringe Therapies 106
    Family Therapy 107

Desirable Helper Characteristics 108

Personal Therapy In Training 110

In-Service Training 111

Social Work Concerns 113

Issues In The Education Of Psychiatric Nurses 115

Sub-Doctoral Training 115

Internship Experience 116

Summary 119

THEME THREE: CREDENTIALING OF PROFESSIONALS 119

6 THE CREDENTIALING OF MENTAL HEALTH PROFESSIONALS 121

Individual Credentialing 123
    Licensure 123
    Certification 127
    Registry/Registration 128

Program Credentialing 129

Credentialing And The Helping Professions 130
    Differences in Educational Requirements for Credentialing 130
    Content of Training 134
    Education, Competence, Both? 138
    Competence 139
    Scope of Practice 142

Credentialing For Consumer Protection *146*

Summary *151*

THEME FOUR: ETHICAL AND LEGAL STANDARDS 153

7 LEGAL AND ETHICAL ISSUES IN THE HELPING PROFESSIONS 155

Terminology *156*

Right To Treatment Or Habilitation *158*

Informed Consent *160*

Research Use Of Clients *162*

Sexual Misconduct *163*

Duty To Warn Or Inform *165*

Confidentiality *167*

Value Conflicts *168*

Training In Legal And Ethical Aspects Of Helping *172*

Additional Resources *173*

THEME FIVE: TECHNIQUES, STRATEGIES, AND PROCEDURES 175

8 CONTROVERSIES IN TECHNIQUES, STRATEGIES, AND PROCEDURES OF THE HELPING PROFESSIONS 177

Social Science Paradigm *178*

Methods Of Studying Persons *182*
    Clinical Assessment *183*
    Psychometric versus Psychodiagnostic Tradition *185*
    DSM-III *190*
    Psychobiological Assessment *193*
    Test Bias and Cross-Cultural Assessment *196*
    Test Bias *199*

Cross-Cultural Counseling And Therapy *204*
    Cross-Cultural Implications of Counseling and Psychotherapy Models *205*

Culture-Bound Theories and Techniques in a Land of Immigrants *207*
Instances of Cultural Diversity *210*
Roots of Intercultural Diversity *211*
Transportability of Models of Counseling and Therapy Across Cultures *214*

Conclusion *216*

THEME SIX: ECONOMICS 217

9 THE ECONOMICS OF THE HELPING PROFESSIONS 219

Fee Setting In Private Practice *220*
Fee as a Therapeutic Issue *222*
Fee in the Counseling Relationship *223*
Medical-Nonmedical Practitioner Fees *228*

Third-Party Payment *228*
Third-Party Payers *229*
Does Third-Party Payment Increase Consumption of Mental
  Health Services? *231*
Will the Poor Benefit from Third-Party Payments? *235*
Who Pays? *237*
Is Psychology a Health Profession? *239*
Third-Party Recognitions of Psychological Services *242*
HMOs, PPOs and DRGs *245*

Cost-Effectiveness *251*
Health Care-Mental Health Care: Separate or Integral? *252*
Results of Cost-Benefit Analyses *252*
Quality of Cost-Benefit Analyses *259*
Lack of Studies of Comparative Effectiveness of Therapy *259*
Productiveness of Various Types of Mental Health Services *262*

Conclusion *266*

Bibliography 271

Index 299

About the Authors 313

THEME ONE: IDENTITY FOR MENTAL HEALTH PROFESSIONS

CHAPTER 1

THE MENTAL HEALTH PROFESSIONS— ISSUES OF IDENTITY

Formalized occupations designed to "treat" or "prevent" emotional psychological, or mental disorders are relatively new in human history. Captured by a euphemism such as the "helping professions," or, perhaps more explicitly, the mental health professions, these occupations are at their oldest probably not more than a century and a half old and in several cases, less than that, coming into being only 40 or 50 years ago.

Part of the basic controversy in the helping professions is, what occupations should be included? Another question concerns which of the occupations among the "helping professions" can claim professional status, by what criteria and under what conditions? A further important question has to do with the degree to which the various occupations defined as part of the helping professions actually overlap in purposes, skills, and preparation. Finally, a basic question is about the characteristics of the behavioral domain in which the helping professions work. Questions of relevance include the following: Are mental illness and mental health simply the opposite sides of the same coin? Is there, in fact, a continuum from wellness to dysfunction along which various of the helping professions can be aligned? Unless answers can be found to such questions, it is difficult, if not impossible, to address other important questions. For example, who ought to provide help and why? Who ought to get help and how?

The controversies cited above will be addressed in this and the three chapters which follow. These comprise the elements of Theme One, the controversy centered in the issue of identity for the mental health professions.

Hurst and Parker (1977) have noted two major functions which a title or, more specifically, a professional identity serves. First, a coherent, well developed identity serves to delimit what is and is not done by those who belong to the profession. As such, clarity of professional identity serves to accurately project or communicate to those outside the profession what can be expected from the profession and from individuals who belong to it. In addition, delimiting the profession acts to shape the roles and activities of its members. A further function of a title of identity is that it serves to distinguish specialties within a profession.

Identity is, in large measure, a function of history and its evolution of claims to competence in particular areas, a language system, and theoretical models. While such matters are essential to establish professional credibility with the users of one's services and with other professions from and to whom one might make referrals, inherent in these elements of identity formation are political factors as well. The characteristics and the timing of an occupational or professional identity is a form of leverage used by professional associations to create the boundaries within which its members may perform their services and the rationale by which to exclude other specialists from performing the same services. Thus, identity issues are at once political and the stuff of controversy among the mental health professions. As emerging professional groups test the boundaries of the professional identities of an older professional group the identities of both groups are subtly shaped and reshaped. Sooner or later issues of territoriality, conflict, and controversy will erupt as assaults on the professional identity of one group by another become too threatening in conceptual, political, or economic terms.

In Chapter 1 are examined the professional identities claimed by different occupations described as the "Core Providers" among the mental health service providers. More important, perhaps, attempts will be made to isolate some of the points of tension and controversy which pervade identity issues among these groups.

WHO ARE THE MENTAL HEALTH PROFESSIONALS?

A fundamental, if not primary, controversy among the "helping professions" is who should be included? What criteria should define such inclusion? Obviously, the occupations included in the mental health professions vary depending upon the criteria used. If one means those occupations the practitioners of which are eligible for financial reimbursement from insurance companies and other third party payers for mental health services delivered, either three or four groups are typically included. The standard groups are psychiatrists, psychologists (usually clinical and counseling), and social workers. However, increasingly psychiatric nurses are considered one of the major "helping professions" eligible for third party payment. By other governmental definitions including training support from the National Institute of Mental Health and various pieces of mental health legislation, these four groups—psychiatrists, clinical/counseling psychologists, clinical social workers, and psychiatric nurses are frequently referred to as "core providers," a term to which we will return when we discuss third party reimbursement more fully later. The origin of the term "core provider" in Federal mental health policy is somewhat obscure and, indeed, it is not the official term embraced by such professional organizations as the American Psychological Association which prefers the term Qualified Mental Health Professional (QMHP). Nevertheless, the term "Core Provider" connotes a conventionally accepted status which will be useful for our purposes here.

Some mental health occupations are usually not attributed core provider status; even so, these groups can legitimately be considered part of the "Helping Professions." These are mental health counselors who are currently the object of proposed legislation amending the Social Security Act which would given them "fifth core provider" status and eligibility for certain types of insurance reimbursement when they render services to clients covered by such plans. Other occupational groups which are ordinarily considered to be part of the "helping professions" are marriage and family therapists, school psychologists, rehabilitation counselors, school (guidance) counselors and employment and/or career counselors. While the latter groups are not typically included under Federal definitions as core providers, eligible, as health care (meaning Mental Health care) providers, for reimbursement under Federal programs (e.g., CHAMPUS, Social Security) as independent mental health practitioners, they may be eligible in certain states for such reimbursement and for licensure as an independent mental health practitioner.

Implicit in the notions of "core provider," independent practitioner, mental health delivery, third party reimbursement are many different issues. One of them is economic. If you belong to an occupation defined as a "core provider" of mental services and you are, in addition, eligible for licensure as an independent practitioner in a state, then you can provide services to clients who can in turn pay for them through various health care or insurance plans. As a result, your access to substantial reimbursement for your services is significantly different from that of a practitioner who can only be reimbursed through fees paid from the client's personal resources. When clients of patients can use insurance or health care funds to pay for psychological services, they are less reluctant and perhaps more able to purchase such services than when one can only use funds from private resources. Thus, in one sense the mental health specialist who is eligible for "third party payment" is more likely to be able to survive in independent or private practice than is a mental health specialist who is not eligible for such funds. The latter are more likely to be found as an employee of some institution in which the delivery of counseling and psychotherapy may or may not be a major organizational mission.

But the issue of third party payment or core provider does not stop with independent practice and eligibility for certain types of reimbursement, it also affects agencies whose principle income is derived from health plans and insurance payments. In order to receive payment for services delivered, frequently these agencies must certify to funding agencies the type of practitioner delivering the services for which payment is received. In short, such persons must be "core providers" or, qualified Mental Health Professionals in some states, eligible for particular credentials/licenses, or they can not be employed in such agencies. In these cases, then, the economic effects upon practitioners may not be as direct as when one is in independent practice as a psychiatrist, psychologist, or clinical social worker but the indirect effect is essentially the same: limited employment opportunities in agencies and reduced income.

A third major issue implicit in core provider status or in licensure is independence of action. As suggested above, a mental health professional eligible for a license in a state as a psychologist or clinical social worker or other mental health specialist can engage in private or independent practice in the same fashion as can a physician, dentist, or attorney. One who is not a core provider or without an adequate credential to engage in private practice is relegated to a status which requires supervision by a person who is so credentialed. Obviously, this imposes a hierarchial status structure among persons in the helping professions depending upon occupational affiliation, training type and level, and other criteria. Such policies also increase the cost of providing mental health services.

The issue of supervision and status is not as cleanly defined as has just been described. For example, rehabilitation counselors, school counselors, and employment service counselors tend to act quite independently within the governmental or educational institutions in which they are employed. They may or may not have intensive supervision and they may engage in many of the same functions or processes as "core providers" or licensed mental health specialists. However, school, rehabilitation, and employment counselors in government agencies and educational institutions tend not to be involved with situations in which the principal source of income is insurance or health plans. They often do not purport to be delivering mental health services, although they probably are in at least part of their responsibilities, and they are typically seen as functionaries whose services tend to be only part of a larger program of education, rehabilitation, or employment and training.

Undoubtedly, then, several of the issues related to the matter of identity among the mental health professions have to do with economics, status, freedom of action, and setting in which the individual specialist is employed. But, however important these are, they do not explain all of the controversy. Indeed, in order to do so, it is useful to consider the independent occupational groups, their history, theoretical roots, and purposes as they define them. It is also important to note what might be described as *the dichotomy between medical or biological approaches versus psychological approaches to mental health or mental illness* as seen from the vantage point of different helping professions. The roots of the controversies which reside in this dichotomy tend to be best seen against the history of psychiatry.

PSYCHIATRISTS

Perhaps in the developed nations, psychiatry is seen as the foremost and most authoritative of the "helping" occupations. With the exception of psychiatric nursing, psychiatry is the only one of the mental health professions to have its origins in physical medicine. Since a psychiatrist must first complete medical training before engaging in psychiatric training, the psychiatrist brings to the analysis of any mental health problem, a unique view of body-mind interaction, the dualism between the soma (body) and psyche (mind) in the etiology (causation) of mental disorders. In the resolution of such disorders, the psychiatrist, as M.D. or physician, can prescribe psychotropic and other forms of medication as a treatment strategy. In general, no other occupational group among the helping professionals can do so.

The origins of psychiatry in medicine tend to confer a status, an authority, as viewed by consumers of mental health services or treatment not enjoyed by other "helping professionals," but this is not to suggest that psychiatry is free of controversy or viewed unequivocally as the most effective of the helping professions.

One of the controversies in which psychiatry is concerned is precisely the degree to which mental illness is physical, chemical, or organic as opposed to psychological or sociocultural. Is mental illness a "disease entity" or is it primarily a problem of skill deficits, poor socialization, and inappropriate cognitions about or labels of life events? Obviously, the way one answers such questions implies differences in treatment strategies emphasizing different balances of chemical or psychological interventions. A number of observers criticize psychiatrists for being too quick and too persistent with medications which reduce symptoms but at the same time mask underlying problems. It is certainly a frequent claim of psychologists that chemical interventions and medications tend often to prolong psychiatric problems and, therefore, that psychologists who deal primarily with the emotional and perceptual, rather than the organic, aspects of mental disorders, are more effective because they can uncover and deal with the underlying causes of the mental disorder rather than the visible manifestations, symbols, or symptoms.

While for purposes of understanding a controversy, one can lapse into dichotomous and, indeed, overly simplistic thinking about mental illness, several observations seem in order. One is that increasingly, research in brain chemistry is implicating physiological factors in many forms of mental illness and addictive disorders. As such factors unfold, more clearly becomes the concept that without the long-term management of appropriate medications, the likelihood of relief or cure based purely on insight or "talking" approaches to mental disorders is not likely. Some balance of chemical intervention and psychotherapy is necessary for treatment success to occur among some forms of mental disorders.

At issue in such controversies is the state of research findings about comparative etiologies and differential treatments related to the large number of mental disorders present in the population. Which are organic, which are functional, which are a function of endogenous or exogenous toxic agents? Which classes of problems require which type of treatment in what combination? While significant research and training strides are occurring in addressing such issues, such knowledge is not always present in the understanding and behavioral repertoire of each "helping professional" whether psychiatrist or psychologist or other mental health specialist.

A related issue concerning psychiatry is a residual of its history from a somewhat different vantage point. From its earliest origins until at least the late 19th and early 20th centuries, psychiatry was preoccupied with the most severe of the emotional and mental disorders. Its primary focus has been psychopathology as it evolves from the original conceptions of demonic possession as the cause of insanity to other views of the origins of the most bizarre and aberrant of human mental disorders. In parallel with such foci has been the use in psychiatry of historical emphases on the most drastic of therapies: lobotomy, electro shock and convulsive therapy, and insulin shock.

Within such a context, psychiatry has been criticized for insufficient attention to the differences *in kind* of abnormal and normal behavior or of imputing a label of mental illness or defectiveness to behavior which is, in fact, explained by social or cultural distinctiveness not mental aberration, thereby causing persons to label themselves as "sick" in order to obtain access to mental health services.

Enter Freud

Undoubtedly one of the most important contributions to the current provision of psychiatric therapy is the psychoanalytic theory of Sigmund Freud. In its totality, Freud's theories represented a personality paradigm in which the effects of the unconscious and historically repressed material upon current behavior provided a comprehensive explanatory alternative to demonic and purely organic views of mental disorders. It moved psychiatry from an emphasis on descriptions of mental illness to an era of interpretation as a base for treatment. In addition, Freud provided a treatment approach involving free association, dream analysis, interpretation of resistance and transference and related techniques which has become perhaps the most classic and the most frequently used psychological approach by psychiatrists. Psychoanalysis has emphasized the importance of the patient, not just the sickness, and the relationship between the psychiatrist and the patient. In this sense, it has had important humanizing effects upon medicine. Combined with the insights of such neo-Freudians as Harry Stack Sullivan and Adolf Meyer, psychoanalytic traditions have stimulated practitioners to listen and try to understand the suffering of their patients, treat personal biography as an essential aspect of illness, and recognize the important clinical implications that result from the meaning the symptoms and treatments hold for the patient (Manschreck & Kleinman, 1979, p. 167).

While perhaps stereotypical, the degree to which psychiatry and the use of psychoanalysis as the psychological treatment of preference are seen as interchangeable, causes other mental health professionals to view psychiatrists as having a limited and, perhaps, outdated vision of psychological treatment. This perspective arises from several factors: First, psychoanalysis is a lengthy and expensive process typically lasting years. Many patients are not able for reasons of money, time, or the etiology of their presenting problem to engage in such a process. Second, the research base of psychoanalysis as compared with other more recent psychological treatments is minimal. Therefore, its opponents contend that psychoanalysis is primarily conjecture rather than scientific or empirical in its validation. Third, as compared with other "helping professions," psychiatrists tend to have less training in psychological explanations of behavior and more on chemical or organic explanations than do other mental health specialists. More will be said about this matter later.

Another interesting criticism of psychiatry (Neill & Ludwig, 1980) is that while until the 1950s and early 1960s, psychiatry had a virtual monopoly on the only "scientific" form of psychotherapy—psychodynamic or psychoanalytic therapy—the meaning, definition, and use of psychotherapy has undergone important transformations in the past two decades which have left many psychiatrists "puzzled, threatened, and angry" (p. 39).

Neill and Ludwig suggested that this transformation has taken place in four important respects.

> First, there has been a shift from viewing psychotherapy as a body of technique to seeing it as a social function. Second, social metaphors have supplanted biological metaphors in the understanding and treatment of mental illness. Consequently, there is a growing consensus that therapeutic transaction or function is pedagogic (i.e., educational) rather than medical in nature. Third, the newer forms of therapy which embody this change in conceptualization are largely incompatible with medical training and etiquette (e.g., equalitarian relationships, treatment of groups). Fourth, there is an increased reliance on this pedagogy as a major source of contemporary values and ethical prescriptions for middle class (i.e., affluent) individuals. These are the changes that have largely undermined the seemingly generic connection between psychiatry and psychotherapy. (p. 39-40)

As these transformations have occurred, one might contend that the provision of psychotherapy has become democratized as the fundamental conceptualization of mental illness has moved from a medical to a behavioral locus. Simultaneously, the term psychotherapy is less and less used to signify a particular theory or process and is increasingly used as an omnibus term embracing a large array of psychotherapeutic interventions. As such interventions find their roots in learning or other behavioral theory rather than in medical, chemical, or organic approaches, the likelihood grows that non-medically trained persons can be seen as having validity as competent professionals in various mental health areas. Also the probability is raised that psychiatrists and other members of the mental health professions are viewing mental illness, symptomology, and behavior in general through different lenses or explanatory systems. In the process, effective communication is reduced, and mistrust as well as allegations of incompetence tend to grow among psychiatrists and others.

Neill and Ludwig suggested that the growing differentiation of psychiatrists and other helping professionals tends to result from several classes of events. For example, through the early 1940s, psychiatry reigned supreme over psychotherapeutics as a result of winning three crucial historical battles: the battle for medicalization of psychotherapeutics (1870 to 1910); the battle for psychiatric monopoly of psychotherapeutics (1890 to 1930) and the battle for medicalization of psychoanalysis (1920 to 1940). As a result of these battles, psychiatry had viewed itself as having "won the day and essentially being in control of the conduct and perspectives defining psychotherapy." However, in the ensuing thirty years three important "revolutions," social or scientific in nature, arose in rapid succession to alter psychiatric perogatives: The psychopharmacological revolution (about 1955), the growing importance of clinical applied learning theory and behaviorism (about 1960) and the community mental health movement (about 1965).

Psychiatry is at odds with other helping professions and, indeed, with broad social mandates for several reasons which go beyond those cited above. A major issue is economic and that concern emanates from the duration and frequency of psychiatric visits by patients. Within this context, whether psychiatrists work within Community Health Centers or in private practice, the principal mode of treatment is one to one psychotherapy of fairly long duration and of high frequency. As compared to group therapy, for example, individual therapy is considerably more expensive. The actual frequency of psychiatric visits tends to depend upon whether the psychiatrist uses psychoanalysis or a non-psychoanalytic form of psychotherapy. Lebensohn (1978) reporting on the results of a 1973 national study indicated that the average number of psychotherapy visits per year for nonanalytic patients was 38, somewhat lower if adjunctive chemotherapy was used, and 140 for analytic patients. At the currently prevailing rates of $50 to $70 and more per hour of treatment, psychoanalytic treatment would cost $7,000 to nearly $18,000 per patient. Nonanalytic psychotherapy is less expensive but on the basis of an average of 38 visits per year at prevailing rates would still cost $1,900 to nearly $2,700 per year. Such figures do not include any costs of hospitalization or other inpatient care or medication. These are only the costs of outpatient or private psychiatric care exclusive of medication.

When the costs of psychiatric care are considered within the context of national health insurance or other third party payments, pressures for briefer forms of psychotherapy, group modes of therapy, or other configurations of the teaming of psychiatrists with non-medical, non-psychiatric professionals increase. Such pressures also exacerbate the defensiveness and tensions between psychiatrists and other helping professionals as issues of therapeutic outcomes and cost-effectiveness become major concerns not only within the helping professions but also in Federal and State Mental health policies.

Psychiatric Identity Crises

What is implicit in much of the above is made explicit by Manschreck and Kleinman (1979): Psychiatry has its own identity crisis.

The ingredients of this crisis take many forms: the psychiatry domain has become diffuse, involving an increasingly wider spectrum of human activity;

> Psychiatry's knowledge base has remained small compared with other medical specialties; too few psychiatrists are engaged in research, and little money is being spent to prepare younger investigators for the demands of psychiatry's growth; the traditional sources of psychiatric identity—psychoanalytic theory and medical descriptive psychiatry—have themselves come under attack. In particular, the persistent 'absence of rigorous and empirical testing of psychoanalytic theory has alienated behavioral scientists and nonpsychiatric physicians to the point that, increasingly, psychiatry is either ignored or denigrated. (p. 166)

Manschreck and Kleinman go on to contend that separate areas of psychiatric activity have developed within narrowly conceived frames of reference "resulting in multiple partial identities" "each of which has its own rules, terminology, data, and a theoretical overgrowth that has obscured its empirical foundations. . ." Hence, we have the "special psychiatries": the psychoanalytic, biologic, social, and community. . . "Psychiatry has become an undisciplined discipline, unable to capitalize on potential intra and interdisciplinary research and to respond to increasing demands for psychiatric services" (p. 169). They contended that an urgent need exists to define a general identity anew which requires, in turn, at least three features: (a) a common language and procedure for assessing psychopathology, (b) a common method for evaluations and use of knowledge from outside psychiatry and (c) a common set of values regarding clinical and research activities (p. 167).

Abroms (1983) extended the discussion of psychiatry's identity crisis by contending that, "one of the major tasks facing contemporary psychiatry is finding a paradigm that retains the valuable contribution of psychoanalysis but that places it in the context of a more comprehensive account of mental illness. Such paradigm must make sense of multiple etiologies and treatments, particularly the combined use of psychoactive drugs, individual dynamic therapy, behavior modification, and family, group, and milieu approaches" (p. 740). Abroms argued that the leading candidate around which to organize such a paradigm for psychiatry is "biopsychosocial eclecticism."

Biopsychosocial eclecticism links biological, psychological, and social determinants in the development of psychiatric disorders and, thus, indicates that the optimal treatment involves interventions in each of these areas. Using a general systems theory model, the biopsychosocial approach arranges the variables implicated in psychiatric disorders in a hierarchy ranging from the micro level of biochemical molecular processes to the macro level of sociocultural events. The assumption is that since each of these levels is interconnected, each may require intervention of some type and that in so doing will result in effects on other levels.

Put somewhat differently, if cognitive and affective stability and productivity are expected to result from psychiatric or other forms of psychosocial treatment, they must rest on a base of biological normality: mood, cognition, and other elements of neurophysiology must be in good working order. Against this context, Abroms (1983) recommended that one view the three forms of perspective and associated treatments as follows:

> The biological perspective looks at disturbed thinking, feeling, and behaving as symptomatic expressions of disturbed neurophysiology. Treatment in this mode involves a medical intervention, such as a drug, or an implanted electrode, aimed at modifying the underlying physical causes. The psychosocial perspective regards disturbed thinking, feeling, and behaving as expressions of faulty learning leading to maturational failure in mating, working, and socializing. Treatment, whether psychotherapy, family therapy, or group process aims to provide new learning to overcome developmental failure through corrective interpersonal relationships and social conditions. Here one operates less in the realm of causes and symptoms than of influences and immaturities. In the existential-moral perspective, what has previously been described by Abroms as social-cultural, one goes beyond causes, symptoms, influences, and immaturities into a realm of pure value, where the ultimate aim is the integrity of the person..... What this amounts to is healing one's character flaws and, in the process, developing a set of guiding ideals about medical, psychological, and moral health that give meaning to life. (p. 743)

Worth noting is that, however enlightened and hopeful such a paradigm is as a way to bring together psychiatry's roots and its current theoretical commitments, psychiatrists trained under different or more unidimensional models are likely to be in controversy with each other about the validity of such an identity for themselves. In addition, the further psychiatry departs from a biological perspective into a psychological and, indeed, moral-existential perspective the more overlap occurs in treatment and identity with other members of the "helping professions" who are trying to establish professional identities unique to themselves.

Given the demands upon psychiatry for service, the lucrative economic context in which it operates, the assaults upon its theoretical and empirical integrity and its fundamental identity crisis, then the existence of controversy between psychiatry and other mental health professions is not surprising. A major focus of such conflicts lies in the interactions between psychiatrists and psychologists. At stake, among other possibilities, are hospital privileges, third-party reimbursement, professional autonomy, and prestige in the eyes of the public (Gabbard & Smith, 1982).

Interprofessional Relationships

According to Gabbard and Smith, issues of power and economics are reality issues but the conflicts between psychiatrists and psychologists "are not determined solely by social and economic conditions... to understand the origins of interdisciplinary conflict, one must look beyond societal inequities to the intrapsychic and interpersonal dynamics which develop in the interprofessional relations between psychiatrists and psychologists early in their careers" (p. 203). While the separate models of training of the various helping professions will be discussed at some length later in this book, the point at issue here is that early contacts with one's fellow mental health professionals "leave lasting effects which lay the seeds of future problems and kindle the fires of conflict" (p. 203).

Gabbard and Smith (1982) effectively portray the psychodynamics which attend the possible interaction between the beginning psychiatric resident and the psychologist trainee as they encounter each other as they participate in the hospital team. For example, they observe that,

> The resident may, in fact, know very little about the actual training experience of the psychologists with whom he is working and may know even less about his attitude and philosophy concerning interdisciplinary collaboration in diagnoses and treatment. This lack of information (characteristic of psychology trainees as well) is a crucial point. A variety of assumptions are made by the resident and by the psychology trainee about the other's knowledge, view of himself, and attitude toward other mental health disciplines... This ambience of ambiguity, poor communication and inadequate personal and professional knowledge of one's colleague provides a fertile field for the development of projection in the interactions between the two disciplines. (p. 204)

The authors also described how the psychiatric resident's self esteem may be threatened by the psychological intern's impressive display of psychological knowledge about test data, research, and diagnostic formulations. The resident's envy and competitiveness may cause him/her to devalue the psychologist's "contribution as an ancillary service such as laboratory data;" or may, if threatened, choose to fight back by speaking 'medicalise' conveying to the psychological intern that the resident has 'his own territory and his own technical jargon which is unique to his background and training;' or, if in awe, the resident may uncritically accept everything the psychologist says thereby deskilling himself and devaluing his own training and knowledge."

On the other hand, the psychologist intern is likely to immediately face the hierarchial structure of authority in the hospital unit in which the M.D. is clearly in charge of treatment and must countersign all documents containing diagnoses in the hospital chart.

> The psychologist may view the psychiatric resident as a neophyte, who has had much less formal education in the area of personality theory, psychopathology, and psychotherapeutic intervention even though the resident is in charge of the patients and has ultimate responsibility for the making of decisions, how daily transference is formed, and the one with whom the primary therapeutic alliance is established.... The psychology intern is likely to envy this authority and to feel that it is unfair to be in a position of lesser authority and responsibility and one where his relationships with the patient is more peripheral, less intense, and less important to the patient. As a result, the psychological intern may react in one of several ways: try to upstage the resident and look more knowledgeable, take a persistent devil's advocate position about anything the resident may propose, become overtly or covertly antagonistic to the resident as a result of displacing his anger at society's values and reimbursement patterns or comply with the resident's wishes but passive aggressively undermine his assigned task to complicate the physician's role. (p. 204)

Gabbard and Smith posited that what these behaviors really suggest is that "each truly wishes to impress the other, to win his colleague's approval and to be appreciated for his or her contribution." However, within the group context of the hospital team interpersonal and intrapsychic wishes and dynamics are likely to be activated which intensify exponentially. As a result, all sorts of prejudices, envy and competitiveness are likely to occur as a result of projective identification and carry a residual into future relationships and interdisciplinary rivalries. Indeed, this kind of scenario between the psychiatric resident and the psychological intern, typically a clinical psychologist, is not unlike that which occurs in different circumstances among other mental health professionals or other members of the helping professions. Within this context, a useful procedure is to consider some of the professional histories and dynamics of each of these. In the next section, we will consider Clinical Psychologists.

CLINICAL PSYCHOLOGISTS

In historical terms, the controversies among helping professionals are most boldly seen in the interactions between psychiatry and clinical psychology. Issues of power, status, reimbursement, superiority-subordination, professional imperialism each are ingredients of the tensions and conflicts between psychiatry and clinical psychology which have accompanied the birth and evolution of the latter in the United States. In the previous section, Gabbard and Smith spoke of the problems likely to occur for psychiatric residents and psychological interns upon their first encounters in a medical setting. The scenario they portrayed of the projective identification and other psychodynamics experienced by the psychiatric resident and the psychological intern are microcosms of the continuing turmoil which has surrounded relationships between psychiatry and clinical psychology.

The term clinical psychologist is attributed to Witmer in his development of the first psychology clinic at the University of Pennsylvania in 1886. Clinical psychologists began to play a visible role in World War I in the administration of Army Alpha and Beta examinations for the screening and classification of inductees. The American Association of Clinical Psychologists was founded in 1917 as the first professional organization for such specialists and it tended to accept the role of clinical psychology as an auxiliary one to psychiatry, not engaged in psychotherapeutics but rather concerned with testing, vocational and educational counseling (Neill & Ludwig, 1980).

According to Sarason (1981), among others, modern clinical psychology was a direct result of the Second World War. As the psychological casualties of the war grew in number and the "ripple effects" of prolonged war, uncertainty, and fear among people at home, extended absences between husbands, boyfriends, or sons and their families became apparent, the need for mental health services became increasingly visible. However, insufficient numbers of psychiatrists were available to meet these needs and relatively few other mental health specialists could be pressed into service.

Thus, in the mid 1940s an interaction arose between the Veterans Administration which needed to provide mental health services to veterans, University medical centers and, particularly, departments of psychiatry, and the National Institute of Mental Health which, in effect, ushered in a new Age of Mental Health (Sarason, 1977).

One of the early aspects of this period was a crash program to train more mental health professionals. Another was the provision of basic research about the causes and treatment of personal disorders. A third was a national mental health policy which provided funds for mental health services, training, and research.

As might be expected at such a historical moment, psychiatrists dominated the formulation of mental health policy for the nation and the allocation of funds by the National Institute of Mental Health (NIMH) to meet policy goals. As part of this milieu, current directions in clinical psychology were shaped. Before World War II, clinical psychology was virtually non-existent in any organized sense. Psychology was primarily academic in orientation and not particularly interested in the provision of clinical services beyond the problem of research and measurement of individual characteristics which were inherent in such situations. In Sarason's perspectives (1981), "psychology had no experience with what was involved in training clinical psychologists, with the creation of settings for clinical practice, and with the culture of existing settings devoted to the clinical scene" (p. 831).

When psychology decided to enter the clinical scene in a major way after World War II it was cordially received by psychiatry because it brought with it research traditions and methodologies not inherent in psychiatry itself. Such functions in addition to diagnostic insights and testing skills deriving from academic research psychology were seen as useful adjuncts to psychiatry. Psychiatry embraced clinical psychology because its own power as part of the medical establishment and within the broad definitions of national health policy were seen by the psychiatric establishment as basically unassailable. Such power was further reinforced by psychiatric stimulation of the criteria for NIMH training grants for clinical psychologists requiring that the latter obtain their field based training in medical-psychiatric settings.

By accepting such NIMH training criteria, clinical psychology's directions were shaped in several ways. One, the training and orientation would be essentially that of a medical model concerned with the severest of emotional disorders and psychopathology. Second, clinical psychologists would operate in a medical setting and culture which was run by and for medical personnel. Non-medical personnel were tolerated as they discharged their particular specialties but these were seen as adjunctive to medical procedures and perspectives. Non-medical personnel could not expect to aspire to the power, status, or financial reimbursements accorded to physicians.

Strangers in a Medical Culture

In a sense, clinical psychologists became strangers in a medical culture which was not of their own making and in which they were seen as subordinate to psychiatrists. They were, in addition, captives in an individual psychology of abnormal behavior in which they were expected to test and, possibly diagnose, but not treat except under the supervision of the psychiatrist.

In essence, in this process two different cultures were amalgamated without systematic concern about such differences: that of the medical-psychiatric world in which empiricism and research were less essential than clinical skills and defined power hierarchies were central to the professional structure which existed; and, that of the academic world of psychology in which autonomy and unfettered pursuit of knowledge through research were central values. It was not long until such value sets were in conflict as clinical psychology began to settle into the realities of the professional niche it had carved for itself within an essentially medically dominated culture.

The Provision of Psychotherapy

One of the early and major conflicts between psychiatry and clinical psychology had to do with the provision of psychotherapy. Until the publication of Carl Roger's book, *Counseling and Psychotherapy,* in 1942, psychotherapy and psychoanalysis or other psychodynamic therapies were seen essentially as synonymous. Roger's book disrupted this view and stimulated the perspective that psychotherapy did not need to be seen in medical terms or be provided by medical practitioners. It made a major impact, which Freud's attempt to advocate lay analysts did not, in its suggestion that counseling and psychotherapy were essentially the same and as such were not the exclusive perogatives of medicine and psychiatry. Within this context, psychiatrists were hoisted on another of their own petards vis à vis clinical psychologists. Psychiatrists had argued the need for large numbers of clinical psychologists to meet the overwhelming needs for mental health services in medical settings. In the face of the wide acceptance of Roger's perspectives could they deny clinical psychologists a treatment role in the provision of psychotherapy? They tried but ultimately failed to do so only after the American Psychological Association and the American Psychiatric Association fought each other in the courts, the legislatures, and the executive branches of state and federal governments. These fights were about who owned psychotherapy, the ability of clinical psychologists to function independent practice, to be seen as "core providers," and to receive third party payment without doing so under psychiatric supervision. These were battles fought in terms of credentialing and licensure, quality standards, protection of the public welfare, and related matters. Obviously they were also battles fought about power, status, and identity. Clinical psychologists were attempting to establish that they were unique in their contributions to mental health and at the same time as good as psychiatrists in providing such services; they were trying to create a level of professional parity.

Clinical psychologists rebelled against the domination of psychiatry, its perceived turfdom, and its use of political processes (e.g., lobbying and other forms of influence) to keep clinical psychology in a subordinate role professionally and, therefore, economically. What is, of course, fascinating and the stuff of controversy is that clinical psychology has in more recent times sometimes resorted to the same behavior in its relationship to counseling psychology and to other groups identified with the provision of mental health services. Clinical psychology having won many of its major battles with psychiatry developed its own brand of exclusivity, monetary orientation, lobbying, sensitivity, and piety about upholding standards and monitoring credentials in relation to the potential encroachment of counseling psychologists and doctoral level practitioners trained in counselor education. These matters will be treated more fully in the next and subsequent sections.

At the moment, clinical psychology seems to have won its major battle for independence from psychiatry although there are continuing conflicts between the two professions. Although both clinical psychology and psychiatrists have moved their provision of treatment to private practice and community mental centers from almost exclusive locus in hospitals, psychologists continue to try to advance their prerogatives in hospitals. Just as the Joint Commission on Accreditation of Hospitals has recently relaxed its standards so that psychologists are no longer restricted from hospital privileges (Taube, Burns, & Kessler, 1984) clinical psychologists continue to strive for parity in providing patient care and having staff privileges equal to those of psychiatrists in hospitals. Clinical psychologists are seeking voting committee membership and clinical privileges to admit, discharge, authorize treatment, and be recognized as the patient's primary (mental) health care provider. Although authority for decisions about patient care still rests primarily with physicians, even non-psychiatrically trained physicians, arguments are beginning to surface in favor of clinical psychologists taking on extended staff privileges. Levy (1981) has summarized such arguments as including continuity of care, freedom of choice, accountability and cost-effectiveness. However, he sees the central issue as "creating a free market situation in which the psychosocial and medical models can compete as equals to see which can provide the better quality of care at the lower price for particular types of patient problems" (p. 24).

Effectiveness of Clinical Psychologists

Levy bolstered his position by arguing from several research studies about the effectiveness of psychologists vs. psychiatrists. Examples of his arguments follow. He stated, "It is now a well-documented fact through clinical research that the most effective way to deinstitutionalize mental health patients is through token economy programs. These programs teach community living skills and self-control over aberrant behavior through step-by-step learning with rewards for successful behavior...Yet, in fact, there are very few token economy programs existent in mental hospitals across the country...The group of health core professionals with the greatest knowledge of token economy programs are psychologists." In addition, "another example of how patient treatment is hurt by the dominance of the medical model over the psychosocial model lies in the provision of psychotherapy to mentally hospitalized individuals..." Research studies show "that days of hospitalization could be cut up to 92 percent" by psychotherapy alone compared to medications alone. Yet, using 1976 as a base year, typically in mental hospitals 90 to 100% of patients receive medications while perhaps 5 to 10% receive psychotherapy from a psychologist or psychiatrist. "This must be seen as a very strong argument for the great importance of providing psychotherapy to hospitalized patients and therefore allowing access to all qualified therapists" (p. 25).

Obviously, the kinds of views represented by Levy make strong arguments for greater psychologist roles in hospitals. At the same time they tend to exacerbate the level of controversy between the two groups as power, territoriality, and economic benefit rather than competence emerge as the major issues which divide such helping professionals.

Parity of Clinical Psychologists

Outside hospitals, clinical psychologists do seem to be achieving parity with psychiatrists. Each and all states have licensing procedures by which Clinical Psychologists can offer their services in private practice. About 70% of the states also have freedom of choice legislation which requires that insurance companies reimburse physicians or psychologists if they are providing services for which either are qualified and for which their licensure permits. In general, the Federal government has recognized clinical psychologists as "core providers" who have the same eligibility to provide psychological services as psychiatrists to persons covered by such legislation as the Rehabilitation Act of 1973, the Federal Employees Health Benefit Program, the Civilian Health and Medical Program of the Uniformed Services (CHAMPUS), the Civilian Health and Medical Program of the Veterans Administration (CHAMPVA), Community Mental Health Center Regulations, Veterans Administration Regulations, Vietnam Veterans Health Care Bill, the Work incentive Program, The Federal Employees Compensation Act, Health Maintenance Organization Regulations, Disaster Relief Act, and Social Security Administration's Bureau of Disability Insurance Regulations. Such widespread access of psychologists to programs as comprehensive as these obviously reduces the monopoly of psychiatrists in providing mental health service. It also defines, inadvertently if not deliberately, many forms of emotional distress as psychological rather than medical and it reflects, again inadvertent perhaps, that psychologists have become quite powerful in their ability to influence federal policies governing the provision of mental health services.

Another perspective on the degree to which psychologists (frequently clinical psychologists) and psychiatrists are achieving parity outside hospitals lies with perspectives on the office-based practices of these two groups. Using data from the National Medical Care Utilization and Expenditure Survey, Taube, Burns and Kessler (1984) estimated that the number of persons seen by psychologists in office-based practice (private-practice), in 1980 was 2,253,000 compared with 2,345,000 persons seen by psychiatrists in office-based practice in the same year. Indeed, by 1980 the number of psychologists in all forms of mental health care delivery equalled the number of psychiatrists. The convergence in the numbers of persons seen in private practice by psychologists and by psychiatrists in 1980 represented the continuing shifts over the past two decades in the locations in which mental health care actually took place. For example, in 1960 the state mental health hospital system was still "the dominant feature of the mental health delivery system, as it has been since the beginning of care for the mentally ill in the United States" (Taube, Burns & Kessler, 1984, p. 1435). In that year, in organized mental health settings, outpatient episodes constituted only 25% of the total episodes and inpatient episodes consisted of 75%. In 1980, these percentages were reversed, and outpatient episodes accounted for 75% of the total. According to Taube, Burns and Kessler, "Growth in the supply of practitioners and in private insurance coverage for outpatient mental disorders spurred a concomitant growth in the office-based practice of both psychiatrists and psychologists" (p. 1435). When one looks at the distribution of ambulatory mental health care among medical specialties alone, psychiatrists account for about half (46%) of the mental health visits, and other specialties, primarily primary care physicians account for half. When medical specialties and psychologists are considered, psychologists account for a third of the visits, psychiatrists another third, and other specialties and nonmedical providers another third (Taube, Kessler & Feverberg, 1984).

In comparisons of the characteristics of persons who make mental health visits to psychiatrists or psychologists in private practice, Taube, Burns and Kessler (1984) found that 66% of all ambulatory mental health visits and 68% of the total expenditures for a year are accounted for by these two provider types (p. 1444). One-half of these persons who are high or frequent users of ambulatory mental health care are seen primarily in psychologists' private practices. With regard to health status, office-based psychiatrists' patients tend to be more impaired than those of office-based psychologists and psychiatrist's patients tended to experience twice the rate of hospitalization as did psychologists' patients. As compared with office-based psychiatrists, psychologists in private-practice tend to see fewer patients over age 55, fewer patients with Medicaid coverage, more patients with a college education, and more employed persons. There appear to be few differences in charges between psychiatrists and psychologists although better insurance coverage exists for psychiatrists' patients, as reflected in both higher government and third-party reimbursement and one-half the out-of-pocket expense, when compared to psychologists' patients. This differential coverage seems to be balanced by a higher rate of discounting among psychologists (pp. 1444-1445).

Such data as these suggest that while both psychiatrists and psychologists in private practice have much to do, points of conflict include psychiatrist resentment that psychologists are "creaming" the "easier" cases and receiving essentially the same payments as psychiatrists; on the other hand, psychologists are likely to perceive the more complete insurance coverage of psychiatrists' patients as unfair to them and as causing them to discount fees to maintain patient loads as inappropriate given their contributions to the mental health care delivery system.

Perspectives on Competence

Another source of conflict between psychiatrists and psychologists lies in the views other helping professionals hold of their competence and indeed how they view each others' competence. Schindler, Berren and Beigel (1981) sent a 33 item questionnaire to psychiatrists, psychologists, social workers, and nurses in various mental health settings asking them to evaluate how large a role psychiatrists and psychologists played in 11 everyday activities, how competent the two professions were to perform the activity, and how much responsibility each should ideally have in carrying out the activity. The 11 activities at issue included those which tend to take place in all mental health facilities: intake screening, psychotherapy, counseling, diagnostics, testing, program coordination (management), supervision and training, consultation and education, staffing decisions, medication management, and testifying as an expert witness. Of the 124 respondents, 47 were psychiatrists, 40 were psychologists, and 37 were nurses or social workers. In terms of actual responsibility, psychiatrists rated themselves as having primary responsibility for all of the activities except psychotherapy, counseling, and testing. Psychologists perceived the division of responsibility very differently. They viewed psychiatrists as being primarily responsible for program coordination, medication management, and testifying as expert witnesses, while reserving to themselves responsibility for testing, psychotherapy, and counseling. They saw themselves having as much responsibility in each of the remaining 11 areas as did psychiatrists.

Psychiatrists rated themselves as more competent than psychologists to carry out 8 of the 11 activities. They saw no difference in their competence to perform psychotherapy and counseling and attributed more competence to psychologists than to themselves only in the area of psychological testing.

Psychologists saw things differently. They rated themselves more competent than psychiatrists to carry out 9 of 11 activities, perceived no difference in their abilities to testify as expert witness, and rated psychiatrists as more competent only in the area of medication management. The other professionals saw no difference in the competency of psychiatrists and psychologists in six of the activities, with psychologists more competent in psychotherapy, counseling, and testing and psychiatrists more competent in diagnostics and medication management.

When asked about the roles psychiatrists and psychologists should ideally play in the 11 activities, there was substantial disagreement among the respondents. Psychiatrists believed that they should have responsibility for all of the activities except psychotherapy, counseling, and testing. Psychologists believed that psychiatrists should have responsibility for medication management only. Nurses and social workers generally agreed with psychologists about who would perform which roles.

Again, such differences in role perceptions and levels of competence are obvious sources of conflict and likely to be deeply held by each group of helping professionals. Such controversies may unfold because of faulty communication, actual differences in training and competence, differences in professional socialization, or parochial tunnel vision. Regardless of the sources of the conflict, however, controversy does prevail and is likely to be a divisive irritant in their relationships. As we will see in the next section, such elements of controversy are also present in the relationships between clinical and counseling psychologists.

COUNSELING PSYCHOLOGISTS

In many state credentialing processes and in many Federal statutes, no distinctions exist between Clinical and Counseling Psychologists or School, Educational, or other types of psychologists for that matter. For purposes of licensure eligibility, they are lumped together as psychologists. This is consistent with a professional view that generic *Standards for Providers of Psychological Services* (APA, 1977) precede and serve as the basis from which specialty standards evolve. In such a view, a psychologist is a psychologist. Specialization is, in a sense, a peripheral issue. Indeed, in much of the literature discussing conflict between psychiatrists and psychologists, no distinction is made about the kind of psychologist at issue although in terms of the roots and functions of clinical psychology, it is obvious that this group is the major protagonists of psychiatrists.

Many counseling psychologists actually serve in positions labeled as clinical psychologist, although in general the training of the two groups does differ. Counseling psychologists tend to be more oriented to prevention, to resolution of the developmental conflicts of essentially normal populations, and to personal self-fulfillment than to remediation, treatment, and severe emotional or psychiatric disorders. Counseling psychologists are less likely than clinical psychologists to have their internship experience in a medical-psychiatric setting and more likely to serve it in a University Counseling Center, community mental health center, child guidance center, or similar setting.

Distinctions in Counseling and Clinical Psychology

One of the classic definitions which distinguishes between counseling and clinical psychology is that proferred by Super in 1955.

> *Clinical psychology* has typically been concerned with diagnosing the nature and extent of *psychopathology,* with the abnormalities of even normal persons, with uncovering adjustment difficulties and maladaptive tendencies, and with the acceptance and understanding of these tendencies so that they may be modified. *Counseling psychology,* on the contrary, concerns itself with *hygiology,* with the normalities of even abnormal persons, with locating and developing personal and social resources and adaptive tendencies so that the individual can be assisted in making more effective use of them. (Super, 1955, p. 5)

This distinction between clinical and counseling psychologists suggests that these are relatively distinct specialties for service delivery within psychology, each with their own value system and priorities vis á vis whom they serve and to what purpose. In fact, the American Psychological Association now provides specialty guidelines for four such groups: clinical psychologists, counseling psychologists, industrial/organizational psychologists, and school psychologists.

With respect specifically to clinical psychology, the specialty guidelines of the American Psychological Association assert that clinical psychological services refers "to the application of principles, methods, and procedures for understanding, predicting, alleviating intellectual, emotional, psychological, and behavioral disability and discomfort. Direct services are provided in a variety of health settings, and direct and supportive services are provided in the entire range of social, organizational, and academic institutions and services" (American Psychological Association, 1981, p. 642). In some contrast, the appropriate specialty guidelines assert that

> counseling psychological services refers to services provided by counseling psychologists that apply principles, methods, and procedures for facilitating effective functioning during the life-span development process. In providing such

services, counseling psychologists approach practice with a significant emphasis on positive aspects of growth and adjustment and with a developmental orientation. These services are intended to help persons acquire or alter personal-social skills, improve adaptability to changing life demands, enhance environmental coping skills, and develop a variety of problem-solving and decision-making capabilities. Counseling psychological services are used by individuals, couples, and families of all age groups to cope with problems connected with education, career choice, work, sex, marriage, family, other social relations, health, aging, and handicap of a social or physical nature. The services are offered in such organizations as educational, rehabilitation, and health institutions and in a variety of other public and private agencies committed to services in one or more of the problem areas cited above. (American Psychological Association, 1981, p. 654)

Others have attempted to distinguish counseling psychology by definitions which attempt to exclude overlap with clinical psychology.

Wrenn (1954) stated that "a counseling psychologist is first a psychologist, with all that this implies, in the way of training in and respect for science, and is next a practicing professional in counseling." The problem with such a definition is that the term counseling is itself controversial. Is it the same as psychotherapy or different? If it is the same, who owns psychotherapy or counseling? Is there some set of explicit and exclusive skills which one needs to offer these processes? What are they? Do either counseling or clinical psychologists have them or do they both? So much for that point!

To attempt to distinguish counseling and clinical psychology on grounds other than the provision of counseling, Ivey (1976), who served as chairman of the Professional Affairs Committee of Division 17 (Counseling Psychology) of the American Psychological Association, reported that psychologists may engage in counseling with the purpose of remediation, prevention, or development but that it was the educative/developmental purpose which was primary as the role for counseling psychologist. Ivey went on to contend that "the counseling psychologist is becoming a broadly-based psychoeducator" (p. 73). In such a role, the intervention target of most concern to the counseling psychologist is the primary group of family or close friends, and the methods of intervention are consultation and media rather than direct service. The content of such intervention includes life-planning workshops, training in listening skills, parent effectiveness training, and family intervention programs. Within such a framework of roles and functions of counseling psychologists is the inclusion of remediation and prevention, direct service, and social change, but these are viewed as being less central than the role of psychoeducator with primary groups.

From a more traditional view, Osipow (1977; 1979) has argued that the core of counseling psychology is direct service, prevention, and vocational development. Other prominent counseling psychologists (Kagan, 1977; Nathan, 1977; Pepinsky, Hill-Frederick, and Epperson, 1978) have agreed with this view. Stone (1986) has analyzed the roots of counseling psychology in vocational guidance and psychotherapy (and their three original perspectives—guiding, healing, facilitating) as these were combined with other trends from the psychological literature—modifying (learning), restructuring (cognition), developing (development), influencing (social), communicating (communication theory) and organizing (community) to create current conceptions of the field.

From these brief examples of definition one can recognize that counseling psychology just as clinical psychology has had its own identity crises and birth pangs. Clinical psychology since the second World War has been characterized primarily in its relationships to psychiatric, medical settings, and problems of severe emotional disorder. Counseling psychology got its major stimulus as an emerging psychological specialty a few years after clinical psychology in the early and mid-1950s. Its roots were in vocational development, guidance, prevention, and normality. More specifically, the historical legacy of counseling psychology derived from three distinct movements: (1) vocational guidance; (2) psychological measurement; and, (3) personality development (Committee on Definition, 1956). The American Psychological Association Committee on Definition (1956) stated that "...counseling psychology draws upon contemporary personality and learning theories. In so doing it employs concepts and tools that are used by clinical, experimental, social, and school psychologists, among other specialties...this specialist is found to be working in the full range of social settings, e.g., school, hospital, business or industry, or community agency " (p. 283). Thompson and Super (1964) reported that at the Greystone Conference at which the specialty was officially established, counseling psychology was seen as having "unity in diversity!" At about the time of the formation of counseling psychology, Hahn and McLean (1955) contended that the distinguishing mark of the counseling psychologist is the breadth of his/her specialization (p. 7). They further noted that, "no group of workers can be accepted as a profession if they duplicate wholly or in major part the functioning and processes of another group under a different name" (p. 10).

Blurring of the Uniqueness of Counseling Psychology

Part of the extant controversy, however subtle or overt, between counseling and clinical psychology is that in many instances practitioners of either of these specialties tend to overlap in function or as the two fields attempt to separate from their roots, they become more and more alike in some training programs and in some settings. For example, while a major emphasis of counseling psychology is expected to be career development, Goldschmitt, Tipton, and Wiggins (1981) reporting on the earlier work of Schneider and Gelso (1972) indicated that directors of APA approved counseling psychology programs perceived the focus of their programs as more on personal concerns and problems than on vocational concerns and problems. Such circumstances may explain Delworth's observations (1977) that graduate students in counseling psychology see themselves as "sort of clinicians and sort of counselors" (p. 43). In a recent occupational analysis of counseling psychology, Fitzgerald and Osipow (1986) find continuing blurring between the roles of counseling and clinical psychologists, counseling psychologists as strongly practice-oriented, self-perceptions of counseling psychologists as professionals who engage in psychotherapy and traditional clinical activities with a reduced emphasis on vocational, academic, and research-focused behaviors. Indeed, Fitzgerald and Osipow indicate that their occupational analysis indicates that counseling and clinical psychology "seem to be converging: Thus, the time may have come for serious consideration of Levy's (1984) proposal for a merger of clinical, counseling, and school psychology into a broader *human services psychology"* (p. 543).

There are other indications of role cross-over between counseling and clinical psychologists. The Veterans Administration which has played a prominent part in stimulating the development of both clinical and counseling psychology as separate specialties provides traineeships for students in each of these specialties, has both types of psychologists on its staff, and outlines the duties of each differently. According to Cleveland (1980) the U.S. Civil Service Position Classification Standards (1968) outlines the duties of clinical psychologists as including psychodiagnostic testing, psychotherapy, and patient-care team participation. In addition the standards indicate that clinical psychologists "are concerned with patient's problems of adjustment to their physical illness, and with vocational rehabilitation" (p. 5). The standards for counseling psychologists include the educational, vocational, and rehabilitation counseling of the physically or mentally handicapped or others in need of or seeking vocational guidance (p. 6). Additional duties involve knowledge about occupations, educational opportunities, and career planning as well as "...help clients modify attitudes, feelings or behavior patterns that interfere with their making progress in educational, vocational, or rehabilitation planning" (pp. 6-7).

Although these distinctions are made by the Veterans Administration in its standards, it allows clinical and counseling psycholgists to perform each other's functions. For example, the Civil Service Standards indicate that:

> Clinical psychologists may engage in vocational counseling as a part of the overall plan of therapy for an emotionally disturbed client. Counseling psychologists may engage in therapeutic counseling with clients whose attitudes are such as to interfere with realistic evaluation and mobilization and use of their personal resources. (p. 9)

Cleveland (1980) studied the perceived status of counseling psychology by querying Administrators in 65 Veteran's Administration (VA) hospitals about the status, roles, and responsibilities of doctoral level counseling psychologists. He found that within these settings was a declining image of counseling psychology as a separate, visible entity and bias operating against counseling psychologists in the areas of hiring, promotional opportunity, and duty assignments. He found many of the counseling psychologists seeking reclassification as clinical psychologists. One of the dynamics operating in this situation is the sheer ratio of clinical and counseling psychologists in these settings. For example, of the 1,300 psychologists employed in VA Departments of Medicine and Surgery, as of 1978, 1,125 were classified as clinical psychologists and 175 were classified as counseling psychologists. Many VA facilities reported no counseling psychologists on their staffs. Thus, the training and the skills of counseling psychologists are certainly less familiar to policy-makers in the Veterans Administration than are those of clinical psychologists. This may be a function of the fact that significantly more APA approved Clinical Psychology training programs exist than APA approved Counseling Psychology programs and thus more clinical students apply for and are employed by the VA. Or, it may be that counseling psychology is not held with as much favor as a quality training program as is clinical psychology. The latter can be seen in some of the remarks of Cleveland's survey respondents who indicated that counseling psychology is frequently associated with Colleges of Education rather than having a complete identity with psychology. This bias seems to pervade many of the observations about counseling vs. clinical psychologists even through respondents contended that there was no quarrel about the competency of counseling psychologists coming from APA-approved counseling programs.

On the other side of the issue some VA administrators criticized clinical psychologists as having no interest in vocational counseling duties and looking down on such activities as being nonprofessional or beneath them. For each of these reasons, the VA administrators argued for the need to cross-train counseling and clinical psychologists to be able to perform each others' duties. When asked whether the VA should continue to maintain separate classifications for clinical and counseling psychologists, the respondents were quite mixed in how they viewed the matter, with 33 of 58 respondents voting to maintain separate classifications and 25 seeing no point in having two different classifications (Cleveland, 1980, p. 317). However, when asked to separate the skills and expertise required of a counseling psychologist but not of a clinical psychologist, they listed in order of priority: (a) vocational testing, (b) awareness of community vocational resources, (c) vocational counseling, (d) knowledge of the world of work, (e) job placement, (f) educational testing, (g) educational counseling, (h) vocational rehabilitation, (i) disability limitations on work. On the other hand, clinical psychologists were expected to have skills and expertise as defined in the following order of priority: (a) psychodiagnostics, (b) projective methods, (c) psychotherapy, (d) knowledge of psychopathology, (e) behavior modification, (f) neuropsychology, and (g) group therapy.

What also seems to be happening is a blurring of techniques and processes between clinical psychology and counseling psychology. For example, even though most of the training of counseling and clinical psychologists is different, both study and practice psychotherapy. The view of psychotherapy originally fought over by psychiatrists and clinical psychologists was a psychoanalytic-psychodynamic orientation derived from Freud, Adler, Rank, and Sullivan among others. This is not the view of psychotherapy espoused for the most part by counseling psychology. The latter tends to be a more eclectic view emphasizing either a client-centered psychotherapy deriving from the work of Rogers, Carkhuff, Gendlin, and others or a behavioral approach evolving from the work of Bandura and Krumboltz or a cognitive psychology emanating from Meichenbaum, Turk, Beck and others. Some evidence exists to suggest, however, that both clinical and counseling psychologists are dipping into the same reservoir of psychotherapeutic interventions and talking similarly about themselves. For example, D.

Smith (1982) found little difference in how clinical and counseling psychologists viewed trends in counseling and psychotherapy, prompting him to suggest that the two specializations are becoming less dissimilar. Fox (1982) has argued that clinical psychology must reorient itself toward general practices that offer services to the many and away from specialty practice that offers services to the few (p. 1051).

In another example of such a possibility, in the inaugural G. Stanley Hall lecture series at the 1980 convention of the American Psychological Association, Jerome Singer (1981), a distinguished Clinical Psychologist, presented a lecture on Clinical Intervention: New Developments in Methods and Evaluation. In doing so, he stated the following: "We are witnessing a shift in orientation—the model of the psychotherapist as a kind of detective searching out root causes of disturbance is being supplemented or even supplanted by the role of the therapist as an educator or perhaps a kind of skills training coach" (p. 108). That sort of notion sounds a great deal like Ivey's 1976 conception of the Counseling Psychologist as a psychoeducator.

Singer, then went on to advocate the importance of the problem-focused, active therapies, principally the behavior therapies, including systematic desensitization, covert aversive imagery, symbolic or vicarious modeling, assertiveness training and vicarious rehearsal procedures, cognitive behavior modification and stress innoculation. Obviously, counseling psychologists do not have a lock on these procedures as definitions of psychotherapy but one would be hard put to read any journal in counseling psychology and not see such techniques represented. Such overlap in the provision of psychotherapy and the interpretation of its meaning portends the potential for considerable conflict between the two specialties in the future.

As clinical psychologists increasingly see themselves as having an educative, skill-training role with populations other than those experiencing severe mental and emotional disorders, it may alter some of the current distinctions in setting, interest, and practice between clinical and counseling psychologists. For example, Pallone (1977) found that counseling psychology is clearly distinguished from other specialties with respect to work settings. He summarized his findings as follows:

> In colleges and universities, counseling psychologists proportionately outnumber psychologists undifferentiated as to scientific or professional specialty by approximately one and a half times, clinical psychologists by more than five times. In health related settings, clinical psychologists proportionately outnumber

psychologists-in-general by more than eleven times, school psychologists by some twenty-six times. In public schools and school systems, school psychologists proportionately outnumber psychologists-in-general by more than nearly seven times, counseling psychologists by more than eleven times, and clinical psychologists by nearly twenty-seven times. (p. 30)

As a result of these analyses, Pallone concluded that "the educational, vocational, and personal adjustment problems of clients are found to be in the repertoire of counseling psychologists alone, among professional psychologists (p. 32). This perspective is essentially echoed by Nathan (1977), a clinical psychologist who states that "the professional contributions counseling psychologists can make are of two distinct kinds, in my judgment. The first, a contribution counseling psychologists can make uniquely, is in the vocational counseling/world of work sphere. No other psychologists are trained in vocational counseling techniques; by the same token, no non-psychologist vocational consultant combines this knowledge of the world of work with skills in vocational assessment and competence in psychological counseling techniques. As a result, the counseling psychologist fills a unique role in our society" (p. 37).

Nathan went on to make another interesting point as follows:

Another professional contribution the counseling psychologist can make is, from my perspective, less unique and, for that reason, less uniquely valuable. That contribution derives from the personal counseling skills many counseling psychologists have chosen to hone into psychotherapeutic ones. In choosing this career option, however, the counseling psychologist joins a variety of other mental health professionals including clinical psychologists, psychiatrists, psychiatric social workers, and psychiatric nurses, some of whom have likely received better training in psychotherapy than the average counseling psychologist... With a modicum of training and adequate interpersonal skills, many persons can do psychotherapy with some effectiveness; but few professionals have the breadth and depth of training in vocational assessment and counseling to which the counseling psychologist can lay claim. (p. 37)

Another perspective on differences between clinical and counseling psychologists is provided by the study of Osipow, Cohen, Jenkins, and Dostal (1979) of the interests of members of Division 17 (Counseling Psychology), Division 12 (Clinical Psychology), Division 29 (Psychotherapy)) of the American Psychological Association and of those who belong to both Division 17 and 12 or 29. It was found that those professionals who belonged only to Division 17 indicated their interests to be primarily in a variety of activities identified as counseling as compared with members of only Division 12 or 29 who indicated more interest in "therapeutic activities" and behavior disorders. Those counseling psychologists who belonged to both Division 17 and 12 or 29 had interests more like those of members of Divisions 12 or 29 only than like members of Division 17 only.

Through whichever lens one views the matter, it appears that counseling psychology and clinical psychology in a number of settings are difficult to distinguish and constantly on the verge of significant controversy. The core of this controversy appears to center around the provision of psychotherapy by many in each specialty. Having wrestled the opportunity to provide psychotherapy from psychiatrists, clinical psychologists have a sense of ownership which is seen by them as intruded upon by some counseling psychologists. The assumption follows that counseling psychologists are attempting to serve the same clients and share in the same economic rewards as clinical psychologists believe should be available to them.

Part of this controversy exists because the terms counseling and psychotherapy have been blurred in their meanings and, thereby, confuse the requirements for training and practice in regard to them. But, part of the controversy exists as well because both clinical psychologists and counseling psychologists have departed from their roots and gravitated to settings and functions which increasingly overlap. Clinical psychologists have begun to stress their contributions to normal populations in educative and skill-building emphases rather than restrict themselves to psychopathology and remediation. Counseling psychologists have frequently been trained in psychotherapeutic techniques, rather than in vocational development and related methodologies, sought settings in which they could be cross-trained as clinical psychologists and deal primarily with chronically emotionally disturbed populations rather than normal populations experiencing developmental dilemmas. These trends exacerbate questions of who is competent to do what, the quality of training in each of the specialties, and, less visibly, issues of power related to credentialing and access to certain kinds of employment.

CLINICAL SOCIAL WORKERS

Clinical social workers, like other members of the helping professions are diverse in their training and in their purposes. Clinical social workers, however, are identified in Federal statutes as "core providers" of mental health services and, therefore, as a key occupation among the mental health professions.

Clinical social workers have to date not been as visible in controversies with other occupational groups in the helping professions as have, for example, psychiatrists and psychologists or clinical and counseling psychologists. Nevertheless, internal controversies in social work are present regarding clinical social work and, as the definitions of the knowledge base and boundaries of such practice expand, it is likely that more visible controversy will emerge between clinical social workers, psychologists, psychiatrists, counselors, and other members of the helping professions.

Social Work

Clinical social work is a relatively new specialization within the older profession of social work. The term apparently entered the language and, indeed, the statute books in the 1960s as social workers were seeking sanctions and legislation permitting them to serve as independent deliverers of direct service to individual clients. An early affirmation of such statutes was reflected in the California State Licensure Law of 1968 (Bandler, 1979) and core provider status for clinical social workers has been reflected in a variety of federal laws regulating who can receive compensation from various sources for delivering mental health services. In some of these circumstances however, the intent is unclear as to whether to recognize social workers in general, psychiatric social workers, or the more inclusive group of clinical social workers by some of the Federal and State statutes. Some States, for example, do not distinguish between social work and clinical social work. Some States recognize the latter as a specialty of the former. In such instances, the practitioner would likely be required to hold certification as an A.C.S.W. from the Academy of Certified Social Workers, which would entail graduation with a Master of Social Work (M.S.W.) degree from a Council on Social Work Education (C.S.W.E.) accredited program in social work, plus two years or 3,000 hours of post-masters practice under the supervision of a clinically trained M.S.W. (Hardcastle, 1983).

Controversies in Definition

Like definitions of other helping professions, definitions of clinical social work are still unresolved and, indeed, controversial within social work (Rosenblatt & Waldfogel, 1983). Nevertheless, several definitions seem to have sufficient credibility within the profession to mark out the boundaries of such "helping professionals." One such definition has been provided by a task force of the National Association of Social Work (Ewalt, 1980). It proposes the following definition:

> Clinical social work involves a wide range of psychosocial services to individuals, families and small groups in relation to a variety of human problems of living. Such practice may be carried out under both private and public auspicies. It is concerned with the assessment of interaction between the individual's biological, psychological, and social experience which provides a guide for clinical intervention. A distinguishing feature is the clinician's concern with the social context within which individual or family programs occur and are altered. Clinical social work, therefore, may involve intervention in the social situation as well as the person situation. Three major principles by which clinical social work produces change or maintenance of functions are (1) through the interpersonal relationship with the clinician; (2) through alterations in the social situation; (3) through alterations of relationships with significant persons in the life space of the individual. (p. 26)

The most recent official definition approved by the National Association of Social Work states that it is "the professional application of social work theory and methods to the treatment and prevention of psychosocial dysfunction, disability, or impairment, including emotional and mental disorders" (Clinical Social Work Council, 1984). This definition affirms that "the perspective of person-in-situation is central to clinical social work practice."

While these definitions, and others, of clinical social work may cause various observers within social work to be concerned about the narrowness or the breadth of the definition, inherent in the definition are emphases which have kept clinical social work from coming into direct conflict with other members of the helping professions. Unlike other groups of the mental health professions, in clinical social work overarching theoretical prominence has been given to sociological perspectives on human behavior rather than to psychological perspectives. The latter are important and given their due in specific treatment processes but the conceptual integrity of social work lies in being principally concerned with individual-environment interaction, what is called in social work parlance, "person-in-situation" (Rosenblatt & Waldfogel, 1983). This fundamental concept brings with it concerns about social systems, group dynamics, small group theory which while not unfamiliar to other helping professionals are seen and emphasized differently.

Social Conditions and Human Behavior

Social work, like each of the other helping professions, has changed over the years but its roots and its conceptual integrity remain focused upon the effects of social conditions upon human behavior. Depending upon what source one reads, a general concensus exists that social work practice received its major stimulus in the United Sates in the latter part of the nineteenth and the early years of the twentieth century. The issues to which social work practitioners responded were the effects of industrialization and urbanization upon the immigrant populations from throughout the world and those American citizens moving from the farms to the cities to seek work and opportunity. Social workers began historically as volunteers in settlement houses and in other charitable organizations, sometimes prompted by religious motives. As they became identified as major instruments of the social welfare policy of the United States, they became paid employees of welfare agencies, attempted to establish a knowledge base and begin formal programs in social work education which in turn began to define the distinctive methodologies of assessment, diagnoses, and case work.

By 1905, specialties in medical social work, psychiatric social work, and school social work began to be formulated and to take on specific professional identities (Johnson, 1983).

The prominence of sociological perspective at the root of the conceptual system for social work is captured in Johnson's observations (1983) that:

> The beginning of a professional social work was a response to the social milieu of the early twentieth century. A time when the new immigrants with their different cultures and life styles were of concern to the larger society was at hand. It was also a time when the progressives were working for reforms that they believed would eliminate poverty. This era saw the development of the social sciences with a belief that application of a scientific method based on the new knowledge could identify the causes of poverty and deviance. It was felt that if these causes could be identified, solutions would be apparent and social ills eliminated. (p. 30)

The Evolution of Social Work

Morris (1979) centered the evolution of social work within the shifting emphases of federal social policy which originally focused upon income maintenance, the provision of health services, housing, education, correction and, after World War I, rehabilitation. As policies in these areas were instituted and agencies developed to implement the policies, the workers (social workers) employed in these agencies tended to offer in a subtle and inadvertent fashion personal services which began to take on a life of their own. These social workers began to perform a variety of counseling and guidance functions "to help individuals deal with troublesome situations." According to Morris, this evolution "can in part be traced back to the historical view that individuals who cannot manage their income, health, housing, and educational needs independently are somehow weaker than the average person and require specialists' assistance" (p. 118).

Morris further contended that this view of "personal services" which became, on an unplanned basis, part of American social welfare policy did so in part as a reflection of policies in England in this regard. In England, income, health, housing and education were long established social programs. But early in this century a fifth social service of equal stature was added and became known as "personal social services" (p. 118). Such services took on several functions. One was to manage a series of services which special groups required but which were not typically provided in the older social programs. These included such services as daycare for children, homemaker services, and referral for clients who had multiple needs for service. A second major function was the provision of psychological counseling since the anxieties, ambiguities, and distresses of modern urban life were perceived to require a "publicly supported" counseling service so that individuals could cope more adequately with such stresses. A third function which emerged as the social welfare bureaucracy became increasingly entrenched and rigid was that of advocacy of the needs of disadvantaged persons and groups.

What one sees in the evolution of social work is that psychological counseling by social workers, while important as part of a larger set of responsibilities, was not seen as independent of the particular social conditions with which a particular client was trying to cope. What is also apparent is that social workers originally were providing their services primarily to the economically disadvantaged, not to the whole range of the population, much in the way that psychiatrists and clinical psychologists originally confined their treatment focus only to the most severely mentally or emotionally disturbed clients.

While the clientele of social workers has broadened over the years, the focus of their efforts on the "person-in-situation" has persisted as a core concept (Rosenblatt & Waldfogel, 1983). For example, Reid (1981) contends that, "the main business of the social work profession is to bring about planned change in individual and social systems and conditions" (p. 127). The interpretation of such notions seem to include assessment and treatment strategies related to understanding the way a person meets the situation and to viewing "casework" as a problem-solving process. Peterson and Anderson (1984) have advocated "single system" research designs as complements to large group, experimental designs as ways to evaluate social work practice. Johnson (1983) compared how the major professional literature dealt with the major concepts characterizing casework, group work, and community organization in social work practice. She concluded that five major concepts were apparent in each approach: assessment, person-in-the-situation, process, relationship, and intervention.

Current Trends

Reflecting both recurrent conflict with clinical social work and the need to carefully examine current trends for the field, Siporin (1985) has addressed current social work perspectives on clinical practice. He suggested that clinical social work has recently emerged from a period of "severe political and ideological struggle" which includes a "rebellion" against the "so-called psychoanalytic therapy establishment by the social reformists and scientific behaviorists" as well as attack by the Reagan Administration which has attempted to emasculate the profession and expel it from many welfare positions.

Although clinical social work area has been under pressure from within the profession and external to it, Siporin suggested that clinical social work is gaining a clearer meaning of its role and its clinical practice. For example, he contended that the traditional person-in-situation perspective is now being reaffirmed in what is known as an "ecological systems model which expresses purposes and values, for interdependence, harmonious complementarity, and productive collaboration by the members or parts of a system to achieve common goals" (p. 200). Within practice theory, the ecological systems framework is utilized for the purposes of assessment, treatment planning and evaluation of intervention. From such a framework, practice principles have evolved which argue that problem-resolution requires a change in the interaction pattern or exchange balance" between people and their life situations; that a basic helping goal should be to improve the adaptive fit between people and their systems; that helping interventions should be systematic in conception and have an impact at the crux or pivot of subsystem interface, so that they are both people-helping and system-changing" (p. 201).

Professional Controversies

Within the contexts in clinical social work of the reaffirmation of person-in-situation or ecological systems models, the reemergence of psychoanalytic-psychodynamic models, and the search for models of therapy which are not simply adopted from psychiatry or psychology but respect the rich heritage of social work, Siporin suggested that other intraprofessional controversies remain. One is the confusion about whether clinical practice in social work is an art or a science or, perhaps, most appropriately a "scientific art." Another is the attempt by the empiricists to turn practice into a research activity and to misunderstand that there is a general lack of relevance of research findings to practice. A further controversy, now being tempered, was the sharp duality between social structure and personality concerns and their interrelations. A final controversy lies with the degree to which morality, spirituality, and hermeneutics, in regard to client needs in a contemporary society which frightens many because of its moral chaos, should become visible and integrate aspects both of clinical practice and of the larger rationale for social work as a profession.

Again, what seems to be apparent historically is that while psychological aspects of social behavior were important ingredients of understanding person-in-situations and that psychological approaches (e.g., behavior modification, reality therapy, crisis intervention) were important to adding to treatment repertoires, they typically remained subsumed by social systems theory. To the degree that such balances prevail, controversies between clinical social workers and other helping professionals are likely to be minimal. However, Reid (1981) alludes to an emerging potential problem in this regard.

> Narrow definitions of relevant knowledge are breaking down in part because of the rapid increase of patently useful knowledge in related fields. An outstanding example has been the phenomenal recent growth of literature on behavioral approaches to human problems. Social workers must come to the disconcerting conclusion that the profession lacks any systematic means of marking effective boundaries around its knowledge base. (p. 126)

As we will discuss later, one of the distinguishing characteristics of a profession is a distinctive knowledge base. To the degree that social workers begin to use a knowledge base and, therefore, a set of treatment strategies which resemble those of psychologists and psychiatrists the more likely territoriality and duplications of effort will arise as sources of controversy.

Certainly another emerging source of potential controversy is who might be served in what ways. As clinical social work is attempting to distinguish itself as a licensure eligible, autonomous, direct, clinical service it is slowly but surely bumping into the job titles and functional descriptions of psychologists, psychiatrists, and others. For example, the National Association of Social Worker's clinical registry gives the following definition: "The clinical social worker is, by education and experience, professionally qualified at the autonomous practice level to provide direct, diagnostic, preventive and treatment services to individuals, families, and groups where function is threatened or affected by social or psychological stress or health impairment" (Rosenblatt & Waldfogel, 1983, p. XXVII). Such a definition begins to look very much like those of psychologists and other helping professionals. As such, it does not delimit the populations who might be served by clinical social workers or the techniques used in providing mental health services in independent practice.

A further indication of possible future conflict in treatment strategies is evident in a study by Hardcastle and Katz (1979) in which one-half the members of the National Association of Social Workers indicated that they provided direct service including casework, group work, generic social work, and *psychotherapy*. Where clinical social workers are visibly practicing psychotherapy as a major function it is likely to stir the ire of other professional groups. For example, in 1981, one clinical social worker in Ohio, despite certification by the Academy of Certified Social Workers (A.C.S.W.) and Registry in the NASW Registry of Clinical Social Workers was charged with practicing psychotherapy without a certificate by the State Board of Psychologist Examiners. Such incidents may well increase in the future. Thus, in reality, definitions of clinical social work practices, processes, and purpose may be expanding and blurring as knowledge bases from psychology are receiving increased attention in social work theory and as the attractions of independent, clinical practice increase as federal funds for agency-based social welfare positions decrease. Indeed, as Reichert (1982) has suggested, the market system with its "fee for service mentality" has changed what had been a partially realized welfare state in such a way that social workers and presumably other members of the helping professions will have no choice but to embrace it.

As Federal funding shifts in emphasis and magnitude in relation to client populations to be served, the potential for controversy between mental health professionals also increases. One such example is that which has occurred between social workers and nurses with regard to home health care (Fessler & Adams, 1985). "Historically, the Community Health Nurse was the dominant, often only, provider of home health care, while social workers are a relatively recent addition to home health care agencies. The needs of the current population of elderly recipients of home health care are increasingly complex and require the expertise of several disciplines" (p. 122). However, Fessler and Adams have described how needs for collaboration in one agency can lead to turf conflicts between nurses and social workers.

> Since, under Medicare regulations, an agency may provide reimbursable services from a psychiatric nurse only if the client is being followed by a psychiatrist, the agency decided to hire instead a half-time social worker for whom Medicare restrictions were less restrictive. The social worker could provide psychotherapeutic as well as case management services with an order from the client's regular physician, so long as the services were required by the acute nature of the client's illness. Psychotherapeutic services for the homebound were only minimally available in the area and not on a regular basis. The social worker's role was envisioned as a therapeutic and consultative one. (p. 113)

As this process unfolded, however, the referrals from nurses to social workers were becoming crisis-oriented only, turf problems were arising, and problems both in communication and in creating a sense of an interdisciplinary team among the nurses and the social workers were becoming obvious. When perceptions of role functions of the various players were assessed, they tended to be seen as overlapping, almost duplicative. Several elements of controversy exist between psychiatric nurses and clinical social workers and, indeed, among any type of interdisciplinary team members. One is that interdisciplinary teams or mental health care systems are comprised of microsystems: in the case cited here, social work and nursing. Because the members of these microsystems have been separately socialized, they do not share common language about behavior, assumptions about functions/techniques or similar problem-solving procedures. They also may carry with them uncertainties about their professional status and about where they fit in a treatment team. They may misunderstand or misinterpret the attempts by other team members to evaluate a treatment condition and create a plan (Lowe & Herranen, 1978). They may be experiencing confusion or apprehension about sharing moral and ethical responsibility with others who are involved in the care of the patient (Abramson, 1984). None of these controversies is inherently unsolvable but they are complex with regard to how members of the mental health professions come together in a therapeutic collective.

While clinical social workers have typically not been controversial among the helping professions because of their outreach to families and to the legal system, and their referral to and coordination of community resources in behalf of particular client needs, social workers have begun to take opposition to the practice of or to the licensing of such groups as mental health counselors and/or family therapists. These matters of controversy will be discussed in subsequent sections.

PSYCHIATRIC NURSES

Psychiatric nurses are the fourth of the generally recognized "core providers." While the subject of mental health nursing and units on psychiatric nursing have been included in the training of general duty nurses since virtually the turn of the century, the differentiation of psychiatric nursing as a specialization is a more recent phenomenon.

According to Carter (1981), "psychiatric nursing arose in general hospitals and in asylums" (p. 363). Just as in psychiatry both World Wars One and Two developed public interest in "war neuroses" and the "ripple effects" of war not only in those in the armed forces but also among the families and friends of servicemen remaining at home. As the mental health needs escalated in both wars, the extreme shortages of psychiatrists and of psychiatric nurses became visible and contributed to the development of various Federal programs designed to expand the available numbers of such mental health specialists.

The American Psychiatric Association was the major influence in the establishment of nursing programs in asylums and in the development of the accreditation requirements for mental-hospital nursing schools. Indeed, it was not until 1965, 60 years after the American Psychiatric Association had taken control of psychiatric nursing education, that the American Nurses' Association gained control of the standards for psychiatric nursing (Carter, 1981).

Just as was true in clinical and counseling psychology, the National Institute of Mental Health, under the influence of psychiatrists, funded various projects related to the education and availability of psychiatric nurses. In particular, NIMH provided support for education and research in psychiatric nursing which moved increasingly toward graduate preparation and clinical specialization in psychiatric nursing. Currently three such specializations are recognized by the American Nurses' Association (1976): child, adult, and gerontological mental-health nursing. In addition, the American Nurses' Association recognizes two levels of psychiatric mental-health nursing practice: (1) the psychiatric mental-health nurse generalist, and (2) the psychiatric mental-health nursing specialist. The first level is basically characterized by baccaleureate level training and the second level requires a minimum preparation level of a master's degree in psychiatric mental-health nursing.

A registered nurse may apply for certification as a mental health psychiatric nurse. The nurse must have had direct practice of relevant nursing care for at least four hours weekly, with two years of mental health-psychiatric nursing experience within the last four years, and access to supervision. On a second level, a certified psychiatric-mental health nursing specialist, in either adult or child and adolescent care, is a registered nurse with a minimum of a master's degree in psychiatric-mental health nursing or a related mental health field, access to supervision, and experience in clinical practice in at least two different treatment modalities. To be certified individuals must pass a qualifying examination administered by the American Nurses' Association (Beck, Rawlins & Williams, 1984).

As psychiatric nursing has evolved from the asylum and the general hospital as well as from private duty psychiatric nursing to community mental health centers and other settings, the role of such specialists has become more comprehensive and more diverse. Psychiatric nurses are involved in custodial care, treatment, and prevention of mental illness. They do intake assessments of patients, determine need for hospitalization or referrals, and sign commitment papers. They establish and maintain the therapeutic milieu in treatment areas, engage in general nursing procedures vis á vis administration and monitoring of counseling and social work, program planning and evaluation, and in the implementation of support systems for patients. Individual, group, and family psychotherapy is frequently practiced by psychiatric mental-health nurses who have appropriate specialized training. They also serve as administrators, supervisors, educators, consultants, health teachers, coordinators and researchers (Carter, 1981, p. 375). Many psychiatric mental health nurses are now in private practice and like psychologists, clinical social workers, and others are attempting to use their "core provider" status as leverage to gain licensure and third party payments on a state by state basis.

Psychiatric Nurse Standards

The standards governing psychiatric mental-health nursing practice as adopted by the American Nurses' Association in 1973 states the following:

> Psychiatric nursing is a specialized area of nursing practice employing theories of human behavior as its scientific aspect and purposeful use of self as its art. It is directed toward both preventive and corrective impacts upon mental illness and is concerned with the promotion of optimal mental health for society, the community, and those individuals and families who live within it. The dependent area of psychiatric nursing practice is implementation of physician's orders. The independent areas are assessment of nursing needs and development and implementation of nursing-care plans, including initiation, development, and termination of therapeutic relationships between nurses and patients. (p. 1)

The standards then go on to contend that:

> The practice of psychiatric nursing is characterized by those aspects of clinical nursing care that involve interpersonal relationships with individuals and groups as well as a variety of other activities. These activities include: providing a therapeutic milieu, concerned largely with the sociopsychological aspects of patients' environments; working with patients concerning the here-and-now living problems they confront; accepting and using the surrogate-parent role; teaching with specific reference to emotional health as evidenced by various behavioral patterns; assuming the role of social agent concerned with improvement and promotion of recreational, occupational, and social competence; providing leadership and clinical assistance to other nursing personnel.
>
> ...Direct nursing-care functions may involve *individual psychotherapy, group psychotherapy,* family therapy, and sociotherapy. Psychiatric nurses engaged in these therapies may employ a variety of approaches, particularly in the rapidly emerging areas of sociotherapy and community health...
>
> ...Psychiatric nurses are more and more involved in providing services aimed toward prevention of mental illness and reinforcement of healthy adaptations in addition to corrective and rehabilitative services. (p. 1)

The concepts discussed above are basically the prefatory material which sets the stage for the 1973 standards themselves. Each of the standards then discusses a particular procedure, its rationale and its assessment. By 1982, these standards had been refined somewhat to include 11 standards and 6 sub-parts under Standard V—Intervention (American Nurses' Association, 1982). The total standards will not be reproduced here, but several significant concepts in them will be highlighted. For example, Standard II—Diagnosis indicates that "The nurse utilizes nursing diagnosis and standard classification of mental disorders to express conclusions supported by recorded assessment data and current scientific premises." Standard V—Intervention includes Standards V-A through V-F which respectively discuss the interventions used: V-A, Psychotherapeutic interventions; V-B, health teaching; V-C, self-care activities; V-D, somatic therapies; V-E, therapeutic environment; and, V-F, Psychotherapy. With respect to Standards V-A and V-F specifically, the standards indicate the following: "The nurse (generalist) uses psychotherapeutic interventions to assist clients to regain or improve their previous coping abilities and to prevent further disability" and, with respect to psychotherapy, "The nurse (specialist) utilizes advanced clinical expertise in individual group, and family psychotherapy, child psychotherapy, and other treatment modalities to function as a psychotherapist and recognizes professional accountability for nursing practice."

Seeds of Controversy

These perspectives and standards represent the seeds for controversy within nursing, the health care system generally, and among other mental health professionals. The Standards suggest that much of the language and many concepts used in psychotherapeutic intervention overlap with those of clinical and counseling psychologists, with those of some psychiatrists, and less so with social workers. As long as psychiatric nurses work within hospitals or, indeed, community health centers, the likelihood of major controversy with other helping professionals is minimal. This prediction seems feasible, in addition, because psychiatric nurses seem to see themselves, according to their standards, as part of a team whether or not they are in a hospital setting. Psychiatric nurses have evolved out of a collaborative and, indeed, coordinated medical team approach and have generalized that behavior within the mental health-psychiatric area in their expectation of collaboration with other "helping professionals" in whatever setting they occupy. How such collaborative behavior will hold up in the crucible of private practice is another matter.

If psychiatric nurses increase their penetration into the realm of licensure and practice as an independent, autonomous mental health specialist, they expand the likelihood that they will be competing with other "helping professionals" for private clients and third party payment for services delivered. As this occurs, turfdom and the economics of the helping professions are likely to become more clearly matters of controversy than is now true.

Nurse-Physician Relationships

Within the health care system generally, and hospitals more specifically, psychiatric nurses find themselves in situations somewhat analogous to those experienced by clinical psychologists. That is, physicians, or more precisely in this instance, psychiatrists have the dominant authority in patient care.

As suggested in the introductory material to the standards, "the dependent area of psychiatric nursing practice is implementation of physician's orders..." While, as was said previously, psychiatric nurses tend to expect to engage in a high degree of interdependence with other professional colleagues in meeting patient or client needs, interdependence is not synonymous with the subordination which is inherent in the nurse-physician relationship. Such subordination creates tensions and is, in fact, controversial for many psychiatric nurses who believe their skills and training specific to dealing with psychiatric patients is equal to that of psychiatrists and certainly superior to that of non-psychiatric trained physicians. Such observations have validity, at least in England, where Marks et al. (1977) have shown that nurse therapists can treat neurotic out-patients as successfully as psychiatrists and psychologists using similar treatments with comparable populations. Often, because males dominate psychiatry and females dominate psychiatric nursing, the controversy becomes a male-female issue as well as a physician-nurse issue (Taylor & Mereness, 1982). In either case, the controversy between psychiatrists or physicians and psychiatric nurses has exacerbated as the focus of education in psychiatric nursing has shifted from custodial care to the treatment of patients.

Notions, earlier identified, which view mental illness as a breakdown of social processes, not just a breakdown of physical or organic processes, psychotherapy as a process not owned exclusively by psychiatry, and a shortage of psychiatrists as compared to the expanding needs for mental health services all combined to escalate the status of psychiatric nursing as an independent and important part of the total mental health system of the United States as well as in other parts of the world (Nichols, 1985). The evolution of beliefs in the informal group process and the therapeutic milieu as treatment strategies led not only to the rise of the community mental health center as opposed to the psychiatric hospital as the appropriate site for patient/client treatment but also sharpened the role of psychiatric nurses as a treatment entity within such therapeutic milieus (Lancaster, 1980). In Britain, for example, a strong movement is present to have nurses trained to provide psychological care for patients in *general* hospitals where the availability of psychiatrists or psychologists is virtually non-existent. While some psychiatrists and psychologists have resisted giving their skills away to nurses either through training or default, a strong effort continues to make nurses front-line psychological workers as a routine provision for the seriously ill, to provide preventive care aimed at reducing the impact of known stresses imposed by the medical subculture and hospital regimes as well as in dealing with the stresses of illness itself. In evolving such a role for psychiatric nursing in general hospitals, six components have emerged to describe the nurses' role in such a context?

1. Monitoring patients' psychological state

2. Representing the client's psychological needs

3. Providing emotional care

4. Providing information to reduce stress

5. Providing counseling

6. Engaging in co-support and case discussions (Nichols, 1985)

Sometimes called nurse-counselors or nurse therapists, the experience in Great Britain of recognizing the therapeutic capabilities of nurses to fill a void in psychological care in general hospitals is a likely prototype for evolving models in the United States. Because of the issues of power, professional hierarchies, training, and economics, such elaboration of the skill overlap of one group of professionals with those of others is not likely to occur without controversy and conflict (Reavley & Herdman, 1985).

Some interesting signs in the United States are that psychologists and nurses are coming into new alliances against the physician-dominated health care system (DeLeon, Kjervik, Kraut, & VandenBos,

1985). The destiny of psychologists, particularly clinical psychologists, who wish full access to hospital privileges and to autonomous practice in behavioral medicine and health psychology is not unrelated to that of nurse practitioners who are attempting to use their clinical skills and understandings to evolve parity and autonomy between themselves, psychologists, social workers, and their medical colleagues. If this critical mass of nonphysician health care providers do cooperate to promote their mutual acceptance as major and autonomous members of the health care system, the issues of controversy which emerge will shift to political settings to sort out the legislative empowerment necessary to client freedom-of-choice and to practitioner clarity about the competence of the various groups contributing to the delivery of health care in institutional and non-institutional settings.

Community Mental Health

As the community mental health movement versus what we might call the institutionalized mental health structure has evolved, the role definition of psychiatric nurses has changed. The term "psychiatric nursing" has typically referred to care provided within an institution and directed toward treatment of individuals designated as "ill" (Lancaster, 1980, p. 7). While such a definition may still be useful, it tends not to capture the broad range of activities which have developed in the past twenty years under rubrics such as community psychology or community mental health. As the latter has unfolded, psychiatric nursing has spawned specializations under such titles as community psychiatric nurse, psychiatric mental health nurse, or community mental health nurse. In combination, these specialties extend psychiatric nursing into the community.

In the case of the *community psychiatric nurse,* for example, treatment is extended into the community, a public health approach is used, and nursing activities include home visits and group and family treatment as well as consultation and education; a primary aim may be prevention of mental disorder. An individual client may still be the object of treatment by the psychiatric nurse but the site for treatment is a location in the community either formally defined in such terms as the community mental health center or less formally as the patients' home.

However, in a specialization such as community mental health nursing, an individual client is not necessarily the focus of treatment, but rather groups of persons who are vulnerable or at risk to mental illness.

In such circumstances, assessment, prevention, education, stimulation of wellness, stress management, mastering community resources or group resources to strengthen that psychological functioning which is intact, integrating concepts of wholistic mental health and systems theory all become the arenas of community mental nursing.

As models of community mental health nursing or community psychiatric nursing unfold, the seeds of controversy with other helping professionals grow. Probably the most likely area for conflict is between community mental health/psychiatric nursing and clinical social work. Both of these groups of helping professionals claim the community at large, populations at risk, group process, bringing together or using referral to community resources as treatment strategies, and systems theory as integral to their raison d'etre and their treatment strategies. Thus, they appear to be moving on a collision course as the numbers of either clinical social workers or community mental health/psychiatric nurses grow. Implicit in such a notion is that what has kept the two groups of helping professionals from coming into major conflict is that the demands for the services of each have significantly exceeded the numbers of helping professionals of either category available to provide such services. If supply/demand comes into better balance in the future, conflicts emanating from matters of territoriality, competence, and training are likely to erupt.

A final area of controversy for psychiatric nursing is within nursing itself. The question is, When is a specialist nurse no longer a nurse? As Taylor (1983) puts the matter: "A major issue is the question of whether the psychiatric nurse is really a nurse like any other or whether by virtue of her specialty she has forfeited her identity as a nurse" (p. 645). According to Taylor, two major factors bear on this issue.

> One factor...is that, despite knowledge and verbalizations to the contrary, health care professionals still practice in a manner that perpetuates a dichotomy between the mind and body. In addition, knowledge and care of the body seem to be more valued by lay persons and professionals alike then knowledge and care of the mind... Whatever the reason, the result is that when nurses or physicians choose to specialize in the care of the mentally ill, they run the risk of divorcing themselves from the mainstream of mental health care delivery. Some persons have gone so far as to state that mental illness, as currently defined, is not an illness at all but rather a reflection of societal problems. Therefore preparation for the care of these persons should not be within the health care disciplines... (p. 646).

Another factor underlying the identity issue facing psychiatric nursing is role blurring. Before the advent of phenothiazine derivatives, the roles of mental health care workers were more clearly defined. The nurse was primarily concerned with the client's activities of daily living, the psychiatrist focused on diagnosing and prescribing, the psychologist focused on testing and research, and the social worker had the client's family as her domain. Very little treatment occurred. When psychotropic drugs made clients more accessible to therapeutic interventions, all mental health disciplines began to claim these interventions as being within their scope of practice. The result was role blurring where members of all disciplines engage in individual, family, and group therapy. The question then arises as to what if anything, differentiates the nurse from the physician, the psychologist, or the social worker. (p. 647)

SUMMARY

In Chapter 1 has been examined the concept of "core provider" in the helping professions. Much of the discussion has considered the characteristics of the four occupations to which that title has typically been ascribed: psychiatry, psychology, social work and psychiatric nursing. Both inter- and intra-occupational controversies have been identified. Chief among these have been history, power, conceptual and language systems, empirical base, and economic opportunities related to independent practice.

CHAPTER 2

NON-CORE MENTAL HEALTH PROVIDERS

Certainly, the four core provider groups described in Chapter 1 are not the whole of the helping professions. While identification as a core provider may confer a status and an entree to economic benefits which not having such designation may reduce, other helping professionals have status that also adds to controversies in the helping professions. To paraphrase the question posed at the end of Chapter 1, what, if anything, differentiates the core provider from the non-core provider? As expected, the answer varies. History, training, institutional allegiance are each involved as one looks at the differences between the so-called core providers of mental health services and those occupations not accorded such status but which either aspire to such recognition or provide mental health services under another rubric.

PROFESSIONAL COUNSELORS

Professional counselors are among the major groups of mental health specialists who are not defined as core providers. These persons often are not trained in psychology programs but rather in university departments entitled Counselor Education. They most frequently are trained at the Master's level, but many of those who call themselves counselors do possess doctoral degrees in Counselor Education, Human Services, Rehabilitation Counseling or related areas.

Professional counselors are found in many settings: community mental health centers, rehabilitation agencies, schools, employment services, business, industry, and private practice. Indeed, some data suggest that mental health counselors deliver most of the mental health services in the nation either under the supervision or independent of other "helping professionals." Available estimates are that one-third to one-half of all mental health services are delivered by counselors who are providing similar treatment to that offered by psychologists (American Mental Health Counselors Association, 1983). In some eighteen states, counselors are able to be licensed as independent practitioners permitted by law to charge for their services from clients and, often, from "third party" payers (e.g., Blue Cross/Blue Shield, Health Insurance plans, etc.). The political press to have counselors recognized as private practitioners is an ongoing issue in some 30 additional states and the press for third party reimbursement is being waged at both State and Federal levels.

Professional "counselors" as contrasted with clinical or counseling psychologists are typically members of the American Association for Counseling and Development rather than the American Psychological Association. Depending upon the specific training received, most counselors tend to be grounded in psychology but are likely as well to have a broad interdisciplinary education including studies in all of the behavioral sciences. In Chapter 5 will be discussed the specifics of their training as compared with that of other helping professions.

Professional counselors are frequently defined by the setting or population which they serve. For example, Mental Health Counselors, School Counselors, Rehabilitation Counselors, Employment/Career Counselors are each likely to consider themselves professional counselors with similar core training and skills even through the application of their training and skills differs. They see themselves as key members of the helping professions and, indeed, because of their numbers and the settings in which they work, they may be the principal providers of mental health services, particularly preventive and developmental mental health services, in the nation.

Professional counselors tend to be organized in their own divisions within the American Association for Counseling and Development. For example, the American Mental Health Counselors Association (AMHCA) represents, as the name indicates, mental health counselors. The American School Counselors Association (ASCA) represents school counselors. The American Rehabilitation Counselors Association (ARCA) represents rehabilitation counselors. The National Career Development Association (NCDA), formerly titled the National Vocational Guidance Association (NVGA), represents career counselors and the National Employment Counselors Association (NECA) represents employment counselors. While these organizations do not constitute mutually exclusive members, they do tend to focus on issues and matters of concern to the settings in which the largest numbers of their members are employed.

Efforts to Become Core Providers

The employment of mental health counselors tends to overlap most dramatically with that of the four groups of "core providers" described in the first chapter. Indeed, AMHCA, in behalf of mental health counselors, has sought to have such professional counselors recognized as "fifth core providers" in Federal statutes dealing with such definitions. Evidence of progress in this respect has taken several forms to date. For example, Senator Denton (R-Alabama) introduced a bill in the U.S. Senate entitled "Recognition of Mental Health Counselors as Independent Providers of Mental Health: Mental Health Service Providers Bill." Congressional efforts have been in place to amend "The Older American Comprehensive Counseling Act of 1983 (HR 2109)" to provide a direct reimbursement provisions clause for mental health counselors as core services providers. Representative Claude Pepper has introduced a bill to amend the Social Security Act to provide reimbursement of the services of Mental Health Counselors under the Medicare Supplemental Benefits and Medicaid Programs. Each of these efforts and similar processes underway are gradually increasing the visibility and, indeed, the sanctioning of mental health or professional counselors within the mental health delivery system of the nation (Beck, 1983).

In addition to efforts to attain "fifth core provider" status at the Federal level, the American Mental Health Counselors Association continues to seek wider sanction of the services of professional counselors at the State level through licensure. Such efforts have been spurred by court cases in favor of counselors. As reported in Van Hoose and Kottler

(1978), for example, in 1974, in the case of *Weldon v. Virginia State Board of Psychologist Examiners,* the court stated that "counseling is a separate profession" from psychology and should be so recognized. In 1975, the case of *City of Cleveland v. Cook,* further boosted the profession by allowing a counselor to practice privately without the blessing of the state psychology board (Van Hoose & Kottler, 1978). In some instances, the approach has been to include professional counselors as one of the eligible providers of mental health services under "Freedom of Choice" legislation (Wilmarth, 1983). Such statutes essentially are reactions to potential restraint of trade by what are sometimes considered to be exclusionary, capricious, or arbitrary definitions of who eligible mental health providers are. In other instances, the effort is focused on getting licensure for the counselor so that he/she can compete for clients and reimbursement in ways equal to that of psychiatrists, psychologists, social workers, and psychiatric nurses.

In view of the legislative efforts made in behalf of mental health counselors and other professional counselors to attain "core provider" status, licensure for private practice, or sanction under "freedom of choice," the opportunities for controversy to arise with other occupations within the helping professions are wide-ranging. In some states, Boards of Psychologist Examiners have opposed counselor licensure. In other states social workers have opposed such licensure (Seligman, 1984). The grounds for such opposition have varied. In some cases, the public issue is whether professional counselors have sufficient education and the right type of training or supervised practice to be considered for licensure as an independent practitioner. In other instances, the matter is duplication of services already available through psychologists, psychiatrists, or social workers (these, of course, become freedom of choice, or restraint of trade issues). Underlying such issues is the matter of economics, territoriality, and definitions of mental illness/mental health. These matters have been addressed previously in Chapter 1 and subsequent sections of the book will treat them more fully.

Certification of Professional Counselors and Their Training

Another area of controversy between professional counselors and other members of the helping professions also needs recognition here. This has to do with professional certification and regulation as an issue separate from state licensure or federal "core provider" status. The

American Mental Health Counselors Association has spawned a separate corporate entity, The National Academy of Certified Clinical Mental Health Counselors. The academy recognizes, "certified clinical mental health counselors," through a process of examination of knowledge, scrutiny of experience and references, and analysis of a work sample. The intent of such certification is to recognize individuals who have met certain predetermined qualifications specified by the Academy to insure that the public health, safety, and welfare will be reasonably well protected. The definition of a Certified Clinical Mental Health Counselor is "an individual certified as having the competency to assist individuals or groups in achieving optimal mental health, through personal and social development and adjustment in order to prevent the debilitating effects of certain somatic, emotional, and intra-and/or interpersonal disorders through the methods and procedures of counseling and psychotherapy" (NACCMHC, undated).

In addition to the certification process of the National Academy of Certified Clinical Mental Health Counselors for mental health counselors, currently three other national counselor certification mechanisms are in place and several others are in various stages of conceptualization. The three in place are the National Board of Certified Counselors (NBCC), the separate specialty for career counselors available after counselors have attained the generic counselor certification from NBCC, and the Council for the Certification of Rehabilitation Counselors. They respectively provide recognition of National Certified Counselors (NCC), National Certified Career Counselors (NCCC), and Certified Rehabilitation Counselors (CRC).

As each of the certification processes for professional counselors unfold, they add visibility and credibility to such persons, provide additional leverage for licensure, and cause potential tension and conflict with other mental health professionals who contend they use similar intervention processes to similar ends.

A further area of controversy between professional counselors and other groups of helping professionals is in the accreditation of counselor training programs. For nearly twenty years, the development of standards for the training of professional counselors has been underway. These have been refined and extended as new emphases or specialties within professional counseling have evolved. In some cases, these standards, which were originally developed by the Association for Counselor Education and Supervision and more recently adopted by the American

Personnel and Guidance Association (now the American Association for Counseling and Development), have been used by other groups such as the National Accreditation Council for Teacher Education (NCATE), State Departments of Education or regional educational accrediting groups to evaluate counselor education programs preparing school counselors. More recently, an independent agency, the Council for the Accreditation of Counseling and Related Educational Programs (CACREP), has come into being to accredit programs across the nation providing Master's and doctoral level training in school counseling, community counseling, and student personnel services. Another national agency, the Council on Rehabilitation Education (CORE) accredits such programs at the master's level for rehabilitation counselors.

The creation of such accrediting agencies gives credibility and sanction to training programs for counselors which do not meet the criteria for doctoral level accreditation of programs by the American Psychological Association or the focus of which is not confined to school counseling and potentially covered by NCATE or which does not think that the latter is sufficiently consistent and rigorous to be the appropriate accreditation process for professional counselors.

The development of such accrediting and certification processes independent of other helping professional groups provides fodder for conflicts and controversies among the helping professions. At issue are matters of power, ownership of training content and processes, as well as independence of identity and regulations which at once denigrate history and territoriality as the prime criteria for professional sanction.

Some Historical Perspectives

The history of professional counselors, particularly mental health counselors, is not unlike that of counseling psychologists and to a lesser degree, clinical psychologists. Both counselors and counseling psychologists have evolved out of roots in the guidance movement, particularly vocational guidance, and they have embraced many of the same psychotherapeutic interventions including psychotherapy. Both mental health counselors and counseling psychologists have emerged from origins in the practice of counseling in schools and universities. Clinical psychologists and mental health counselors share roots in the treatment of mental illness. However, as national mental health policies have shifted funding from institutional settings, particularly educational settings, increasingly to community settings and, more recently, to private practice, professional counselors, particularly those who wished to engage in longer-term and more in-depth procedures with children, youth, or adults than educational settings permitted sought other settings, including autonomous practice in which to employ their skills. They also sought an identity which was not lodged in psychology per se.

Under the impetus of the Community Mental Health Systems Act of 1963, other community-based programs concurrent with the deinstitutionalization of the mentally ill, as well as the growing national emphases on counseling of substance abusers, Employee Assistance Programs and on health psychology, fitness, wellness, stress management and prevention of mental distress, by the mid-1970s a larger number of master's level graduates of counselor education programs were finding employment in community and nonschool settings. Essentially, these counselors were shaping a professional identity outside of the traditional professional organizations. The American Psychological Association, for example, had been primarily supportive of doctoral level practitioners who had graduated from departments of psychology, while the members of the American Personnel and Guidance Association were primarily master's level professionals, comprised largely of school counselors, vocational counselors, college student development specialists, and rehabilitation counselors who typically practiced within institutional and governmental settings in which mental health care was not the principal mission or goal. To serve the professional mental health counselor, who previously had no clear organizational home, in 1976, the American Mental Health Counselors Association came into being as a Division of the American Personnel and Guidance Association (now the American Association for Counseling and Development). From its founding 50 members in 1976 it had grown to 500 members by March 1977 and it now constitutes the largest of the 12 divisions of the more than 50,000 members of the American Association for Counseling and Development with a membership of more than 9,000 members.

From their organizational beginnings in 1976, the priorities of mental health counselors have consistently included "licensure, third-party payments, full parity with other mental health professionals, and the treatment of special populations in community and private settings" (Weikel, 1985). In one sense, each of these priorities was a hope, not a reality in 1976. There was no licensure for professional counselors other than that of a psychologist. There was no separate counselor certification. The likelihood of obtaining access to third party payment as a counselor or parity with other mental health professionals was small. In the past decade all of these goals have been achieved in multiple States and, as has been suggested previously, national organization, leadership, and visibility has escalated. Political efforts to reflect the contributions of mental health counselors to the national mental health care agenda have received intensified and comprehensive political attention directed at obtaining fifth core provider or service provider status through amendments to titles XVIII and XIX of the Social Security (Medicare Act), a new hospice bill revision of the Older American Act of 1965 and to other legislation as dicussed previously.

In response to its support for the contributions of Master's degree level service providers, the American Mental Health Counselors Association is typically comprised of about 70% with Master's degree, 20% with doctoral degrees, and the remainder student members. Membership is not confined to professional counselors and includes psychiatrists, nurses, psychologists, social workers, pastoral counselors, and others. While 10 years ago, most of the members of the American Mental Health Counselors Association worked in community mental health centers, today the largest number of the members work in private practice (22%), 13% work in private counseling centers, 13% in colleges and universities, 11% in community mental health centers, and 4% in community agencies. Smaller proportions of the membership work in rehabilitation agencies (5%), state or local government (4%), parochial or private institutions (3%), secondary schools (3%), elementary schools (3%), junior college (2%), business and industry (2%), the federal government (2%), and "other settings" (13%)(American Association for Counseling and Development, 1983).

Given its expansion in membership and success in gaining recognition, the mental health counselor profession is clearly seeking licensure in all 50 states in the next decade. It also seeks third-party payments and nondiscrimination in federal legislation and by private insurance carriers. Beyond those matters other emerging issues are related to the role of "mental health counselors in business and industry through Employee Assistance Programs and other modalities; Health maintenance organizations; hospital privileges for counselors; the counselor's role in diagnosis; and other interprofessional liaison" (Weikel, 1985, p. 459).

Current Controversies

Obviously, the forms of controversy engendered by the march of professional counselors to full parity with other mental health service providers in virtually any setting or private practice include a wide-range of possibilities. They include whether a mental health provider trained at the Master's level (even a 60 semester credit hour degree) is the equivalent of a doctoral level provider; does the scope of practice of professional counselors overlap that of psychologists so fully as to precipitate violations of state psychological statutes; are adequate distinctions possible between professional counselors, psychologists, and social workers to legitimize separate licensure; with what other groups of mental health practitioners do mental health counselors have most in common or with whom are they likely to create professional alliances and coalitions; are professional counselors generalists or specialists. If the latter, what are their most distinctive competencies and with whom are they most capable of working?

These forms of controversy are both matters of professional identity and of political reality. Clearly, as professional counselors gain visibility and credibility they compete for positions previously occupied by other mental health providers. In some states, the principal protagonists are counselors and psychologists; in other states, it is counselors and clinical social workers or, even, counselors and marriage and family therapists. The issues in any of these states are those of sharing an economic pie allocated in whatever form to the provision of mental health care and which of these groups can most effectively influence the state legislature to accommodate its interests.

Emergence of Professional Validation

The issue of professional identity is somewhat different. The controversy here relates to how professional counselors differ in their techniques or intervention strategies from other mental health providers? How do they define their client population and to what ends? As Brooks and Weikel (1986) have suggested, in one sense it has become almost impossible to separate the development of mental health counseling as a profession from its organizational expression in the American Mental Health Counselors Association. Be that as it may, however, mental health counselors have since 1976 attempted to clarify and differentiate their identity from other groups. Among the most significant of these efforts was the development in 1981 (Palmo, 1981) of a definition which was subsequently included in 1984, in part, in the *Occupational Outlook Handbook* (U.S. Department of Labor), an official government document, acknowledging both the existence of the mental health counselor as a separate occupation and, as some observers would contend, a de facto recognition of its core provider status.

The accepted definition of mental health counselor is as follows:

> The mental health counselor performs counseling/therapy with individuals, groups, couples, and families; collects, organizes, and analyzes data concerning client's mental, emotional and/or behavioral problems or disorders; aids clients and their families to effectively adapt to the personal concerns presented; develops procedures to assist clients to adjust to possible environmental barriers that may impede self-understanding and personal growth; utilizes community agencies and institutions to develop mental health programs that are developmental and preventive in nature. Trained to provide a wide variety of therapeutic approaches to assist clients, which may include therapy, milieu therapy, and behavioral therapy. Employed in clinics hospitals, drug centers, colleges, private agencies, related mental health programs or private practice. Required to have knowledge and skills in client management, assessment and diagnosis through a post graduate program in mental health or community mental health counseling. (Palmo, 1981, p. 1)

In at least relative terms, this definition suggests that the mental health counselor can be distinguished from other mental health providers because of an interest in the client's environment and in his/her interaction with significant others including family; in the use of testing and data collection; in the use of counseling (or psychotherapy) to promote self-understanding and promotion of personal growth; in the emphasis on a developmental model rather than a pathology model of behavior and on prevention; in the attempt to use a psychoeducational model designed to build client strengths and teach them life skills as a major therapeutic tool. Clients are not typically viewed as sick or experiencing an underlying pathology in their personality structure. Clients are more likely to be seen as people in transition or in crisis as they are attempting to deal with such conditions, to muster available personal resources, and to move toward new areas of growth and development.

Obviously, controversy can arise as any other group of mental health providers project themselves into any given phrase of the definition of mental health counselor and experience feelings of ownership. While mental health counselors might reasonably argue that it is the whole configuration of processes and assumptions that make mental health counselors distinct, other groups of providers may argue quite differently. Such is the stuff of controversy.

FAMILY THERAPISTS

A potential source of controversy, conflict, or tension within the helping professions is the growing autonomy of family therapy as a specialization independent of other members of the "helping professions." Family therapy has, in some cases, been a part of the training of psychiatrists, clinical psychologists, pastoral counselors, and others. But, the growing issue within the family therapy movement is whether family therapy is a technique which might be included in the repertoire of essentially any helping professional or, and this is the critical issue, a paradigm shift requiring a complete systems view, related techniques, and fully trained practitioners in their own right.

The fact that family therapists are becoming increasingly formal in their professional organizations is a sign that family therapy, while open to many different types of conventional mental health practitioners, is taking on its own rapidly evolving professional identity as a discrete occupation among the helping professions.

Three forces, or mechanisms, now describe the professional movement in family therapy. One is that the American Association for Marriage and Family Therapy (AAMFT) has put into place a process of accrediting (or certifying) individuals through admission to clinical membership in the AAMFT. The second force is a national movement to achieve licensure on a State by State basis which recognizes the competency of Marriage and Family Therapy Education (Bloch & Weiss, 1981). This Commission has developed model curricula and standards by which to evaluate training programs seeking accreditation (Commission on Accreditation for Marriage and Family Therapy Education, 1979).

Each of these steps toward professionalization is cause for controversy between family therapy and other mental health service providers. Again, issues of history, power, training, and economics each arise as points of contention about the validity of independent status for family therapists.

Controversies with Other Groups

An explicit area of controversy with certain helping professions is family therapy training. As suggested above, training in family therapy at a sophisticated level is now more or less a part of the training of psychiatrists (perhaps all physicians should have such training), psychologists, social workers, and psychiatric nurses. But, in addition, the new profession of family therapist has its own entry point and academic pathway.

To date, training in family therapy is a diverse mix of institutional settings in which training in family therapy is provided. These include free-standing family institutes; medical schools; hospital-based general psychiatric residency and clinical psychology internships; doctoral programs in clinical psychology, sociology, child and human development, and family therapy; social work programs; entry level master's degree programs in marital and family therapy; family casework agencies; and pastoral counseling training centers (Block & Weiss, 1981). In these settings one finds a profusion of purposes: Enrichment, Training (Bachelor's, Master's, Doctorate, Non-degree granting), Mixed (Training or Enrichment), and accredited or not. Where enrichment is the major purpose, the typical student is a trained mental health professional of some sort who wants further training in family therapy. But, specific Master's and Doctoral level programs have as their intent the training of family therapists as a new professional with a different view of behavior and intervention than is common in many traditional clinical mental health programs. Such family therapy graduate programs are probably most directly competitive with existing doctoral programs in social work and clinical psychology. These, of course, sow seeds of conflict with such professional groups. In addition, however, doctoral training programs emphasize family therapy in clinical psychology, sociology, human development, and marriage and family counseling (Bloch & Weiss, 1981). The fact that family therapy at the doctoral level has penetrated so many of these disciplines threatens discipline bound professions, raises questions of theoretical dilution and acknowledges that no longer does any single profession claim sole expertise in this new orientation and technology. It also affirms that family therapy does operate from a new and different conceptual set than is apparent in other helping professions.

Thus, the conceptual perspectives and language system of family therapy becomes another issue or controversy among the helping professions. As currently experienced, family therapy training rests upon an "ecosystemic, biopsychosocial" base rather than a medical model with its linear definitions of illness and treatment. Therefore, cure is not defined in terms of intrapsychic change in the patient but as maintenance and functioning within the family and community (Meyerstein, 1981). In such a view

> the focus moves from the "figure" (the individual client or even nuclear family unit) to "the ground" (the social network in which it is embedded)... This approach is concerned with how people manage psychological, as well as concrete issues of daily living with one another at home and in their community.

Ecological family therapists are more than just client advocates. They actually teach families how to relate to outside systems, using the interaction generated as grist of the therapeutic mill... The ecological therapist becomes somewhat of a 'social engineer who creates a network of natural helpers in the neighborhood as resources, such as relatives, peer groups, and friends to help jointly a high-risk client and family... (Meyerstein, 1981, p. 481)

"The systemic paradigm authorizes interventions at the family level in regard to dysfunctions of an individual" (Block & Weiss, 1981, p. 146). Obviously, such excerpts only touch the highlights of this new paradigm of family therapy. But, even from this standpoint of a somewhat different language system, the concepts expressed and the therapeutic purposes smack of the systems theory and small group processes espoused by the clinical social worker and of the therapeutic milieu of the psychiatric nurse. In addition, in its rejection of the medical model, this paradigm puts at odds the conceptual frames about mental illness espoused by the psychiatrist and to a lesser degree by the clinical psychologist. These, too, are the seeds of controversy.

While something of a digression, it is worth noting that the American Association for Marriage and Family Therapy (AAMFT) may have competition, if not some internal sources of controversy, from other organizations dealing with family issues. For example, also concerned with family matters is the American Association of Family Counselors and Mediators (AAFCM) incorporated in 1983. The AAFCM, according to its descriptive material, was formed: "(1) to improve the quality of counseling and mediation services generally available to individuals and families and for extending these services to many more people and families; and (2) to enable the public and employers to identify those practitioners who exhibit a high degree of competency in mediation." To the latter ends, the AAFCM grants Registration and Certification (1) in Family Mediation, (2) in Community Mediation, and (3) for Supervision of Mediators. While no apparent relationship exists to the AAMFT, the AAFCM is apparently addressing in its training, credentialing, code of ethics and publications an important subset of the skills generally involved in some cases of marriage and family therapy. While distinct from therapy per se, mediation as a process of conflict resolution represents a tool for the negotiation of issues in a family or community in dispute and its practitioners also represent economic competition for other marriage and family therapists. While still emergent as a profession and as an organization, issues of economics, power, and status may become controversial within and among the marriage and family therapists and family mediators in the future.

A final potential area of controversy between professional counselors and family therapists is their simultaneous attempts at the State levels to achieve licensure and at the federal level to achieve "core provider" status. Indeed, Bloch and Weiss (1981) contend that governmental acceptance gives official acknowledgement that marital and family therapy represents a fourth mental health discipline or core provider status as we have previously discussed it. "It validates that the field has a separate body of therapy and techniques for which a distinct training process is appropriate" (Block & Weiss, 1981, 145-146). Professional counselors, social workers, and psychiatric nurses might well disagree with this assessment.

SUMMARY

Two broad groups of mental health practitioners—Professional Counselors and Family Therapists—tend to be aggressively challenging traditional concepts of who the "core providers" of mental health services should include. Each of these groups is seeking Federal and State sanctions which permit them to act as independent practitioners or deliverers of mental health services. Like the "core providers," they have developed individual certification, accreditation of training programs, ethical standards, conceptual systems, and growing empirical bases. In some states they have achieved licensure. As their power and visibility grows, probably the controversy now surrounding their competence and viability as independent practitioners will grow.

CHAPTER 3

ARE THE MENTAL HEALTH PROFESSIONS, PROFESSIONS?

As has been suggested throughout Part 1, the various occupations making up the mental health professions as we have defined them are in the throes of establishing their individual and collective identity. Such a task requires essentially three foci: the degree to which any specific occupation (e.g., psychiatry, social work) meets the criteria for a profession; the degree to which the occupations which in the aggregate make up the "helping professions" converge to qualify as a profession; and, the degree to which other professions or the broader public views the "helping professions" as professions either in individual or collective terms. Each of these three domains is the center of potential controversy among the helping professions although the particulars of such controversy are not easy to establish.

Probably the least difficult way to think about the "helping professions" as professions is in terms of what are essentially sociological and, indeed, conventionally accepted definitions or criteria of what constitutes a profession. Many perspectives on this matter tend to agree in the essential elements of a profession. Two examples of statements of criteria will suffice for our purposes here.

CRITERIA OF A PROFESSION

Barber (1965) has suggested that the essential attributes of a profession include:

1. A high degree of generalized systematic knowledge.

2. Primary education to community interests rather than self interests.

3. A high degree of self control of behavior through codes of ethics internalized in the process of work socialization and through voluntary associations organized and operated by the work of specialists themselves.

4. A system of rewards (monetary and honorary) that is primarily a set of symbols of work achievement and thus ends in themselves. (p. 18)

Greenwood (1957) viewed the attributes of a profession as including some subtle differences from those proposed by Barber even though the two perspectives are in essential agreement. The criteria for a profession according to Greenwood include (1) systematic theory, (2) authority, (3) community sanctions, (4) ethical codes, and (5) a culture.

When these criteria are applied to the "helping professions" by separate occupation, the following observations seem appropriate.

Knowledge Base

Each of the occupations described in Part 1 tend to profess a base in systematic theory. Psychiatry, psychology (clinical or counseling), social work (psychiatric or clinical), nursing (psychiatric, community mental health) tend to receive an intellectual edge on this criterion because they are seen as identified with an established disciplinary base or core of knowledge: medicine, psychology, social work. The newer mental health occupations—professional counselors, family therapists—tend to be more interdisciplinary in the core of knowledge which they espouse and are without the disciplinary history of the older mental health occupations.

However, several additional things need to be said. While each of the helping professions has tended to develop by consensus a basic core of knowledge important to its practitioners, some in each mental health occupation disagree about the core and, more importantly, about the need for specialized knowledge in particular settings or with particular populations. In addition, while psychiatrists and, to a lesser degree, psychiatric nurses acquire their basic identity from medicine as the disciplinary base, the knowledge base required in either psychiatry or psychiatric nursing is considerably different from medicine in its traditional conceptualization. Further, it seems useful to observe that the core knowledge of each of the mental health occupations tends to overlap in some magnitude. For example, each of them treats psychotherapy as an intervention technique. Similarly, each of them treats growth, learning, and other conceptions of the factors influencing human behavior and mental problems as important knowledge although the depth and basic explanatory models are likely to differ from occupation to occupation.

We will be discussing the knowledge base of each of the mental health occupations more specifically as we consider the training of these practitioners in Chapter 5. Suffice it to say here that each of the occupations described in Chapters 1 and 2 does seem to adequately meet the criterion of a base in systematic theory and, also, when generalized in an aggregated sense. The stuff of controversy across mental health occupations is which theoretical explanations or intervention knowledge is seen by others as the most current, empirically based, or appropriate? In some instances, the question is not so much whether the particular mental health occupation has an adequate knowledge base but are the practitioners adequately trained to use that knowledge base with clients, patients,and other users?

**Community Interests
versus Self-Interests**

As we will see when we talk about credentialing in Chapter 6 and the economics of the helping professions in Chapter 9, the lines between community interests and self interests tend to blur. We will not explore the reasons for such blurring here although Federal mental health policy changes which reduce support for mental health agencies or institutional programs and therefore stimulate a market economy in the delivery of mental health services by private practitioners is undoubtedly a major factor in the rising concern about self interests of mental health professionals. To be fair one would observe, however, that the line between community interests and self-interests is no more blurred for the mental health professions than it is for physicians, attorneys, and other occupations whose responses to community interests for health care, legal assistance, or other such matters can lead to substantial economic return to the practitioner.

Apparently the philosophical and ethical statements of each of the mental health occupations does reflect a basic intent to serve community interests as these are reflected in the mental health needs of individuals, families, or other groups. The degree to which this occurs is, of course, a potential arena for controversy within the professions and between them and the society at large.

Authority or Regulation of Practitioner Behavior

In Chapter 6, as we deal with credentialing we will deal with a particular view of professional authority—that which relates to the regulation of who can practice the delivery of mental health services, in what settings, and in what ways. Credentialing in its broadest view can be separated into those mechanisms—e.g., licensure, certification, registry—which regulate individual practitioners and those mechanisms which accredit or approve training programs which prepare practitioners.

Without exception, each of the occupations discussed in Part 1 have accreditation mechanisms in place, either through professional association or governmental auspices, which approve training programs with respect to some set of standards reflecting the appropriateness of the knowledge base, faculty qualifications, and supervised practice provided by the training program for student candidates. These accreditation mechanisms can deny approval to training programs on the basis of existing standards and therefore put the graduates of such programs at risk vis á vis future personal credentials as a practitioner or in terms of employment. The regulation of training programs by professional standards and accreditation mechanisms is essentially absolute in psychiatry and nursing, in clinical and counseling psychology and in social work, and less than absolute but increasingly so in professional counseling and in family therapy. These differences in absolute power have to do with legal sanction, history, and other matters. For example, psychiatry as a medical specialty is recognized in law throughout the nation. No educational program or institution could allege that it is training psychiatrists without the approval/accreditation of the American Psychiatric Association or the American Medical Association. The authority of the professional association to regulate who is trained to be a psychiatrist and how, is established in convention and in law. It has a history defined in precedent and when controversy about the power of such accreditation has been raised it has been adjudicated in courts of law. Persons can not simply choose to call themselves a psychiatrist or charge fees for such services without the appropriate training and credentialing. If they do they will be arrested for fraud, endangering those they treat or on other legal bases. If bona fide practitioners subsequently violate the ethical standards of psychiatry, they can lose their credential to practice if such a violation is severe enough to warrant such sanction. This is a professional regulation expressed as well in the law. In such cases, the power of the profession and, indeed, the authority of the profession to regulate professional practice is absolute. Essentially the same situation is true in nursing and relatively so in clinical or counseling psychology in most states.

Social work has its own accrediting mechanisms for training programs although not every training program which alleges that it trains social workers is accredited. In the latter case, the issue becomes one of what happens to graduates of social work programs which are not accredited and whose graduates can not then become certified as an A.C.S.W. In this case, the problem is not in the accreditation standards but in the power of the professional association to close programs which do not meet such standards for the training of social workers. Currently such power does not accrue in an absolute sense to the American Association for Social Work. The other part of the power equation is the legal sanctions which occur if one calls oneself a social worker but is not so trained. It depends upon the State. In those States where Clinical Social Workers receive licensure, improper use of the term "clinical social worker or social worker" in describing oneself is a legal violation and can lead to fines or imprisonment.

A similar situation to that of social work now exists within professional counseling and in family therapy. In both cases, standards, and mechanisms exist for the accreditation of training programs which prepare counselors or which prepare family therapists. However, in neither occupation does power exist to close training programs which do not meet the standards developed and promulgated by the respective professional association. Persons violating the ethical standards of these associations can be removed from professional membership. However, because of the confusion which attends the use of the term counselor or family therapist, no legal sanctions can be levied against persons who use these terms except in those states where separate licensure exists for counselors or for family therapists. While such licensure and the related legal sanctions are growing from state to state, in relation to the regulation and sanctions available to psychiatry, nursing, or psychology, the degree of professional regulation available to social work, professional counseling, and family therapy is not yet comparable. For the most part, the status of professional regulation is not a matter of professional intent but of statutory recognition of such power. Clearly, the professional associations representing social work, counseling and family therapy have developed ethical guidelines, accreditation standards, and other mechanisms designed to regulate the professional behavior of their members. However, they have not yet received the authority and legal sanctions to regulate, on a universal basis, the use of their titles for performance in the work place as is true for the other mental health occupations. The lack of such statutory regulation concerning counselors and family therapists, in particular, leads to other kinds of controversy in regard to such areas as third party payment, independent practice, parity versus subordination in mental health teams and so forth.

Community Sanction

The status of community sanctions for the various mental health occupations has been suggested in the previous section and will again be discussed in those parts of the book dealing with credentialing and economics. Basically, legal protection of title and function is a community sanction. So is third party payment or licensure or certification. To varying degrees each of the mental health occupations identified here have received such sanctions. The older discipline based occupations—Psychiatry, Psychology, Nursing—tend to have more complete and unequivocal sanctions while the other occupations—social work, counseling, and family therapy—have received many evidences of community sanction although the application of such sanctions is unevenly distributed.

A Culture

Each of the mental health occupations has a professional culture to which its practitioners tend to be socialized while in training. Psychiatry, psychology, nursing, and social work tend to be the most focused and consistent in their training, knowledge base, and supervised practicum and internship processes. Professional counseling also has a culture but until recently it tended to be that of the institutions in which counselors worked—schools, rehabilitation agencies, colleges—rather than a separate, professionally defined culture. The latter is emerging rapidly as a requisite to the statutory sanctions counselors are seeking in behalf of independent practice, licensure, and related affirmations of professional identity.

Family therapy seems to be evolving its culture in ways analogous to counselors. Until recently, family therapy tended to be viewed as an add-on, a specialization acquired by persons who were trained as a psychiatrist, psychologist, social worker, pastor or other professional. In that sense, a separate professional culture was not as likely or as possible as is now emerging. As family therapy is taking increasing steps to have its own separate, professional identity it must evolve a professional culture and belief system which while relevant to those who come from other mental health occupations to add the skills of family therapy to their repertoire does not depend on the culture of these other occupations as its only raison d'etre.

System of Rewards Symbolic of Work Achievement

Perhaps less equivocal than any of the other criteria, each of the mental health occupations does have a system of rewards symbolic of work achievement. These vary, of course, in their source and their character but they exist throughout the helping professions. Frequently and almost invariably these are mediated through the Professional Associations representing each set of occupations. Sometimes the reward is in a title or status conferred: Fellow, Diplomate, Professional Member; sometimes it is a plaque, certificate or term, e.g., Eminent Career Award, Eminent Practitioner, "Distinguished Achievement." Sometimes it evolves in a differentiated way through the credentialing process: "permanent certification," Full rather than Provisional licensure, sometimes it is reflected in a University Chair or research professorship in psychiatry, clinical or counseling psychology, social work or counseling. Each of these symbolic rewards tend to accompany some form or level of economic reward.

While symbolic or even monetary rewards are not typically controversial in themselves, their comparability tends to be. For example, is being a Fellow in the American Psychological Association as prestigious, or as difficult to achieve, as in the American Psychiatric Association? Does being a Fellow in Division 17 (Counseling Psychology) of the American Psychological Association represent the same level of distinction or difficulty as in Division 12 (Clinical Psychology)? Is it more prestigious to be the President of the American Psychological Association or the American Association for Counseling and Development? While only partial answers can be given to these questions in objective terms, the rest of these answers represent a subjective evaluation of many aspects of prestige, power, and economics among the helping professions.

CONCLUSION

This analysis of how generally accepted criteria necessary to becoming a profession fit the "helping professions" is obviously subjective and equivocal. Nevertheless, several of the occupations—psychiatry, psychology, nursing—tend to have achieved all criteria in a comprehensive fashion. In general, so has social work. Professional counseling and family therapy have met the criteria less comprehensively. The differences between having met all criteria for a profession and having met most criteria may seem to be a subtle difference. In practice, the differences are the substance of controversy, particularly when the major criterion unmet by professional counseling, social work, or family therapy is in the regulation of who can be trained, who can use a title, who can do the work described as that of counselor, social worker, or family therapist. In essence, what is missing in these terms is legal sanction supporting the unique identity and therefore, the parity of these occupations with others qualifying as professions. In turn, such a deficit complicates issues of eligibility for certain sources of reimbursement, independent practice, and associated rewards reserved for the fully sanctioned professional provider of mental health services.

CHAPTER 4

THE ULTIMATE QUESTION OF PROFESSIONAL IDENTITY: WHAT IS MENTAL HEALTH AND WHO SHOULD PROVIDE IT?

Related to the matter of the professional status of various mental health occupations, but possibly more controversial, is the question of who shall provide mental health services? In a sense that question has pervaded all of Theme One. It is a question of competency, training, sanction, and other elements which have been discussed thus far. But, it is also a function of another question which has not yet been asked. That is, what is mental health or mental illness? Without looking at the controversy inherent in these terms, possibly most of the inarticulated confusion which underlies the status of various mental health occupations would be missed.

Frequently, mental illness and mental health are treated as though they are discrete and dichotomous entities. In this sense, they also are treated as homogeneous entities. In casual terms one is either ill or well, sick or healthy. But, regardless of how easily the layperson can think in such terms, these concepts are at the core of professional controversies about who should receive mental health services, for what purpose, and by whom?

Obviously, such questions can be answered in power, status, and economic terms as we have suggested throughout Theme One. However, the more basic and scientific answers to such questions emanate from what is known about the nature of mental illness, mental health, or other perspectives on mental behavior.

Nature of Mental Illness

Deviant human behavior, abnormal mental behavior, psychopathology, whichever term you use, has been chronicled in literature, in the theater, in the popular press throughout recorded history. Its manifestations have fascinated the public and the social scientist for centuries. Many explanations for aberrant behavior have been advanced through the years—e.g., demon possession, sin, lunacy, disease—particular in western societies which have essentially tended to isolate or distinguish the person experiencing some form of emotional or mental disorder from other "normal" persons. Such efforts have manifested the linear, causal, categorical thinking which has dominated western scientific thinking but not, for example, that of Eastern Psychology. Unlike the psychology of the West, Eastern Psychology tends to see variations in "mental health" or "normality" as part of individuality and as dynamic. In this view, people are not typically mentally ill *or* mentally well. They are continuously both as they move from reactions to one event to another. This notion is exemplified in western thought by such perspectives as those of Glasser (1970) when he stated: "most people, even those with effective egos, have many different types of ego defects. We are all at times a little neurotic, a little psychotic, and have elements of character disorder and depression. Few of us escape some manifestation of psychosomatic disease at one time or another...

We have these ego defects transiently as our ego is constantly adjusting to variations of internal and external stresses" (p. 58).

In efforts to understand variations in human behavior, social and behavioral scientists have tried to classify such behavior into distinct categories or entities which could be helpful in assessment and treatment as well as in understanding. Two of the most comprehensive directories of such classification structures are the World Health Organization's *International Classification of Disease* (1977), now in its ninth revision, which includes a comprehensive discussion of mental disorders and the American Psychiatric Association's *Diagnostic and Statistical Manual of Mental Disorders* which first appeared in 1952 and in 1980 appeared in its third major revision as, the *DSM-III*. The *Diagnostic and Statistical Manual of Mental Disorders* has changed over its thirty-five year history in diagnostic criteria used, descriptions of the disorders, and in the etiology (or causes) of the disorders described. For example, in the first edition of the DSM, the term "reaction" was used throughout the classification system as a reflection of the dominant role played at that time by Adolph Meyer's psychobiological view that mental disorders represented reactions of the personality to psychological, social, and biological factors. The term "reaction" is no longer used in *DSM-III*. Rather, "diagnostic terms are used that do not imply a particular theoretical framework for understanding the nonorganic mental disorders" (American Psychiatric Association, 1980, p. 2).

Perspectives of DSM-III

More particularly,

> In DSM-III each of the mental disorders is conceptualized as a clinically significant behavioral or psychological syndrome or pattern that occurs in an individual and that is typically associated with either a painful symptom (distress) or impairment in one or more important areas of functioning (disability). In addition, there is an inference that there is a behavioral, psychological, or biological dysfunction, and that the disturbance is not only in the relationship between the individual and the society. (American Psychiatric Association, 1980, p. 6)

The *DSM-III* goes on to contend that "a behavioral or psychological problem may appropriately be a focus of professional attention or treatment even through it is not attributable to a mental disorder" (p. 6). In addition, it is stated that

> for some of the mental disorders, the etiology or pathophysiological processes are known. For example, in the Organic Mental Disorders, organic factors

necessary for the development of the disorders have been identified or are presumed. Another example is Adjustment Disorder, in which the disturbance is a reaction to psychosocial stress... For most of the DSM-III disorders, however, the etiology is unknown. A variety of theories have been advanced, buttressed by evidence—not always convincing—to explain how these disorders come about... Undoubtedly, with time, some of the disorders of unknown etiology will be found to have specific biological etiologies, others to have specific psychological causes, and still others to result mainly from a particular interplay of psychological, social and biological factors. (p. 7)

When reduced to its essence, *DSM-III* is a reflection that psychiatry is basically descriptive, not definitive, in its current understanding of mental disorder. Its current state of science is such that a consistent, differentiated classification of mental disorders can not be made on qualitative (discontinuity between diagnostic entities, exclusive or separate from other classifications), or quantitative (differences on a severity continuum) grounds, or on their etiological bases (what causes the disorders). What is unstated in such a classification is that however speculative such classifications of mental disorders are, because of the prestige of psychiatry itself, the classification system is used inadvertently or directly to determine what types of mental disorders are reimbursable by insurance, who should or should not be institutionalized, and the effects of "mental disorder" upon allegations of criminal behavior in courts of law. In essence, the descriptive language of mental disorders pervades the society and becomes a popular as well as a professional "shorthand" for sickness and stigma, not health. While DSM-III tries to dilute such effects by indicating that the classification of mental disorders does not classify individuals but rather the disorders that individuals have (p. 6), the nuances and caveats in such statements tend to get lost in the application of the classification structure throughout the mental health delivery system, the criminal justice system, or the common parlance.

To return to the matter of understanding of the causes of mental disorders as reflected in the *DSM-III,* one can define these into several classes. For example, the mental disorders for which the causes are most clear tend to be the organic mental disorders. The organic factors or etiological agents are "a primary disease of the brain. It may also be a substance or toxic agent that is either currently disturbing brain function or has left some longlasting effect. Withdrawal of a substance on which an individual has become physiologically dependent is another cause of Organic Mental Disorder" (p. 102). A second set of mental disorders in which growing evidence of organic or chemical factors seem to be causative are called the organic brain syndromes. Included in organic mental disorder are dementias arising in the senium and presenium (e.g., Alzheimer's and Pick's disease, brain tumor, Huntington's chorea) and substance induced disorders (e.g., intoxication, delirium, delusion, hallucinois, or affective disorder arising from alcohol, barbituates, opioid, cocaine, amphetamines, PCP, hallucinogens, Cannabis, etc.). Organic brain syndromes include delirium, dementia, amnesia, intoxication, and withdrawal. Increasingly, the Schizophrenic disorders are seen as having organic factors in their etiology but that matter is not yet clear.

Also disorders are present in which the etiology is not clear and to which organic factors are not seen as primarily predisposing. For the most part, these are seen as responses to psychological or social factors. Included here are the broad category of neurotic disorders comprised of such groups as the affective, anxiety, somatoform, dissociative, psychosexual, impulse control, and adjustment disorders. Also a series of conditions are present which are not attributable to a mental disorder but that do yield to treatment. These include malingering, borderline intellectual functioning, antisocial behavior, academic problems, occupational problems, marital problems, parent-child problems, uncomplicated bereavement, and other interpersonal, life circumstance, or family problems.

What is controversial in the previous classifications is suggesting that all of the mental and behavioral disorders or problems included in DSM-III, or its predecessors, are forms of "mental illness" or the result of "disease entities." A growing number of observers are taking very different views. For example, persons holding humanistic views are much more likely to see psychopathology as resulting from normal learning processes occurring in pathological social environments (Albee, 1982). Certainly as one departs from defect explanations for behavior, the mental health occupations appropriate to dealing with the behavior become less restrictive and less "psychiatrized."

Opponents of Mental Illness

Among the pioneering opponents to labeling all behavioral problems "mental illness" is Thomas Szasz. His book *The Myth of Mental Illness* (1961) began a significant process of demystifying mental illness and its treatment which continues to the current day. It is at the roots of the controversy which swirls around notions of mental illness/mental health and who should treat them.

In the preface to his book Szasz made several observations which relate to our current discussion. For example, his rationale for writing the book:

> I became increasingly impressed by the vague, capricious, and generally unsatisfactory character of the widely used concept of mental illness and its corollaries, diagnosis, prognosis, and treatment. It seemed to me that although the notion of mental illness made good historical sense—stemming as it does from the *historical* identity of medicine and psychiatry—it made no *rational* sense... Although dissatisfaction with the medical basis and conceptual framework of psychiatry is not of recent origin, little has been done to make the problem explicit, and even less to remedy it. In psychiatric circles, it is almost indelicate to ask: "What is mental illness?" In nonpsychiatric circles mental illness all too often is considered to be whatever psychiatrists say it is. The answer to the question Who is mentally ill? thus becomes: those who are confined in mental hospitals or who consult psychiatrists in their private offices... The question, 'What is mental illness?' is shown to be inextricably tied to the question What do psychiatrists do? (p. ix)

Szasz's major contributions lie in his ability to shift the paradigm of what psychiatry is about and the historical definitions of mental illness to alternative models. For example, "It is customary to define psychiatry as a medical specialty concerned with the study, diagnosis, and treatment of mental illness. This is a worthless and misleading definition. Mental illness is a myth. Psychiatrists are not concerned with mental illnesses and their treatments. In actual practice they deal with personal, social, and ethical problems in living" (p. 296). Within such a context, Szasz viewed mental illness not for the most part as a structural illness, but as a functional illness—indeed, it is behavior imitating illness.

Szasz suggested that the diversity in so called mental illness is analogous to different foreign languages or forms of communication through which the individual attempts to achieve certain end-goals of domination and interpersonal control (p. 9). Thus, "psychiatry, a theoretical science, consists of the study of personal conduct—of clarifying and explaining the kinds of games that people play with each other; how they learned these games, why they like to play them, and so forth" (p. 7). "Man is confronted by the imperative need to relinquish old games and to learn to play new ones... This fundamental game-conflict leads to various problems in living. It is these that the modern psychotherapist is usually called upon to 'treat'" (p. 308).

The concepts provided by Szasz have been extended and redefined by other observers. As Gorenstein (1984) observed, "the mental health field is still unable to establish, except as a matter of faith, whether or not there is such a thing as mental illness..." Gradually, though, the views of Szasz and like-minded commentators have had a subtle but detectable impact on a field that remains staunchly medical in orientation. The standard terminology of the past—"mental disease," "insanity"—is now considered archiac by most mental health professionals. Even "mental illness"...is increasingly avoided in the scientific literature" (p. 50). Thus, mental health theory seems to be moving rapidly away from reliance on "disease entities" as an explanation of behavioral problems. Indeed, "problems in living" are increasingly being viewed in terms of the behavioral or skill components by which they are comprised. The resulting approaches to either treatment or primary prevention views skill training as a primary intervention modality. The assumption is that skills can be taught as a means of eliminating interpersonal deficits or being prepared to anticipate or overcome problems or barriers in the future.

Primary Prevention or Treatment. Albee (1982), like Szasz, saw mental illness differently from the traditional psychiatric/medical perspective and his is a strong advocacy of primary prevention in mental and emotional disturbance. A variety of his views of these matters follow.

> ...careful studies concur in estimating that 15% of the population—32 to 35 million Americans—constitute the 'hard core' of the emotionally disturbed. These are persons with depression, alcoholic addiction, incapacitating neurotic anxiety, organic brain conditions, associated with old age, and the several functional psychoses. But in any given year, the *entire* mental health delivery system (mental hospitals, clinics, individual practitioners) is able to see only about 7 million persons. Many of these 7 million persons do not come from the 'hard-core' group. Many are middle-class people with problems in living—persons undergoing marital disruption, those who have lost a loved one, those who are out of work, those with identity problems. so the mental health community actually see fewer than one in five of the seriously disturbed people, and only a small proportion of the larger group of people with problems. (p. 1043)

Albee continued

> Clearly the logistics of this whole situation demands increased efforts at primary prevention. But logic and good sense rarely guide the formulation and development of social policy. Too many vested interests depend heavily on an ideology that finds mental illnesses inside each affected individual and that advocates one-to-one therapy, including the use of psychotropic drugs and other organic forms of treatment. We are witnessing an increasing medicalization of psychiatry, along with strong and growing opposition to efforts at social change aimed at alleviating the environmental stresses that are responsible for the higher rates of emotional disturbances among the poor, the powerless, the disenfranchised, and the exploited.

> ...An important reason for neglect or resistance to preventive approaches to mental conditions is the heavy emphasis on social and environmental change required (p. 1045)... If our purpose is to reduce the incidence of the different conditions or life styles we refer to as mental disorders... There are several strategies for accomplishing our purpose: the first of these is to prevent, to minimize, or to reduce the amounts of the organic factors that sometimes do play a role in causation (e.g., lead poisoning, brain damage from automobile accidents)... A second strategy...involves the reduction of stress... (p. 1046). Another area...involves increasing the competence of young people to deal with life's problems, particularly with the problems of social interactions, and the development of a wide range of coping skills... Increases in support systems and self-esteem have been shown to reduce psychopathology (p. 1045)... Those who argue against the concept of mental "illness" do not deny the existence of behavior that can be called abnormal or pathological. They simply hold that abnormal behavior can be learned through perfectly normal processes—and what can be learned can be unlearned or prevented. (p. 1050)

From such a perspective, *personal competence* is seen as a series of skills which an individual either possesses or can learn through training. The acquisition of certain skills may generalize to facilitate the development of competence in other aspects of one's life (Danish, Galambos, & Laquatra, 1983). Termed by some observers as "life development skills," these objects of intervention include *cognitive* and *physical* skills; interpersonal skills such as initiating, developing, and maintaining relationships, e.g., self disclosing, communicating feelings accurately and unambiguously, being supportive, and being able to resolve conflicts and relationship problems constructively; and *intrapersonal* skills such as developing self control, tension management and relaxation, setting goals, taking risks, etc. (Danish, Galambos, & Laquatra, 1983).

Undoubtedly these conceptions of life coping skills are gaining in credibility as research is unfolding about the importance of specific types of skills or the barriers to the particular kinds of social or occupational settings which can be overcome by the possession of particular skills. These types of research demystify the problems in living at issue: e.g., interpersonal relations, work adjustment, mental harmony. In so doing, content evolves to develop therapeutic activities tailored to individual or group needs for specific attitudes, information, or skills.

Projects in several countries deal with the facilitation of "life coping" skills in people whether these are specifically defined in terms of assertiveness training, decision-making, psychosocial development, obesity or smoking control, anger management, stress inoculation or similar emphases. The end result of such efforts is to increase the controversy about what is mental illness and who should deal with its behavioral imitations.

A related controversy which arises in this context is that which centers around treatment or prevention. As certain mental disorders are seen to arise from genetic, organic, or chemical factors, prevention in the commonly accepted sense of that term is probably not possible. Treatment through medication and related processes are preferred. However, as behavioral or learning deficits are seen as the root of mental disorders, then treatment is seen as primarily educative in focus and prevention becomes not only feasible but possibly imperative. Perhaps even more feasible is the evolution of "mental health promotion" and mental health wellness. Primary prevention is activity designed to reduce the incidence of a disorder or the likelihood of its occurrence in a population at risk.By contrast, mental health promotion is activity designed to increase people's sense of competency, coherence, and control so they can live effective and satisfying lives in a state of social well-being (Perlmutter, 1982, p. 7).

As each of these notions unfold they put at some risk other paradigms within the mental health field; they also shift the status or power of those engaged with different purpose in the spectrum of treatment, prevention, promotion. They cause new definitions of professional roles to be advanced and questions to be raised about whether mental health promotion or prevention can or should be conducted within the locations primarily concerned with mental illness (Perlmutter, 1982). As such perspectives ensue, an ongoing and circular argument is stimulated about the wisdom of pursuing primary prevention at all, given the scarce resources for mental services (Lamb & Zusman, 1979). Also at issue in this debate is the lack of available evidence that primary prevention and/or mental health promotion, in fact, reduce the incidence of mental illness.

Other controversies are inherent in primary prevention and mental health promotion. One is measurement of the effectiveness of primary prevention. Another is that, if primary prevention is to be effective, a necessity is to define both the factors that predispose and those that precipitate mental illness. Since, as Bloom (1981) among others has suggested, these precipitating factors are likely to be multiple not singular for any given individual, this promises to be a formidable task. A further controversy is what are we trying to prevent: diagnosable mental illness or "unhappiness, feelings of distress or social incompetence" (Lamb & Zusman, 1979). Unless clear agreement can be obtained as to what the target of primary prevention is intended to be, no clear agreement will be obtained as to what the indicators of effective primary prevention need to be, how they could be measured, or what the acceptable levels of primary prevention are which should result. Finally, perhaps, is the question of the boundaries of mental health and where prevention, particularly primary prevention, fits into such a concept. Should mental health services, for example, be directed only to persons with diagnosable mental illness or to people as well who have problems in living, or indeed, those who have no definable problems but instead want to maximize their quality of life and self-fulfillment. However one defines such matters will ultimately raise additional controversies about which mental health "helping professions" become the central or core providers of such services and the professional identity which results.

Health and Wellness

Against these areas of controversy, new specialties and new sites for delivering mental health care are emerging. Examples of the first are health psychology, behavioral medicine, prevention, for example, of drug abuse in the workplace, and counseling for health. Examples of the latter are the community or the workplace either directly in vivo or in some adjunctive setting.

Among the major changes in the American culture and therefore in the provision of mental health service is in the active pursuit of wellness. As applied to the dichotomous thinking between mental illness and mental health as discussed at the beginning of this chapter, Grossman (1981) cited estimates that 96% of federal expenditures in health care are for treatment and only 4% for efforts in prevention. On the other hand, some signs suggest that future federal efforts will be directed to changing that balance. A variety of federal reports including that of *The Surgeon General's Report on Health Promotion and Disease Prevention* (Department of Health and Human Services, 1979) have suggested that 50% of all deaths can be attributed to an unhealthy life style. Seven of the ten leading causes of death are largely behaviorally determined. In young people ages 15 to 24, 75% of deaths are the result of accidents, homicides and suicides. Thus, federal policy has begun to recognize the need to make prevention a national priority as it deals with smoking, smokeless tobacco, alcohol and substance abuse, diet, exercises, and other health matters.

Applying the skills of mental health providers to the promotion of health and wellness includes helping persons develop problem-solving skills, manage anxiety and stress more consciously and with more control, assume personal responsibility for their lives, gain an internal locus of control, and increase their feelings of power or reduce their feelings of powerlessness. These involve the skills of interpersonal communication, anger management, assertiveness training, decision-making, values clarification, relaxation. Krumboltz and Menefee (1980) suggested that the decade ahead will require counselors to concentrate to a greater degree on prevention rather than on remediation, to give increased attention to helping people develop self-control and the skills they need to regulate their behavior, and to adopting a more integrated approach to the three facets of thinking, feeling, and acting. Similarly, Thoresen and Eagleston (1985) have contended that good health and chronic disease exist essentially as matters of habit as well as contexts in how people routinely go about the business of everyday living. Therefore, they contend that counseling psychologists can use their skills both in the promotion and maintenance of good health and in the prevention and treatment of disease.

Rosen and Solomon (1985), editors of the eighth book which has evolved from the Vermont Conferences on the Primary Prevention of Psychopathology, have identified a variety of basic issues in the prevention of psychopathology: promoting social competence and coping in children and in adults, facilitating infant development, prevention through political action and social change, and promoting positive sexuality. As the contributors to this volume on health psychology examine the health care continuum, two major emphases are identified: prevention and modification of early risk factors for disease and development of coping strategies necessary for psychological adaptation to chronic illness. The thrust of the first emphasis, as was suggested previously, is that

> most of the major causes of premature death and morbidity in the United States have behavioral antecedents. For example, smoking is a significant independent risk factor for cardiovascular disease and several forms of cancer. (p. vii)

A second perspective on these matters is that

> over the past decade we have seen a dramatic escalation in medical care costs...Prevention activities offer the greatest hope for a decline in incidence rates and a concomitant improvement in the general health of our population...Such activities suggest possible solutions to the problem of rising health care costs.

Finally there is

> increasing evidence of the relationship between ways of coping with illness and psychological functioning. Serious physical illness, especially illness involving

painful and disabling conditions, is a major life stress for most individuals. Considering that such illness and disability burdens the individual with threats to self esteem and to normal functioning in social, familial, and vocational spheres, it is not surprising that psychopathology is a common outcome in illness situations. It is within the "preventionists" realm to consider strategies to assist chronically ill individuals to adjust to the stress of physical disease. (p. viii)

The importance of a prevention or promotion model for dealing with mental health or wellness as contrasted with trying to remediate mental illness is seen in another perspective. Estimates are that 15% (Kiesler, 1980) to 35% of the population (Dohrenwend et al., 1980) is in need of mental health services in any given year. Using the conservative estimate of 15% of the population, that means 33 million people need some form or another of mental health service. If all the available licensed and certified psychiatrists and psychologists were to provide psychotherapy on a full-time basis offering it 3 times a week to each client, they could provide such service to only 2% of those needing it (Kiesler, 1985). Thus, the deduction can be made that not only is the need necessary to redefine mental illness in behavioral terms and to define mental health as a target of mental health services, but also is the need necessary to recognize that the current controversies—economic, territorial, and others—serve to reduce the availability of core and noncore providers to contribute, each as they are prepared, to the provision of mental health services, the demand for which significantly exceeds their collective capability. such a notion is itself highly controversial. It suggests the need for mental health providers to apply their skills of conflict resolution, cognitive resolution, cognitive restructuring, treatment, and prevention within and across all of the professional groups which comprise the "helping professions." It suggests the need to demystify mental illness and mental health so that both a continuum of behavioral deficits and a continuum of mental health responses inherent in psychiatry, psychology, social work, nursing, mental health counseling, and marriage and family therapy can be conceptualized and played out in public policy.

PROFESSIONAL IDENTITY: A REPRISE

In the first four chapters, we have examined many forms of controversy relating to the professional identity of specific occupations dealing with mental health in the United States. Some of these controversies are internal to a particular occupation; others are the source of tension and conflicts among different groups of mental health practitioners.

Some of the controversies arise from history, some from economic issues, some from the dynamics of power and territoriality. Some conflicts emanate from the political process as it is manifested in legislation and statutes favoring one group of practitioners rather than another or as it conveys an image of prestige or status within the helping professions.

Controversies among the helping professions also arise from conceptual or meaning and language systems. Different mental health occupations have tended to use different theoretical or explanatory systems to interpret human behavior and act upon it. Such phenomena have invariably given rise to which system is the most correct one, the most scientifically or empirically valid one, the most comprehensive one. In some cases, the controversies which have ensued have focused upon the overlap in techniques used (e.g., psychotherapy) rather than in the differences in meaning or definition attributed to such terms.

Perhaps the root of the controversy in the helping professions has to do with definitions of mental illness or mental health or both. Embedded in such controversies are concerns about biological versus psychological interpretations of behavior. Questions about whether mental illness exists as an entity and about the etiology of its various manifestations. The farther models of mental disorders depart from biological or disease entities, the more difficult it is to sustain some of the hierarchial models of the helping professions in which psychiatrists and clinical psychologists are viewed as at the zenith in training, prestige, and skills and other groups of mental health professionals arrange themselves in a descending order of autonomy, competency, and training. Increasingly, a paradigm emerges in which a range of mental health occupations clamor for parity in providing mental health services based upon the possibility of bringing different skills and insights to different categories of persons experiencing mental illness (as defined primarily in terms of organic and chemical imbalances which require medication maintenance in conjunction with other therapeutic regimens), problems in living (as defined in the need to acquire skills and learning pertinent to various life transitions in which they are engaged), and needs for life enhancement (as defined in terms of holistic health and wellness). Thus, such mental health professionals, while overlapping to some degree in the intervention processes used (e.g., psychotherapy) and even in populations served, will be seen to differ significantly in their purposes and in their contributions to treatment, education, or prevention ranging across a continuum from mental health "wellness" to mental health illness, the latter defined in quite precise and circumscribed terms.

THEME TWO: EDUCATION AND TRAINING

CHAPTER 5

THE EDUCATION AND TRAINING OF PERSONS IN THE MENTAL HEALTH PROFESSIONS

The various themes discussed in this book suggest that many forces and factors combine to create controversy within and among mental health professions and between those professions and the general public, third party payers, and policy makers. Matters of history, perspectives on one's helping role and its relative importance to the contributions of other mental health providers, boundaries of the professional field, perspectives on the conceptual roots of a specific profession and the important content which undergirds its practice, the intervention procedures, and the ethical context in which they are conducted each represent sources of controversy among mental health professionals.

Although the content and nature of controversy exist in many guises, probably that existence is nowhere more clear than in the education and training of persons in the mental health professions. The length, content, and "apprenticeship" (practica, internships) requirements of training which various groups of mental health professionals undergo is a source of considerable tension vis ā vis credentialing expectations, prestige, remuneration, autonomy, and other matters which appear to afflict mental health professionals with controversy and conflict.

Education and training is the crucible in which mental health professionals are socialized to the belief systems, the "world views," the ways of conducting oneself politically, economically, socially, and clinically which give a particular profession its distinctive qualities and purposes. In these senses, education and training represent the switching mechanisms between the past—the heritage of a professional group—and the future. Education and training are where traditions formed by each professional group's history and images of its future are embedded in the student professional's psyche. Through education and training the professional culture is conveyed, shaped, and reinforced.

In Chapter 5 are discussed how and where education and training occur across the mental health professions. Content and form as well as the "culture" of professional training are discussed. Points of controversy which emerge from such systems and sub-systems will be identified in terms of major issues which characterize certain mental health groups more than others or which tend to be pervasive issues of concern to education and training across the mental health professions.

A major contextual issue which has historically framed training controversies in the mental health professions flows from some of the identity issues described in the first four chapters. Specifically, a subtle but enduring concern continues about whether mental health professionals should be trained within a medical setting and a medical mode. Psychiatrists and psychiatric nurses are. Many clinical psychologists and clinical social workers are. Some counseling psychologists are. Virtually by tradition, training in a medical setting suggests that the client or patient is seen in diagnostic and remedial terms, as a person who suffers from a deficit or dysfunction of some sort which needs to be corrected. While something of a caricature, such a view obviously affects the socialization of the mental health practitioner as he/she identifies the critical "treatment" variables, the prime causative factors in mental illness or distress, and other factors affecting professional identity. Such a view obviously contrasts with a "wellness" or even a "problems-in-living" perspective as a *raison d'etre* for providing services. As such, the place, medical or non-medical, of training and internship is undoubtedly a major ingredient in controversies within the mental health professions. Other issues are present as well.

In any profession, inevitably conflicting ideas occur regarding appropriate curricula, experiences, emphases, and balances between aspects of didactic, clinical, and personal development training. In the helping professions, these differences exist both between component disciplines *and* within each discipline. In this chapter, we discuss several of the more problematic issues. Among these are The Medical Model and the Education of Mental Health Workers; The Scientist—Practitioner versus the Practitioner; Clinical versus Counseling Psychology; Differences in Training; Specializations; Desirable Helper Characteristics; Personal Therapy in Training; In-Service Training; Social Work Concerns; Issues in the Education of Psychiatric Nurses; Sub-Doctoral Training; and the Internship Experience.

MEDICAL MODEL AND EDUCATION OF MENTAL HEALTH WORKERS

The so-called medical model has been extremely influential in the education, training, and mode of operating in the mental health professions. It stems from a tradition of medicine that placed emphasis on disease rather than on health. As summarized by Thoresen and Eagleston (1985), the model has been severely criticized over the years. Specifically:

> It is based on the "germ theory" explanation of disease (that is, each disease is due to a single cause, such as a particular bacteria or virus) and is not useful in explaining the multiple causes or guiding the treatment of chronic diseases.
>
> It relies too heavily on the effectiveness of differential diagnosis when there is poor reliability among those diagnosing physical and mental disease.
>
> It seeks a single "best" treatment that eradicates the cause; yet chronic diseases have many causes and may not be completely curable.
>
> It results in the dehumanization of health care due to an overreliance on sophisticated technology and overspecialization of health care providers.
>
> It promotes authoritarian relationships between practitioner and patient in which the locus of responsibility typically is removed from the patient.

It acknowledges only the physical factors in disease and does not address the social, psychological, and behavioral dimensions of disease, illness, or health in terms of etiology, prevention, and treatment.

It is actually a model of disease care delivery—not health care delivery—and virtually ignores efforts to improve health and prevent disease, especially multidisciplinary efforts. (p. 33)

Consequently, various alternatives to the medical model have been proposed, including diverse holistic, wellness, cognitive, social learning, and preventive models. While all of the mental health professions now at least give lip-service to the concept of prevention (for example, the community psychiatry and community psychology movements and the policy aspects of social work), no clear translation of that philosophy into education and training aspects seems to be in effect. For instance, McNeill and Ingram (1983) surveyed APA- and non-APA-Approved graduate training and internship programs and concluded that psychological education was seriously deficient in providing training in preventive principles and interventions and in offering experiences within community mental health settings.

The response to the weaknesses of the medical model has been for some to leap from the narrow and the perhaps overly empirical to the overly broad and the spiritual, where one transcends mind and body and enters some higher reality. How to bridge the obvious gap between narrow, disease-oriented organic views of man at one extreme and the pollyannish reduction of all experience to feeling and mysticism at the other extreme is a current challenge and controversy in the education of mental health professionals.

SCIENTIST-PRACTITIONER VERSUS PRACTITIONER

Within the field of psychology, the primary issue now being considered is the matter of the Ph.D. versus the Psy.D. This issue has been debated for a number of years and is usually characterized as the difference between models of psychologists: scientist versus scientist-practitioner (professional) versus practitioner (professional). In the 1940s, the so-called Boulder Conference resulted in the promulgation of a combination scientist-practitioner model to replace the then prevalent notion of the non-applied laboratory scientist. Thus, the science of psychology (research) was to complement the practice of psychology (therapy). In the 1960s, the Committee on the Scientific and Professional Aims of Psychology, chaired by Kenneth B. Clark, concluded that neither function was being effected to a large degree in university training programs, and the committee recommended a new degree, the Doctor of Psychology, in which research consumption rather than research productivity would be the goal. In the 1970s, the American Psychological Association held a training conference at Vail, Colorado in which the Psy.D., representing the professional training model, was endorsed as an alternative route to producing a *bona fide* psychologist. In 1987, APA will sponsor still another national conference on issues pertaining to university-based graduate education in psychology in which concerns will be addressed such as what constitutes a generic core of knowledge and the continued exploration of whether or not scientist and practitioner should be educated separately.

The disagreement between "academic" psychologists and "applied" psychologists goes back several decades. For example, from 1937 to 1945, applied psychologists withdrew from APA. The basic conflict continues to the present. Research training is the primary focus of the debate. The emphasis on research training emanates basically from the need for Ph.D. trained clinical, counseling, and school psychologists to achieve some separate status in the mental health professions, independent of the dominance of psychiatry. After all, it is reasoned, both psychiatrists and psychologists assess and counsel; only the psychologist receives research training. The fact of the matter is, however, that psychologists in practice (and many university psychologists) do relatively little research and dangerously little consumption of research (Bornstein & Wollershein, 1978; Cohen, 1979; Kelly, Goldberg, Fiske, & Kilkowski, 1978). Frank (1984) suggested that this lack of research productivity may be due in part to

> ...the attitudes of faculty (who might undercut the value of research in and for clinical psychology), the role models students encounter during the course of their training (who most often do not reflect the scientist-practitioner model in what they do, either in the university or in the practicum settings), and the positions psychologists secure after graduating (which, ordinarily, pay for direct service to patients, not to research). (p. 429)

Further, Frank went on to maintain that, in addition to these practical differences, academic clinical psychologists (scientist-practitioners) differ from those psychologists interested in only clinical practice "with regard to abilities, interests, a variety of aspects of personality, and even the possibility of differential cerebral dominance" (p. 429). Although

Frank's data are not complete and his conclusions are stretched, the fact is that more complete data might well prove him correct. Data from a study by Weiss (1981), for example, strongly suggests that the "frequency and nature of contact with faculty members is significantly related to the amount of professional role commitment" (p. 13). If this be so, Frank may prove to be accurate.

Others such as Goldfried (1984) affirm that the researcher-practitioner problem might be solved by insisting that research take place within practice-oriented work settings and deal with the "stuff" of practicing clinicians so that the results of research have immediate impact on practice. Findings of a national survey by Perl and Hahn (1983) offer both good news and bad news to those who advocate the scientist-practitioner model. They found that the majority of psychology graduate students indicate that they are interested in doing research, that they plan to do research, and that with training in and experience with research, an intensified level of interest occurs. On the other hand, for clinical and applied psychology students, their main identification is still with the role of practitioner. The paramount argument for the Psy.D. presented by those who advocate its use is that the subject matter of the field and the application of that content have exploded to such a degree that insufficient time is available to train for research competency as well as clinical skill. One wonders if the same argument could be made for, say, a Ph.D. chemist (where the so-called half-life of knowledge is much shorter than in psychology), and one wonders what the role of in-service education as a lifelong endeavor might be in balancing the equation. Montgomery (1977, p. 96), an Australian psychologist, offered a clean and neat heuristic model of the differences in orientation of the various training model combining the theory-research dimension with a level of training dimension to yield nine alternative models.

Whichever model is the more effective at this point is moot because very little, if any, research evidence is persuasive in holding one model superior to the other. Partly, this condition is due to the fact that we are not sure how to assess professional competence or that our current methods for evaluating training models are valid (Stern, 1984).

TABLE 5.1

CLINICAL TRAINING MODELS

Level of Training	Practical Experience Versus Theory and Research		
	Highly Experimental		Theory Research
Low	A. Bachelor's degree, non-degree courses (stress on practice' in-service training; courses for non-psychologists	B. Bachelor's degree with psychology major including field observation and work introduction to research)	C. Bachelor's degree, usually honours level (may be able to do research in applied area)
Medium	D. Master's degree or postgraduate diploma (by coursework and fieldwork; no thesis)	E. Master's degree or postgraduate diploma (by coursework, fieldwork and research thesis; some Australian programs	F. Master's degree often honours level (mostly by research thesis, little or no coursework or fieldwork; typical Australian master's)
High	G. Professional doctorate (mostly by practicum and internship; research consumption, e.g., D.Psy. at Univ. of Illinois)	H. Scientist-Practitioner (Coursework practicum, internship, research thesis; e.g., most U.S. clinical Ph.D.'s)	I. Research Ph.D. mostly or exclusively by research thesis, little or no coursework or practicum; typcial Australian Ph.D.

CLINICAL VERSUS COUNSELING PSYCHOLOGY

Also within the field of psychology is the question of whether one type of applied psychologist is "better than" other practitioner psychologists by virtue of being "different from" them. Because of the increasing number of doctoral-level trained counseling psychologists and the steady rise in the number of APA Approved Counseling Psychology Programs, the confusion is mainly between counseling and clinical psychologists. On paper, at least, and historically, the differences are easily limned. In current practice, however, these differences become obfuscated.

As we have seen previously, counseling psychology has its roots in educational and vocational counseling and its major institutional identification with Veteran's Administration Centers and college and university counseling centers. The counseling psychologist was to tend to clients who represented concerns within a "normal" range of problems, was to use trait and factor methodology, and was to have comprehensive knowledge and skills in vocational psychology. As the years progressed, the boundaries became blurred between clinical and counseling psychologists: the community psychology movement caused clinical psychologists to be more concerned with all individuals—those within a normal range as well as those who were deviate—and the training of counseling psychologists and the plying of their trade became more applicable to abnormal populations in a variety of settings that had previously been the sole domain of the clinical psychologist.

Hence, to perceive great differences in training required of clinical and counseling psychologists is now difficult. The differences are currently so minimal that some have suggested that clinical and counseling psychologists be homogenized into one specialty—human services psychology (Levy, 1984; Watkins, 1985). This specialty would include "all professional psychology specialties concerned with the promotion of human well-being through the acquisition and application of psychological knowledge concerned with the treatment and prevention of psychological and physical disorders" (Levy, 1984, p. 490). Further clouding an already indistinct picture are the claims of "professional counselors" who are largely graduates of counselor education programs and who assert that they have the equivalent of training in psychology. For this latter group, Lanning and Forrest (1984) conducted a fascinating study which determined that counselor education is now moving toward training agency/community counselors while the counselor educators themselves have had their principal training and work experience in public schools and colleges. Nevertheless, the core programs they would establish now are not greatly different from those found in most graduate psychology programs.

Although presently no agreement exists as to the core of courses in either clinical or counseling psychology, the influence of APA accreditation standards and conventional wisdom have combined to make programs, in fact, more similar than dissimilar. A typical program, of course, includes enough hours of practica and internship to satisfy APA and subsequent licensing agents (usually 750-1,000 practicum hours and 2,000 internship hours). A research-statistics core is also apparent in the non-Psy.D. programs, as are courses in the areas of social, developmental, cognitive and physiological psychology, history and systems, and, usually, psychopathology. A psychological assessment core is also evident as is some sort of group intervention course and a psychotherapy (counseling) base. Ethical issues and supervision training are typically built into programs, whether offered as separate courses or assimilated into other courses. These areas then, *de facto,* constitute a core in both counseling and clinical psychology.

The major differences in training of course, lie in the area of vocational psychology, with counseling psychology still typically requiring at least one course in this area and clinical psychology not doing so. In recent years, some de-emphasis of the role of vocational psychology in the preparation of counseling psychologists has occurred, a development that has seemed to many, including the present authors, to be unwise. Myers (1982) for example, makes the following recommendation:

> Training programs in counseling psychology should rediscover the importance of work (and workplace) as an influence on human well-being and seek to stimulate student interest in the psychological aspects of work. (p. 44)

Simultaneously (and ironically), the practice of occupational clinical psychology appears to be a new focus that holds a great deal of attraction for clinical psychologists (Manuso, 1983).

Beyond the core, few agreements exist regarding what should be stressed in the training of psychologists. In addition, a number of areas are now being offered to students as "concentrations," "minors," or "specializations." The following section outlines some of the suggestions and specialties currently available or advocated. We discuss these differences in terms of the major orientation of a program, the "tools of the trade," and the populations to be served.

DIFFERENCES IN TRAINING

One Orientation or Multi-Orientation

Most programs provide their students with training in the basic counseling skills of attending and responding, usually by means of some programmatic method, such as that of Ivey, Carkhuff, or Kagan. Beyond this rudimentary training, great differences exist in terms of the view or views of psychotherapy which are espoused. Most programs expose their students to a wide range of orientations, from cognitive through self-insight to psychodynamic; the students are encouraged to adopt one orientation and to be able to apply it and explain it consistently or to adopt several for use in particular types of situations or when confronted with certain types of problems. A few programs hold to a single orientation and advertise themselves as producing individuals in the light of whatever that mode happens to be. So long as prospective students know what they are "buying," nothing is wrong with this latter orientation.

Tools of the Trade

As we have seen in a previous chapter, perhaps no aspect of the training of psychiatrists and psychologists receives more attention than assessment. Most, if not all, agree that students should receive instruction and supervision in administering and scoring tests, making inferences on the basis of test results, and sometimes, communicating test findings. The usual way these goals are accomplished is through classroom instruction, observation and modeling of assessment procedures, and supervision and criticism. Now the disagreements: what tests should be taught to whom and who should teach them?

In psychiatry, most observers, such as Berg (1984), believe that psychiatrists should not be practitioners in testing but should know only enough about testing to allow them to be sophisticated consumers of the psychologist's consultative service. Presumably, a social worker would need not possess even this much knowledge of assessment. In psychiatric consultation teams (so called P-L, for psychiatric-liaison teams), for example, the psychologists would do psychological testing although not be limited solely to that role.

For a number of years now, projective techniques have been in general disfavor and their validity has been less than impressive (Thelan & Ewing, 1970; Piotrowski & Keller, 1984). Yet, required coursework and familiarity with projectives is a virtual *sine qua non* in every preparation program in clinical psychology and increasingly in counseling psychology. Piotrowski and Keller's survey of clinical graduate programs asked respondents to list the five projective and five objective personality measures with which Ph.D. psychologists should be familiar ("familiar" not being further defined). The results in descending order of mention: *projective* (Thematic Appercetion Test, Rorschach, Sentence Completion, Human Figure Drawings, Bender-Gestalt, Children's Appercetion Test, House-Tree-Person, Holtzman Inkblot Technique, and Word Association); *objective* [Minnesota Multiphasic Personality Inventory, California Psychological Inventory, 16 Personality Factor (PF) Questionnaire, Depression Inventories, Anxiety Inventories, Eysenck, Edwards Personal Preference Schedule, Personality Research Form, and Locus of Control]. Perhaps the most interesting response of all was to the question: "Based on research findings, do you feel that the extent of projective test usage in various applied clinical settings is warranted?" Of the respondents, 22% replied yes, 23% somewhat, and 51% said no. Contrast these responses to the same question posed in relation to objective personality test usage: yes (58%), somewhat (34%), and no (8%).

If the majority believes projectives to have little validation and if their use has been predicted to decrease for the last two decades, why are they still taught and widely used? Some believe that those teaching the courses are not sufficiently skilled to help students extract from the tests what is presumed to be the wealth of psychological information in them or that insufficient time and practice are given over to help students master the tests. Or, perhaps a self-perpetuating cycle exists: internship sites and certain employing institutions require student to have a projective background for selection. Or simply, perhaps, we teach what we are taught. Based on one study (Lubin, Larsen, & Mataruzzo, 1984) the tests that clinicians are taught are those that they recommend for others to use. Finally, perhaps newer methods of interpreting projective techniques bring them closer to objective test interpretation (e.g., the Exner system for interpreting the Rorschach) and provide now or will provide in the future stronger research validation.

Psychologists also are typically expected to be trained in assessment of the entire age range, from infant to senior citizen. To do so raises the question as to whether such a large range allows for intensive knowledge of any segment of that range. Elbert's (1984) survey of training in child diagnostic assessment in clinical programs concluded that intelligence and personality were the primary dimensions being assessed and that relatively few instruments were being taught. She stated

> ...training in the specialized assessment of children is primarily focused on the formal assessment of intelligence and personality functioning. Such training is limited to a comparatively few test instruments, with cursory coursework exposure and minimal experience in test administration of other measures. (p. 131)

One assessment subspecialty that appears to be on the rise is clinical neuropsychological testing. Students are increasingly provided instruction in such specialized instruments as the Halstead-Reitan, Luria-Nebraska, and Luria-Christensen. As with any relatively new development, however, apparently a disparity exists between the qualifications of those teaching the instruments and the desired outcomes. On the basis of research into clinical neuropsychology training, McCaffrey and Isaac (1984) concluded

> ...the formal educational background and clinical experiences of most instructors of clinical neuropsychology in graduate training programs falls far short of the minimal training guidelines proposed by INS (International Neuropsychological Society) for students currently receiving training in clinical neuropsychology. (p. 32)

SPECIALIZATION

A number of specialty areas have been advocated, ranging from courses, to practicum placements, to a series of integrated didactic and practicum experiences. Some of these areas have traditionally been the "territory" of one or another of the helping professions, but now all are being advocated by elements within each profession, for each profession, thus contributing to the obfuscation of traditional role boundaries. Each of these areas is briefly discussed.

Gerontology

Social work has always had a concern with the aged, and psychiatry has also focused its attention on this population because of the number of hospital beds in state institutions occupied by the elderly. Late to come has been psychology. VandenBos, Stapp, and Kilberg (1981) determined that only 2.7% of all psychological health services go to the aged and 7 of every 10 psychologists never work clinically with the aged. A number of programs, however, now offer gerontological training as a subspecialty in clinical or counseling psychology. This training typically takes the form of a course(s), such as Life Span Development, and/or a practicum in working with the elderly, and usually entails close cooperation with other disciplines and agencies, such as social work and medicine. Topics commonly addressed are "normal" psychological, social, and physical development; special problems (e.g., terminal illness, loss and bereavement, etc.); assessment of the elderly; and intervention with the elderly for common psychological syndromes, such as depression, dementia, incontinence, etc. (Lewisohn, Teri, & Heatzinger, 1984).

Cross-Cultural Counseling

To what extent should ethnic minority content and experience be provided to those in training for the helping professions? As we have observed, psychiatrists, social workers, counselors, and psychologists are typically functioning in both a multicultural and a multiracial context. How much of their preparation (if any) should be devoted to issues pertaining to generic concerns of minority groups and how much (if any) to specific concerns of specific minority groups? How does training bring about cultural sensitivity (or can it)?

One survey of clinical psychology programs (Bernal & Padilla, 1982) determined that about 40% of them are offering one or more courses specifically related to working with minority populations. Results of a broader series of surveys of psychiatry, psychology, social work, and nursing programs (Dunston, 1983) suggested that elective courses are the primary avenue by which future mental health professionals are trained to work with minorities, that faculty members themselves have taken relatively few initiatives to enhance their own knowledge and skills in this area, that relatively few minority students are preparing to become mental health professionals, and that possibly one's entire pre-service clinical work can be done in a setting in which one does not come in contact with any minorities.

Psychiatry also is paying more attention to cultural factors in training, mainly on the grounds that lack of knowledge of cross-cultural or racial factors impedes clinical progress because of misdiagnoses and inappropriate psychotherapeutic methods, among other factors. Hispanics, Blacks, orientals, Native Americans, a number of large immigrant groups (e.g., Russians), and foreign student populations are all presumed to be sufficiently culturally different to require some specialized attention in residency programs. Not the least problem in such cases, of course, is for the therapist to recognize his/her own cultural, racial, and xenophobic responses to be sure that they are not getting in the way of a therapeutic relationship.

If the truth is that most mental health professionals come from the white middle class (Sue, 1981) and that the *modus operandi* of counseling is basically geared to the white middle class (Atkinson, Morten, & Sue, 1979), then the assumption is that specific and systematic training is required to alter the attitudes of therapists toward minority populations, and that new technologies of counseling are required to enhance working with these groups. *A priori,* such an argument appears sensible. On the other hand, some evidence exists to suggest that race, for example, is not so important a variable in "successful" therapy as we may believe (Ewing, 1974; Christensen, 1984). Until more definitive and persuasive research is forthcoming, those who provide specific cultural and racial training at the pre-service level will be doing so on the basis of faith.

**Sexual Orientation,
Sexuality, and Gender**

Both the American Psychological Association and the American Psychiatric Association, by voting of the membership, no longer consider homosexuality a mental disorder. Nevertheless, some professionals believe that gays and lesbians require specialized counseling, and consequently, that "training in counseling lesbian/gay clients (should) become a standard feature of APA-accredited training programs in clinical psychology, and that competence in counseling lesbian/gay clients (should) become a prerequisite for state licensure, and that the availability of continuing education regarding therapy for lesbian/gay clients (should) continue for practicing clinical psychologists" (Graham, Rawlings, Halpern, & Hermes, 1984, p. 482). Similar advocacy can be found in the literature of social work, psychiatry, counseling psychology, counselor education, and school psychology.

While this view represents an extreme within these professions, many professionals believe that therapists should have a sensitivity to the unique concerns and needs of those with atypical sexual orientations. If homosexuality is no longer a mental disorder (certainly in terms of politics although the clinical question is still moot for many), then no need is present for therapists to adopt a curative stance; rather, the idea is to work with lesbians and gays to help them "self-actualize" (Woodman & Lenna, 1980). At the very least, the argument is that therapists should be aware of and subsequently eliminate in themselves any homophobia or heterosexism, should recognize and understand homosexuals as a minority group with lifestyles different from those of the majority culture that is frequently hostile to them, and should be cognizant of how sex orientation or identity may affect the psychological assessment of homosexuals.

Beyond sexual orientation is the broader issue of sexuality. If sexual object preference no longer indicates disease (or, is at least independent of mental health), general sexual dysfunctions are still surely the focus of therapists' concerns. Female problems of body image, arousal, and orgasm and male problems of impotence, premature ejaculation, exhibitionism, fetishism, sadism, and other abnormalities are foci for counseling. Other events stemming from incest, molestation, and rape are traumatic occurrences that usually result in need for therapy. Thus, the recommendation is that those in the helping professions receive training in "sexual development, behavior, and problems" (Kirkpatrick, 1983, p. 33). Usually, such courses include biologic information, sexual development issues, and normal and abnormal sexual behavior.

In terms of gender, some advocate specific training activities to help safeguard against therapists' sexism—the stereotypical notion that only certain work and home roles and personality behaviors are appropriate for either sex. Sexism, racism, ageism, and other forms of irrational behavior still obviously exist, but one is heartened by their diminished manifestations. Executive orders and legislation have served as a comforting protection in effecting change, but part of the credit also must go to the assertive efforts of training programs to alter attitudes.

Substance Abuse

Schlesinger (1984), based on a study, determined that most graduate psychology training programs provide their students with "at least some exposure to substance misuse issues, and that programs focus on alcoholism and misuse of other drugs'' (p. 131). Corrigan (1979) has reported similar results for social workers and Stainbrook (1976) has indicated that medical schools likewise offer some instruction in substance abuse. Some institutions require such training; others offer elective courses. As with any other specialized aspect of training, instruction typically focuses on providing students with theoretical knowledge of the effects of substance abuse on the person, the family, and society and on achieving self-awareness by therapists of their own attitudes, and/or developing intervention techniques to work with substance abusers. Interestingly, one counselor education program uses its students to counsel court-referred clients as a part of a community DWI education and awareness program (Wigtil & Thompson, 1984).

Fringe Therapies

A number of therapies exist which relatively few practitioners have adopted. These are not generally included in standard training programs, but one can find at least a few persons urging that each should be included. For example, a fairly well-developed movement seeks to ally various aspects of the arts with psychotherapy. Thus, we have music therapy, poetry therapy, art therapy, dance therapy, bibliotherapy, sociodrama, psychodrama, and so on in an attempt to merge the fine and performing arts with the healing arts.

A second group of fringe therapies seeks to align physical interventions with salubrious mental changes. Consequently, we have such movements as Rolfing, reflexology, Tai Chi, acupuncture, elements of chiropractic medicine, and so forth that seek to capitalize on what is generally acknowledged to be a mind-body connection.

A third group of fringe therapies can be grouped under the general rubric of "pop" therapies. Included in this category are such movements as Est, scientology and various other religious-oriented groups, diverse Eastern mystical cults, any of a hundred systems represented in self-help books and their money-making off-shoots, and so on.

Also some fringe assessment techniques purport to measure psychological characteristics of the person and/or to offer advice based on these characteristics. Examples are graphology, palmistry, phrenology, astrology, psychic phenomena, and so on.

What each of these fringe therapies has in common is that none is subjected to very rigorous evaluation. Consequently, other than the desultory subjective testimony of some individuals who have experienced one or another of these modes, we have no evidence that any of them achieves what it purports to achieve. On the other hand, some traditional and respected therapies similarly lack documentation of positive results.

Family Therapy

Another common area to which several of the helping professions give their attention is that of family therapy and its attendant foci (e.g., couples counseling, marriage counseling, marital therapy, etc.). No agreement, however, exists as to what skills and knowledge are required and can be taught and what methods are best to learn which skills (Mohammed & Piercy, 1983). Some programs use case demonstrations, some employ didactic or clinical work, some utilize seminars, some rely on supervision as the primary teaching technique, and some use all of these approaches. Within psychiatry, Sugarman (1984) pointed out that one of the problems is that of definition—that the current emphasis on family therapy may be nothing more than old wine in a new bottle, since good clinical work has always entailed a focus on the family. Others, of course, see family therapy as *sui generis* in terms of both content and process. This problem of definition of family therapy extends to other helping profession discipline as well.

Although a few university-based programs are devoted to marriage and family therapy, most education and training takes place within extant program that are broader in scope but that adhere to standards promulgated by the American Association of Marriage and Family Therapy (AAMFT). The basic concept is that in addition to the development of good clinical skills, therapists need also to acquire substantive knowledge unique to marriage and the family. Nichols (1979) advocated a progression of education: first, training should produce therapists who can work with individuals; next, knowledge should be gained of mate selection and marital interaction, accompanied by supervised clinical work with marital partners; and lastly, the trainee should work with family units and systems. Most programs tend to short-cut this proposed sequence and try to develop all skills simultaneously; and some programs see no need for family therapists to have skills in individual psychotherapy.

Within the fields of counselor education and psychology, a great deal of enthusiasm is present for training in marriage and family therapy; and an increasing number of courses is being made available to students, although these formal courses are still relatively fewer than would be suspected, judging from the support for them in the professional literature (Liddle, Vance, & Pastushak, 1979). Within those courses that do exist, the foci generally are on both family developmental issues and clinical treatment approaches. *A priori,* a formal, coherent programs of courses and clinical experiences would seem to be an improvement over the relatively *ad hoc* nature of most family therapy training in the past; further more protracted study appears preferable to a short course approach.

Liddle (1982) defined the issues in the field of training family therapists as

1. *Personnel.* Who should teach and be taught family therapy?

2. *Content and Skills.* What should be taught?

3. *Methodology.* How should the content and skills be taught?

4. *Context.* How does the setting influence training and how does training influence the setting?

5. *Evaluation.* How should training be assessed? (p. 82)

One other consideration is that of non-specialized training in family therapy; that is, how much do non-family therapists need to know about family-related issues and how do they acquire that knowledge? Wendt and Zake (1984), for example, offered guidelines for the optional training of school psychologists in family systems theory. Should such training be optional or required? Similar posers pertain to almost any relatively specialized area of study within any of the helping professions.

DESIRABLE HELPER CHARACTERISTICS

Because of the intense competition to gain entry into advanced degree programs in most of the helping professions, a reasonably large pool of applicants is available from which to choose individuals who, after proper education and training, will become competent professionals. One would think that with this many degrees of freedom of choice, the "hit" rate would be almost perfect. Unfortunately, because research studies have not identified what an effective professional is in any definitive sense, the difficulty comes in knowing for what to look in the selection of those to be educated for a helping profession, and we have only nebulous criteria for determining professional competency.

Lacking any sort of clear guidelines in terms of personality characteristics, interests, biodata, or other information from the non-intellective domain, we usually rely predominantly on intellective data: past performance in academic course work and standardized test scores, such as those yielded by instruments like the GRE, MAT, MSAT, and so on (Ingram & Zurawski, 1981). Because the group for whom we are attempting to gain predictive efficiency is so homogeneous, difficulty occurs in obtaining any variables that correlate highly.

Consequently, the interview is frequently utilized in an attempt to bring some clinical judgment into what otherwise is a relatively mechanical, actuarial process of selection. To do so presumes some notion about what constitutes desirable helper characteristics. Unfortunately, the literature in this regard is not at all clear. Although interviews in the admissions process designed to estimate the clinical potential of applicants may have an effect on selection (Nevid & Gildea, 1984), they have not been demonstrated to relate to prediction of success as a counselor or therapist.

Shertzer and Stone (1980) attempted to extract some sense from the literature of what characteristics define a "good" counselor. Although they pointed out a lack of consistency of findings, they nevertheless concluded:

> Tolerance for ambiguity, maturity, self-understanding, ability to maintain an appropriate emotional distance from the counselee, and ability to maintain good interpersonal relationships are characteristics demonstrated to be associated with counselor effectiveness. While psychometric data reflect that, as a group, counselors exhibit greater needs on variables such as succorance, intraception, exhibitionism, affiliation, and the like, non-intellective measures have not consistently discriminated between so-called effective and ineffective counselors. (p. 114)

Effectiveness, of course, depends on how it is defined. For example, if the ability to make accurate clinical predictions is the criterion of effectiveness, Watley & Vance (1964) have demonstrated rather convincingly that about the only variable that seems to differentiate good from poor clinical predictors is abstract reasoning ability as measured by such tests as the MAT or GRE Verbal—traditionally defined intellect. This characteristic is not one of those offered by Shertzer and Stone. The prediction task, or course, is a relatively cognitive process and might be expected to correlate highly with measures of academic aptitude. A study of counselor education by Hosford, Johnson, and Atkinson (1984) also determined that MAT or GRE Verbal scores were significantly related to faculty-ranked academic success of 77 counseling students but were not related (nor was any other criterion, background experiences, or interview data with faculty and students) to faculty rankings of either counseling competency or anticipated success in the field. Thus, the question of the non-intellective characteristics desired in mental health professionals is still moot and will likely remain an open issue until such time as we are able more clearly to define the standard of what constitutes the "successful" helper.

Ford (1979) summarized the situation in this manner:

> ...several studies have demonstrated that trainees' scores on psychometric personality measures (e.g., MMPI, Omnibus Personality Inventory, Edwards personal Preference Scores, Myers-Briggs Type Indicator; Dogmatism Scale; Tolerance of Ambiguity Scale) and aptitude or vocational preference tests (e.g., Strong Vocational Interest Blank), trainee-supervisor similarity on such personality scales, trainee's past academic achievement (e.g., GRE scores; GPA, letters of recommendation), and trainee's performance on analogue measures of the target skills (i.e., simulated counseling interviews; discrimination of optimal counselor responses on a written multiple-choice test; written responses to audiotaped client statements) are *not* significantly predictive of the trainees' abilities to effectively conduct therapy interviews after receiving training (i.e., supervisor or peer-related therapist competencies; observer-rated FC communication levels). (p. 115)

PERSONAL THERAPY IN TRAINING

A number of the helping professions either require or strongly urge trainees to experience personal therapy as a part of their education. Almost all psychoanalytic and a number of psychiatric programs do so; it is strongly recommended in many clinical psychology programs; and it is less strongly advocated for counseling psychology and social work programs. Such advocacy or requirement is related to the presumed salutory effect of therapy on trainees' self-awareness and self-understanding, the release of neurotic defenses, and improvement of general personality integration.

As yet, no definitive research has emerged to suggest that either personal therapy or its absence is beneficial in the training of clinicians.

Some believe that to help people in their struggles in life, one has to have participated in that struggle (Hill, 1978). Very little evidence, however, is present to indicate that this is so (Garfield & Kurtz, 1976). Some preliminary data support the idea that one's own therapy has an influence on aspects of life, for instance, on one's theoretical gender orientation—masculine, feminine, or androgeneous—(Gerson & Lewis, 1984), but very little demonstrated relationship is present as to effective therapeutic outcome. Some believe that requiring personal therapy of trainees is a violation of their rights and that an understanding of self that is sufficient to be an effective helper can be attained without a trainee's experiencing the cost, time, and potentially stigmatizing effects of therapy. For example, some believe that a comprehensive supervisory relationship can produce such a result.

This is not to say that distressed clinical trainees should go without assistance. Impaired clinicians, even in the training stage, are a potential danger to themselves and to others, whether that impairment stems from alcohol or substance abuse, psychiatric disorder, or disturbed interpersonal relationships. In general, any severe mental or physical impairment requires remediation via treatment, and most training programs will be alert to recognize such problems and to take appropriate steps to ameliorate them (Nadelson, Salt, & Notman, 1983). One study (Schultz & Russell, 1984) determined that Directors of Training considered 8% of their child psychiatry trainees to have "significant emotional disturbance" and an additional 7% to have other difficulties ranging from financial to marital. Training in most programs designed to produce practitioners in the helping professions is typically a stressful process and maladaptive responses should be readily observable.

IN-SERVICE TRAINING

Assuming that within a discipline agreement can be reached regarding what is taught, we are still left with the whole area of in-service education and training. Some professions mandate continuing life-long education; others strongly recommend it as one way of attempting to remain professionally alive and growing.

Whether the instruction is effected by professional organizations, colleges and universities, professional schools, proprietary educational institutions, agencies, hospitals, or whatever, most helping professions award continuing education credits for such approved endeavors. Among the foci for such education have been training for: writing behavior-based client objectives (Hinman & Marr, 1984); specific ethnic groups in specific techniques, such as behavior therapy (Stumphauzer & Davis, 1983); teaching helping relationship skills to other types of health care providers (Arnold et al., 1983); a specialty, as in child psychology (Ollendick, 1984); and various types of helping professionals in psychotherapy (Hooper & Roberts, 1976), to cite but a few of the many examples possible.

In some helping professions, continuing education—as distinct from basic education—is a highly structured, well-developed, organized activity. Such is the case, for example, with Regional Rehabilitation Continuing Education Programs (RRCEP), sponsored by the federal government and designed in accordance with the ten geographical regions stipulated by the United States Office of Education. These programs identify and assess training needs of practicing rehabilitation counselors and then engage in appropriate educational activities to meet the needs. This program is voluntary; other professions, in some states, have mandated continuing education such as state branches of the American Medical Association, through its Division of Educational Policy and Development, Division of Physician Credentials and Qualifications.

The American Psychological Association has a voluntary continuing education program, although many states require continuing education as a condition of renewal of a psychologist's license. The National Association of Social Workers also has a voluntary program, although a certain number of clock hours of continuing education is recommended over a period of years. Some states have continuing education requirements for licensing of social workers. Other specialties, such as pastoral counselors and marriage and family therapists, also have recommended continuing education programs.

Welch (1976) has outlined three delivery modes for health-care continuing education. One is the continuing education model in which approved workshops, seminars, etc. carry credit; as we have observed, a set number of credits may lead to continued licensing or recertification. A second model is the examination model, whereby the practitioner must take and pass periodic examinations (or perform work samples) to demonstrate competency for perpetuation of licensure or certification. The third model is the peer review model, in which a practitioner's record of clinical practice is compared with an established criterion of care for a profession as a whole. Wilson (1982) has argued that such a system is reactive rather than proactive and is, therefore, of less value as a continuing education model. In general, Vitulane and Copeland (1980) pointed out that "There appears to be little evidence of a positive relationship between either the number of continuing education credits accumulated or the scores on an examination and actual competency demonstration in practice" (p. 893). The reader will recall that similar findings pertain to pre-service education.

In psychology, the topic of respecialization further complicates the continuing education picture. Respecialization—allowing Ph.D.s in developmental, cognitive, social, physiological, and other types of psychology to become eligible for clinical practice—must be achieved by means of a formal graduate program, including course work and internship. This opportunity for lateral change of specialty within psychology is offered by approximately 20% of the APA clinical training programs (Stricker, Hull, & Woodring, 1984). Although some argue that it is an easier way to get into clinical work, usually such respecialization amounts to a career change rather than a "back door" entrance to clinical practice.

SOCIAL WORK CONCERNS

The education and training of social workers presents a number of problems different from those in the other helping professions. Not the least of these concerns is the fact that social work is one of the few helping professions that offers a professional degree at the baccalaureate level. The BSW is a degree that enables the recipient to become employed in entry level positions in social work; some charge that it takes jobs away from more highly trained MSWs because employees find that BSWs are less costly to hire. Further, critics of BSWs and entry-level practice argue that the MSW may offer much redundancy in preparation for those who achieved the BSW rather than majored in one of the liberal arts or sciences. Such duplication, when not used deliberately for reinforcement purposes, appears wasteful.

A second problem in social work education is one of semantics. For a number of years now, social work educators have cavilled over such terms as "generic" versus "generalist" versus "specialist" (Anderson, 1982). These debates are symptoms of the controversy of how much social work education should be a core or common base for all social workers and how much social work practice preparation should be specialized. Similar lack of agreement on meaning extends to definitions of "research" in social work (Heineman, 1981; Hudson, 1982; Schuerman, 1981).

The latest Curriculum Policy Statement (1984) of the Council on Social Work Education tries to address some of these confusions. It mandates graduate level training, but it does not distinguish clearly what knowledge and skills are needed for advanced as opposed to beginning professional practice. It advocates that practitioners be able to accomplish research and use research in their practice—in a relatively crude way. It encourages MSW programs to do everything possible to prevent repetition. It urges a common core prior to any specialization. Finally, it fosters an interaction between social work practice and social work education. The specifics of how many of these changes are to be effected are vague (Hokenstad, 1984).

Another problem in social work education has been the distinction made in policy skills versus practice skills. At the MSW level, students typically "majored" in one or the other, and emphasized casework, group work, or community organization. Newer ideas suggest that elements of both should pertain in the education of all students. Within each of these "tracks," debate continues regarding breadth versus depth (Leighninger, 1980), and whether social work is simply a collection of specialties or a coherent profession. Brooks (1982) surveyed 83 preparation programs and tabulated the frequency of specialized areas available in the curricula of these programs. The nine highest were health and mental health (28.5%), family and children's services (22.4%), aging (12.7%), corrections (9.7%), school social services (6.1%), poverty and minority issues (4.8%), public social services (4.8%), mental retardation and disabilities (3.0%), and alcohol and drug abuse (3.0%). Somewhat broader categories are possible by looking to focus of employment: industrial social work (Kurzman & Akabas, 1981), the aged (Monk, 1981), family, mental health and health.

In general, then, social work appears to be a more inclusive and a less well-shaped profession than some of the other helping relationship areas that are more sharply defined and focused.

ISSUES IN THE EDUCATION OF PSYCHIATRIC NURSES

Psychiatric nursing, as we have observed, is a relatively new specialization within an old profession. it has thus not yet agreed upon a set of educational experiences that constitute an acceptable basis for entry into the profession. In fact, currently two avenues are open to one who wishes to become a psychiatric mental health nurse. One is to receive a baccalaureate in nursing (focusing in all areas) and then specialize in psychiatric nursing at the graduate level (the master's degree). This route has existed since 1967 and leads to certification by the American Nurses' Association (ANA) if the applicant also passes a specialty examination. A second approach, however, was created by ANA in 1977, whereby nurses who are experienced in psychiatric nursing (a minimum of 5 years) may take the certification examinations and be credentialed as psychiatric nurses.

Within the undergraduate curriculum, all registered nurses are supposed to receive some psychiatric nursing training, although a number of observers feel that such training is not present in many programs (Hipps, 1981). At the graduate level, no agreement exists on what knowledge base should be required for certification (Tousley, 1982). This relative training disarray is further complicated by the fact that applicants to psychiatric nursing master's programs are relatively few in number, and outside funding for training is being withdrawn (Dumas, 1983). All of these factors have led Pearlmutter (1985) to conclude that "nursing-education continues to struggle with the problem of how to most effectively educate nurses for increasingly specialized and complex functions" (p. 59).

SUB-DOCTORAL TRAINING

The terminal degree in social work is a master's degree. Similarly, the master's is a "bankable" degree in areas such as school counseling, school psychology, rehabilitation counseling, college student personnel, psychiatric nursing, and several others. In counseling psychology, industrial/organizational and clinical psychology, however, the terminal master's degree has less currency. As Perlman and Lane (1981) stated the case: "There is a strong tenor within psychology that the master's level psychologist is a second class citizen" (p. 73). Yet, these clinicians appear to be at least as well-trained as MSWs, since they typically take a core of traditional psychology courses and practica, and must demonstrate research skills. Blume and Perlman (1981) concluded that with "appropriate controls," master's level clinicians trained in psychotherapy, consultation, research, administration, and standardized projective and occupational testing were perfectly capable of functioning as psychologists with adjective-identified specialties (e.g., Associate Psychologist, Applied Clinical Psychologist, etc.).

The argument within psychology is essentially about how much is enough and parallels, in many respects, the BSW-MSW debate, including arguments about redundancy, depth, and breadth.

INTERNSHIP EXPERIENCE

The most common procedure for internships is to have them take place after all course work is completed (although obvious exceptions exist to this procedure) and after preliminary practica are successfully handled. Some programs allow students to work with clients (relatively innocuously, to be sure) directly from the first semester of training, while others insist on some knowledge background and simulated experiences prior to seeing actual clients, no matter how benign the presenting problem. Some internship settings consider training a specified and paramount goal; others take interns but regard the training function as peripheral, at best (such settings are *not* likely to have the imprimatur of the relevant professional organization, however). Most internship settings provide a variety of experiences or "rotations," such as adult-clinical, child-clinical, neuropsychology, forensic, gerontology, chemical abuse, in-patient, etc., and utilize a variety of techniques (group work, individual work, assessment, consultation, in-take, etc.).

Frequently, communication between internship settings and sending educational institutions is less than complete and effective. Because the clinical skills sometimes have no relationship to past academic performance, an important procedure is for both sender and receiver to have comprehensive and frequent feedback. Another issue in internships is that of funding. Although the internship setting is getting "cheap," although relatively raw labor, some feelings are frequently expressed that the sending educational institution, the government, or some other source external to the placement should fund the intern. Weiskopf and Newman (1982) have predicted a possible increase in unpaid psychology internships (or a decrease in the number of positions available) if funding continues to be a problem, and they have proposed a more cost-efficient system.

Schmalz (1983) reported on one survey of psychology internships in the Province of Ontario in Canada. The typical intern's work week "involved spending 16 percent of his/her time in supervision, 37 percent in direct service and 47 percent in other activities such as report writing, meetings, training seminars and research. The bulk of the typical intern's time was spent doing psychology therapy and writing reports" (p. 23).

No standardization of psychological internship training exists, except as generally defined by a setting's being an APA Approved internship site. An APA Internship site must (1) meet specific criteria, (2) be visited by an appointed APA evaluator, (3) and then be approved by an APA committee. But such criteria do *not* say *what* experience must be provided. For example, if you do an internship in a college counseling center you may never see a test. Similarly, in social work there are no universal standards for practicum experiences. Larsen (1980) suggested a competency-based, task-centered approach to practicum instruction in social work, including:

1. Specifying concrete skills to be mastered in the practicum (e.g., using appropriate open-ended responses, responding accurately and emphatically, maintaining focus, being authentic, etc.).

2. Providing systematic group training sessions that include didactic instruction and modeling by the instructor and practice by students.

3. Requiring students to document the use of specified skills through weekly process records and audiotapes.

4. Establishing and monitoring specified learning tasks (expressed in behavioral terms) designed to increase student mastery of skills.

5. Using specified skills as criteria for grading in the practicum. (p. 88)

Psychiatric internships and residences offer a "good news-bad news" scenario. Gilmore and Perry (1980), for example, reported on a study in which psychiatric interns were seen to go through a stressful attempt to cope with a changing professional identity, a period of "professional adolescence." They view this process in four phases:

1. a phase of helplessness when the interns over-identify with the patients and view themselves as totally incompetent and delegate exaggerated process to others;

2. a phase of aggrandizement when the interns inflate themselves with magical expectations for cure and admiration;

3. a phase of despair when the interns grieve over the lost omnipotence in themselves and others; and

4. a phase of transformation when the interns set more reasonable expectations for themselves and others, accept their limitations, and continue to grow by finding positive aspects of their work and colleagues with which to identify. (p. 1209)

Such stages or phases are probably equally instructive when applied to the internship and/or practica experiences in other helping professions.

Finally, some rather surprising findings emerge from a study of 22 individuals who entered psychiatry with an internship, compared with 22 persons who went into psychiatry without an internship (Lindy, Green, & Patrick, 1980). Faculty rated individuals in each group in terms of such variables as responsibility, insight, teachability, and knowledge, as well as on their overall performance in inpatient, consultation, and emergency psychiatry. No significant differences were found in terms of these dimensions. The only significant differences discovered were in the realm of outpatient psychiatry—and these favored the non-internship group! The investigators suggested that internship experiences may deaden empathy responses, a suggestion that certainly merits further study.

SUMMARY

As has been illustrated in Chapter 5, controversies in education and training are primarily intraprofessional but many controversies are interprofessional. Regardless of where they reside, such controversies embrace concerns about the balance of research and didactic instruction, the place of training or apprenticeship, the models of professional socialization to be emulated. Each of these areas of controversy ultimately is shaped by the peculiar history and meaning system of the professional group for whom the education and training system provides entree. In either single dimension or combinations of dimensions, education and training of mental health professionals have within them the seeds of controversy.

THEME THREE: CREDENTIALING OF PROFESSIONALS

CHAPTER 6

THE CREDENTIALING OF MENTAL HEALTH PROFESSIONALS

Regardless of the professional identity, the competencies, or the education and training one has acquired, the fundamental question is, can one receive the legal or professional sanction to practice as a mental health professional? The latter is a credentialing question. It is also an economic question, a question of gatekeeping, a question of professional differentiation, a legal question. Credentialing of mental health professionals has become a major source of controversy among the "helping professions."

Credentialing is not only a matter for individuals, it is also a matter for institutions. Increasingly, for individuals to be able to receive an appropriate credential—license, certificate, registration—the first necessity is for institutions from which they received their education to have been accredited or to have received program approval. Thus, a complex interaction of evaluations, professional and legal sanctions, and other mechanisms have emerged to protect the consumer from ill-prepared or incompetent practitioners. But, these mechanisms also have been preserved for the protection of professional rights, economic benefits, identities, and other secondary effects. They have created professional in-groups and out-groups; hierarchies of prestige and status within the mental health professions; and unevenness in who can provide mental health services from one state to another.

In the first five chapters, the issue of the credentialing of professional helpers has been raised in relation to other issues of power, economics, territoriality. These processes, assumptions, and sanctions symbolized by the rubric, credentialing, are important sources of controversy among the "mental health professions" and among the "helping professions," legislatures, health care insurers, and the general public. Of concern are questions of occupational regulation, restraint of trade, who benefits from regulation, practitioner competence, who will credential, access to certain forms of reimbursement, professional prestige, independence in professional behavior, and many other lesser matters.

Credentialing, then, is not a benign, bureaucratic mechanism by which one pays a fee and secures a certificate attesting to one's freedom to practice one's profession. It is rather the external symbol of gatekeeping and the crucible through which professional politics, special interests, identity conflicts, and related elements are played out.

Although the common usage of the term would suggest so, credentialing is not a singular process. Rather, credentialing tends to encompass several types of testimonies to individual qualifications, eligibility to use a title, or authority to perform specified occupational tasks as well as the mechanisms which acknowledge that institutions or programs are qualified to prepare certain types of practitioners. The credentialing of individuals typically takes the form of *licensure, certification,* or *registry*. The credentialing of institutions usually involves *accreditation* or *program approval*. Although these terms are frequently used interchangeably, they generally connote separate mechanisms having different legal authority and status. Therefore, an important issue is to consider the language and the content of credentialing for individuals and for programs as primary sources of controversy in their own right.

INDIVIDUAL CREDENTIALING

Licensure

Licensure of an occupational group is the most restrictive and most powerful of the current credentialing mechanisms. It is, therefore, the most coveted by members of the "helping professions" or, indeed, other occupations.

According to the U.S. Department of Health, Education and Welfare (DHEW, 1977), licensing is "the process by which an agency of government grants permission to an individual to engage in a given occupation upon finding that the applicant has attained the minimal degree of competency necessary to ensure that the public health, safety, and welfare will be reasonably well protected." Shimberg (1982) indicated that licensing laws are often referred to as "practice laws" or "practice control" (p. 15). This is so because in agreeing to regulate an occupation by licensing its practitioners, state licensing laws typically define the "scope of practice" which is covered by the licensing statute.

Shimberg and Roederer (1978) characterized the power of licensing as awesome. This description prevails in their view because "licensing makes it illegal for anyone who does not hold a valid license to engage in the occupation, profession, trade, etc., covered by the statute. Thus, the power to license can be used to deny individuals the legal opportunity to earn livelihoods in their chosen fields" (p. 1). Put somewhat differently, Mackin (1976) stated "that having power over a person's subsistence amounts to having power over a person's will, occupational licensing can control people's subsistence by denying them the opportunity to practice an occupation. We must review that control to insure that the license does not wrongfully control a person's will" (p. 511).

The major intent of occupational licensure is to protect the public from practitioners who are incompetent or likely to injure or exploit their clients for personal gain. Such a rationale is, on its face, reasonable and appropriate. However, more than 800 occupations are regulated by different states and/or the federal government. These occupations include a broad spectrum ranging from psychologists to egg candlers, pilots to pet groomers, physicians to barbers and cosmetologists. Except under the very widest interpretation, to conceive of each of these 800 occupations as equally likely to injure the public or exploit it through some form of charlantanism or quackery is hard to do. Indeed, most occupational regulation does not evolve from public outrage or complaint but instead is stimulated by persons within the occupation itself (Shimberg & Roederer, 1978).

Here lay the sources of much of the controversy attending licensure. Who benefits from licensure? The public? Or, the occupational practitioners? If the public, in what ways? If the public does not stimulate the regulation of a particular occupation, why do its practitioners wish to be regulated? Undoubtedly, some benefit to the public accrues when an occupation weeds out or suspends incompetents, frauds, or the unethical. Such possibilities of quality control reside within the licensing process in most instances. The public tends to assume that it will be protected by government and, therefore, takes statutes licensing physicians, nurses, and related health care specialists pretty much for granted. However, since most occupational regulations are proposed and lobbied for by members of the occupation to be regulated, licensure is likely to be sought for reasons other than altruism or protection of the public.

That reason is found in the implications of Shimberg and Roederer's use of the term awesome to describe the power of licensing. Inherent in such processes is essentially the definition of an occupation by identifying the scope of practice its licensees are permitted to engage in. Also inherent to the process is regulation of who can and cannot be admitted to the occupation.

> Licensed practitioners gain an exclusive right to deliver services. They may then ask the Board, made up of fellow practitioners, to use its power to restrict entry into the field by setting high education and experience requirements, giving difficult tests, and erecting barriers to keep out practitioners from other states (or, indeed, from other emerging occupational groups). Thus, the licensed group may establish monopoly conditions which enable it to control the availability and cost of services and restrict competition...Such practices often operate to raise costs to consumers. (Shimberg & Roederer, 1978, p. 3)

An interesting note is that one of the major sources of legal actions taken against psychologists, for example, is by other psychologists who have been denied licensure.

Depending upon how broad the scope of practice of practice is, a particular occupational group acquiring licensure eligibility can essentially control how many people and under what conditions they will practice their occupation or profession. By so doing, they can prohibit other occupational groups the opportunity to engage in their scope of practice and thereby restrain free trade in the delivery of particular services to the public. This outcome obviously carries enormous economic implications for those who are licensed, for consumers, and, on the negative side, for those practitioners who may have considerable training and experience in relevant practices but not be licensable for some reason: They may come from another state or nation which does not have licensure reciprocity; they may have training different from that required for licensure in a particular state; they may have different or less experience than that required for licensure eligibility.

Ordinarily, licensure of an occupation is a prerogative of the state legislature. Upon agreeing to license a particular occupational group and define its scope of practice by statute, the typical procedure is to create a board of examiners to implement the licensure statutes. The State Board of Examiners is generally comprised of persons representing the occupation to be regulated. Indeed, such Board members are frequently nominated by the professional associations or occupational groups who stimulated the statute in the first place and in so doing are likely to be largely responsible for how the scope of practice is described. In essence, then, licensing becomes a process of self-regulation by an occupational group. Within the parameters of the State statute under which a particular Board operates, it can determine what type of examination will be used to determine competency, who will be eligible to take the examination (usually this prerogative is expressed as what type of training and experience makes one licensure-eligible and therefore permitted to take the examination), how complaints of incompetence or ethical violations will be handled, and what penalties or sanctions will be imposed upon those who violate the licensure standards or the legal guidelines on which the licensure statutes was promulgated.

Shimberg and Roederer (1978) suggested a number of guidelines for the development of licensure laws which for the purpose of this book, when not met, are also likely to be the stuff of controversy. They include in paraphrased form:

> Licensure requirements and evaluation procedures should be related to safe and effective practice. However, such requirements and evaluation procedures are not uniform across states or across occupations being regulated. Sometimes requirements for particular types of education and training, age, residency are not related to effective performance on the job. Therefore, they become exclusionary unless alternative ways are

established by which persons who wish to become licensed can demonstrate their competency.

Persons from out-of-state holding licensure or wishing to be an applicant for such licensure should have fair and reasonable access to the licensure process. Unless state reciprocity is available for persons already having licensure in another state wishing to work in a new state, this person will have to go through the licensure process as if he or she had never been licensed elsewhere or been in the field, the licensure examination may test information which this individual has never studied or studied many years before. In such instances, the licensure examination may be primarily an academic exercise with little direct relationship to effective practice. Thus, unless ways are provided to give credit for one's prior occupational experience or to demonstrate one's competency other than by taking a knowledge test of theories and other such information, some practitioners from other states or nations will be unfairly excluded from practice in the receiving state.

Frequently, when a licensure statute is adopted in a state all of the persons in the occupation at that time are "grandfathered" in without the need to be examined or otherwise demonstrate their competency. Therefore, some incompetent practitioners are licensed and, at the least, newcomers to the occupation are likely to be held to higher standards than older members of the occupation.

When licensure is granted to a practitioner it should be valid only so long as the holder can provide evidence of competency. In general, competency concerns of licensure boards are confined to matters of initial competence, not continuing competence. As a result, some group of practitioners may become at high risk to be inadequate due to a deterioration of skills or for other reasons. A system needs to be in place, as it is in some States for some mental health occupations, to identify and either upgrade the competencies of such persons or terminate their license.

The public, the consumers, should be represented on licensure boards. In general, licensure boards are comprised of representatives of the occupations regulated, not the consumers of such services. While this is changing, the participation of the public is and has been minimal, often by law, in the decision-making process concerned with matters affecting their welfare.

When an occupation is to be licensed, its scope of practice should be designed in such a way as to avoid fragmentation and inefficiency in the delivery of services. When the scope of practice is too broad and therefore highly restrictive as to who can be licensed, it fails to recognize that many groups in a system (such as the health care system) have overlapping functions. Excluding overlapping from licensure through overly broad scopes of practice leads to a proliferation of licensure requests, fragmentation of service delivery, and underutilization of available practitioners.

Certification

A second category of credentialing, less restrictive and less powerful than licensing, is certification. Certification, because it is less restrictive, is less likely to be the source of controversy between an occupation and the public or among overlapping occupations such as those found in the helping professions. Shimberg (1982) described certification as "government title control." According to him,

> Certification is the process by which a governmental or nongovernmental agency or association grants authority to use a specified title to an individual who has met predetermined qualifications...Unlike licensure, the law does not prohibit individuals from engaging in the regulated occupation. However, it prohibits some from using a given title or from holding themselves out to the public as being certified... (p. 10)

Certification identifies competent practitioners who are typically in occupational areas assumed to be less risky to health and safety than those which warrant licensure. Frequently, certification is extended to occupations where the practitioner is not likely to be in independent private practice but is likely to work within an educational or agency setting in which other practitioners and supervisors are available (school counselors are such an example).

Certification is not only offered by governmental agencies, such as State Departments of Education, but is also increasingly provided by non-governmental agencies. Frequently, professional and trade or occupational organizations establish standards and mechanisms by which to recognize individuals who have specialized expertise or who have attained performance levels beyond some preset standard. For example, the American Board of Internal Medicine identifies physicians who pass specialized examinations in internal medicine and have other experiences as "diplomates." The National Board of Certified Counselors grants the title of National Certified Counselor to those who pass its examinations and a review of professional training and experience. Similar titles derive from passing examinations of the National Academy of Clinical Mental Health Counselors and other professional certification groups. While such certifications are independent of governmental agencies they attest to the voluntary effort of practitioners in their respective occupations to maintain and extend their knowledge and skill in their field. In some cases, these voluntary certifications have important implications for occupational opportunities and mobility since they have acquired a level of credibility in their own right.

Registry/Registration

A third credentialing mechanism is sometimes called registry and, in other instances, registration. Actually, the two terms can have rather different meanings. For example, registry may mean to have one's name, title, address, etc., included in a directory of persons who have successfully completed the requirements of licensure or certification. The National Council of Health Care Providers publishes a registry of psychologists who have been licensed in their states and who meet other requirements attesting to their competence. The National Board of Certified Counselors (NBCC) publishes a registry of National Certified Counselors (NCC). Such registries allow consumers or agencies in need of practitioners who might serve as referral sources for them to identify in a given geographical area the names of persons who have met certain types of professional standards and are therefore likely to have particular types of knowledge or skill.

The term "registration" or "registry" can also have another meaning. In some states it can mean that a practitioner has filed his/her name, experience, training and other information pertinent to profession practice with a designated state agency charged with monitoring or regulating practice. In such instances, the practitioner participates in a "public disclosure" process by contending that he/she has the requisite skills or training to hold themselves out to the public or to use the title of some occupation (for example, marriage and family counselor, rehabilitation counselor, financial planner). The state may then publish a registry of such persons, their qualifications, and the services they intend to offer. If consumer complaints arise or if persons are found to have misrepresented in their public disclosure their training or other qualifications, the state agency can impose sanctions upon such people as are provided by law or regulation.

While registration is not yet common across the nation, registry is increasingly so. Neither of these mechanisms to date has been particularly controversial because they are not typically seen to have the legal force, exclusiveness, or economic implications that licensure has and less so certification. Some individual cases have occurred where persons who for various reasons have not been permitted to be included in a registry have experienced some personal and legal conflict. However, on balance, while these mechanisms tend to provide minimum protection for the public, they do not have the power or the comprehensiveness of coverage or the restrictive characteristics likely to stimulate wide spread controversy.

PROGRAM CREDENTIALING

In addition to licensure, certification, registry or other forms of credentialing for individuals mechanisms also exist to credential programs or institutions. The major one of relevance here is program approval or accreditation. Basically, program approval or accreditation occurs when a governmental agency and/or a professional association applies a set of standards to a training program which purports to train a particular type of specialist, professional, or other. The standards are likely to include many criteria such as quality of faculty, the nature of the training facility, availability of equipment, curriculum content, instructor-student ratios, supervisory practices, resource availability, program objectives, placement record, and related elements. If a visiting evaluation team finds that the program being evaluated is in compliance with or meets such standards, and forwards a recommendation to approve the program to the responsible government agency or professional association, the program is likely to be "accredited" or receive "program approval" for a specified period of time, usually not more than five years, after which it must be re-evaluated.

The effects of program approval are several. Persons trained in an accredited or approved program are likely to be endorsed for certification or considered to be licensure eligible on the basis of their training.

Thus, they are likely to receive priority access to credentials and employment opportunities which persons not trained in approved or accredited programs will find difficult if not impossible to achieve. In addition, approved or accredited programs are more likely to attract superior applicants, be eligible for external fiscal support for research or training, and accrue other benefits (prestige, etc.) as compared to non-approved programs.

Again, in such instances, controversy settles on the content of the standards used to evaluate programs, the criteria by which programs are permitted to be considered for program approval or accreditation, the favorable or exclusive treatment accorded to the program's graduates and, indeed, the presumptions implicit in the governmental agency's or professional association's prerogatives in fostering such an accreditation structure.

CREDENTIALING AND THE HELPING PROFESSIONS

Thus far in Chapter 5 we have discussed the emphases which differentiate one form of credentialing from another and the fact that some mechanisms credential individuals and other mechanisms credential programs or institutions. These individual/institutional credentialing processes are not necessarily mutually exclusive but they warrant separate treatment in order to understand the context in which credentialing operates.

Most of what has been described in this chapter could apply to the regulation of any occupation, not just those which make up the "mental health professions." The task in the remainder of this chapter, however, is to be more specific about controversies in the helping professions precipitated by the credentialing of people and programs. Because licensure is the most powerful and restrictive of the credentialing mechanisms discussed, it is also the mechanism around which most controversy swirls.

Differences in Educational Requirements for Credentialing

One of the major issues which is a recurrent source of controversy in the "helping professions" is how much education and training a practitioner needs to be able to engage in independent practice. This major issue tends to be driven by state licensure processes which permit the practitioner to be an independent professional and see clients for fee outside of an institutional base. The arguments are less intense in relation to certification which is used in this chapter primarily as "title control" rather than "practice control."

Psychiatrists in the United States have historically been M.D.s, persons who have acquired the Doctor of Medicine before they have participated in the specialization of psychiatry. While a moot point, the authority which comes from being called "Doctor" likely carries some residual into discussions about how much education other members of the helping professions should obtain in order to receive a credential to practice.

Since 1974, the American Psychological Association (1984) has defined a "Professional Psychologist" as one who has a doctoral degree in Psychology. Before 1974, persons with master's degrees in Psychology could be so identified. However, increasingly the American Psychological Association has contended that persons with less than a doctoral degree should work under the supervision of a professional psychologist and be identified as a *professional associate* or *psychological assistant*. Such persons, depending upon their training and experience, can deliver virtually any of the psychological services which a professional psychologist can deliver. However, the APA Standards for Providers of Psychological Services contend that in a psychological service unit, the professional psychologist should be legally and ethically responsible for what assistants do, review the delivery plan designed for specific users with them, and review and countersign all reports prepared by an assistant.

Social workers typically have as their major academic credential, the M.S.W. (Master of Social Work), rather than the Doctor of Social Work. While some social workers have the latter degree, the clinical registry of both the National Association of Social Workers (NASW) and the National Federation of Societies of Clinical Social Work (NFSCSW) require a master's degree from a Council on Social Work Education (CSWE) accredited graduate social work program; two years or 3000 hours of post-master's clinical social work practice under the supervision of an M.S.W. social worker; membership in the Academy of Certified Social Workers; or a license in a state with ACSW standards (Hardcastle, 1983, p. 828).

Psychiatric nurses tend also to use the master's degree as the appropriate level of academic preparation for credentialing. Relatively few nurses, other than those in academic positions, possess a doctor of nursing or comparable degree.

Similarly, Mental Health Counselors and Marriage and Family Therapists tend to advocate the appropriateness of the Master's degree as the level of academic training necessary to receive a credential to permit one to engage in private practice. In each of these instances, many, perhaps most, mental health counselors and marriage/family therapists have doctoral degrees in guidance and counseling, psychology, or some other behavioral science. But, although that may be true, a major source of controversy among the helping professions is the necessary and sufficient level of academic training to be an independent, credentialed deliverer of mental health services. The more basic question is, does an M.S.W. or a Master's degree in Counseling requiring 60 academic semester credits plus a specified amount of supervision constitute the equivalent of a Ph.D. plus supervision in counseling or an M.D. plus specialization in Psychiatry? The American Psychological Association would say No: that persons with master's degrees in psychology, or in other behavioral sciences for that matter, cannot be considered full professionals qualified to obtain credentialing as an independent practitioner. The American Association for Counseling and Development in behalf of its Division of Mental Health Counselors would say that a master's degree, essentially one that is two years in length with appropriate practicum and other supervised experience, is adequate. The National Association of Social Workers and the American Nurses' Association would likely agree as would the American Association of Marriage and Family Counselors that the Master's level of training is appropriate for independent practice.

While the level of academic training and supervision required for licensure/certification as an independent mental health professional is a serious issue among the "helping professions," where State licensure statutes have been enacted and, particularly where licensure for counselors, marriage and family therapists, psychiatric nurses, or clinical social workers have been separated from that of psychologists, the Master's degree tends to be the minimal level acceptable. For example, in an analysis of the eight states which regulated marriage and family therapy in 1980, every one of them permitted the applicant to possess either a relevant Master's degree or a doctorate (Sporakowski & Staniszewski, 1980). While some states, e.g., Virginia, provide umbrella legislation which includes marriage and family therapists and other professional counselors in the same statutes, in those eighteen states where licensure for professional counselors exists, the academic level required is also a Master's degree plus specified supervision and experience. In a study of the perceptions of counselors and psychologists of this matter, Snow (1981) found that counselors and counselor educators favored the Master's or Master's-plus level more frequently than psychologists who were likely to favor the doctorate or the Master's-plus rather than the Master's degree as the minimal academic level necessary to obtain a counseling license for private practice. Obviously, both the perceptions and the reality of such differences in levels of training provide the seeds for controversy.

An interesting "window' on the doctoral/subdoctoral controversy has been provided by Colliver, Havens, and Wesley (1985). Their findings suggest that like most other controversial issues, the issue of whether or not doctoral level practitioners are the unequivocally preferred types of mental health professional is open to debate. In 1979 and in a followup survey in 1983, these researchers queried directors of public mental health agencies throughout the U.S. about the employment opportunities, salaries, duties, and skills of doctoral and subdoctoral clinical psychologists and MSWs. They found that while subdoctoral (MA level) clinical psychologists were rated lower than doctoral-level clinicians and MSWs on adequacy of academic training, clinical effectiveness, and contributions to the functioning of the agency, the ratings received by subdoctoral clinicians were also positive on all dimensions and over half of the agency directors surveyed indicated that they believed the discontinuation of training at that level would have a negative impact on the services provided by their agencies. Colliver, Havens, and Wesley suggested that

> it could be argued that continuation of subdoctoral-level training is a disservice to the graduate students who eventually will be asked to perform the same services with the same patient populations as Ph.D.s and MSWs, only with lower salary, status, and recognition. (p. 639)

However, they go on to contend,

> Given their consistently positive ratings on all dimensions of competence, it would seem inappropriate and even irresponsible to propose the abolition or disenfranchisement of subdoctoral-level clinical psychologists and clinical training programs... To do so would be a disservice to the public mental health system, to the patients they serve, and to the students who choose terminal clinical training programs because they are unable or unwilling to enter doctoral-level programs. (p. 639)

Content of Training

Another focus of controversy surrounding the matter of the credentialing of "helping professionals" is the content of training. As suggested previously, each of the states which offers licensure for counselors, marriage and family therapists, psychiatric nurses, or clinical social workers, specifies the level of training, experience, and supervision required. Ordinarily, the Master's degree is the academic level specified. The situation in psychiatry and in psychology is different.

Psychiatry is entered only via professional training in medicine and such entrance is strictly regulated by state law and closely mediated by the American Medical Association (AMA). In such instances, no real variability exists in the credentialing system for psychiatrists.

Psychology, like medicine, has achieved a national licensure/certification system. In 1977, Missouri became the 50th state and the 51st jurisdiction (the District of Columbia) to have a licensing statute for psychologists in force (Koocher, 1979). The difference between psychiatry and psychology, however, is that the latter does have variability or play in who is eligible to become licensed as a psychologist. In other words, the 51 jurisdictions which license psychologists do not fully agree "about who ought to be a psychologist" (Koocher, 1979, p. 696). In some states, Master's level persons are still eligible for licensure as psychologists even though the American Psychological Association (APA) has asserted that the doctoral degree should be the minimum standard for a professional psychologist (American Psychological Association, 1984).

What is of more importance to the controversy in psychology is where the individual applying for licensure obtained his/her degree? From a Department of Psychology or from a Department of Counseling and Guidance, Counselor Education, or Education? States vary with regard to whom they admit to the licensure examination based upon the answer to this question. As a result, it sometimes occurs that a person fully licensed as a psychologist in one state and successfully practicing for a number of years in that state may be denied permission to take the licensing examination in a neighboring state (Wellner, 1977, 1978). In one sense, this difference reflects the status of State Boards of Psychologist Examiners as bodies promulgated by each state legislature which are independent of other state bodies and, indeed, from the control of the American Psychological Association. In such circumstances, the American Psychological Association is advisory to but not controlling of the standards and definitions used by the individual state boards.

While undoubtedly many reasons can be given as to why state boards differ in who they consider to be eligible for licensure as a psychologist, a major issue is the content of the doctoral program as clearly comprised of psychology, or instead, "as psychological in nature." The latter phrase is much more permissive than the former phrase. As Phillips (1982) has suggested,

> Most states define the title psychologist in terms of education and training background; they usually require a doctoral degree in psychology from a recognized program *or* its equivalent. These equivalency clauses often refer to training that is 'primarily psychological in nature' and this phrase can be interpreted in many ways. A recent survey conducted by the American Association of State Psychology Boards (AASPB; Note 1) concluded that 'primarily psychological in nature' has been interpreted loosely and broadly. (p. 919)

Under equivalency clauses, persons graduating from programs not clearly identified as psychology and not having the traditional Ph.D. are seen by some states as offering equivalent training. This leads some observers (e.g., Bennett, 1980) to argue that persons with Ed.D. degrees rather than Ph.D. degrees have degrees in education, not psychology. In her view such persons ordinarily do not have undergraduate backgrounds in psychology and possess academic potential lower than psychology graduates. While she acknowledges that some individual exceptions do exist to such perspectives, she maintains that licensing boards must operate on generalities and that such generalities are sufficient to cause concern about whether the background and training of an Ed.D. truly is equivalent to background and training in a Ph.D. or Psy.D. program in psychology. She maintains that the Ed.D. is a degree in education, not in psychology.

Stigall (1977) has examined the situations in which state licensure boards are challenged when they deny admission to candidacy to persons on the basis of interpretation that their academic credentials did not meet statutory criteria of a doctoral degree primarily psychological in nature. Ordinarily, such challenges by persons denied candidacy for licensure lead to litigation in the courts. In the several court cases from which findings are now extant, the outcomes are mixed but they suggest that licensing boards cannot be capricious and arbitrary in their judgments. These court cases have stimulated the American Psychological Association and its Committee on State Legislation to revise its Guidelines for State Legislation and to bring to more specific focus its recommendations on education and credentialing in psychology. As a result, since 1977 a clearer definition of what constitutes training in psychology has been advanced by the American Psychological Association (Wellner, 1977) and incorporated in its essence in the 1979 and 1980 Criteria for Accreditation of Doctoral Training Programs and Internships in Professional Psychology (American Psychological Association, 1974, amended 1980). These criteria follow.

A. CRITERIA FOR MEETING THE DEFINITION OF A "PSYCHOLOGY PROGRAM"

Principle: The Foundation of Professional Practice in Psychology is the Evolving Body of Knowledge in the Discipline of Psychology

The following criteria will be used to identify and designate educational programs as psychology programs.

1. Programs that are accredited by the American Psychology Association are recognized as meeting the definition of a professional psychology program. The criteria for Accreditation serve as a model for professional psychology training.

2. Training in professional psychology is doctoral training offered in a regionally accredited institution of higher education.

3. The program, wherever it may be administratively housed, must be clearly identified and labeled as a psychology program. Such a program must specify in pertinent institutional catalogs and brochures its interest to educate and train professional psychologists.

4. The psychology program must stand as a recognizable, coherent organizational entity within the institution.

5. There must be a clear authority and primary responsibility for the core and specialty areas whether or not the program cuts across administrative lines.

6. The program must be an integrated, organized sequence of study.

7. There must be an identifiable psychology faculty and a psychologist responsible for the program.

8. The program must have an identifiable body of students who are matriculated in that program for a degree.

9. The program must include supervised practicum, internship, field or laboratory training appropriate to the practice of psychology.

10. The curriculum shall encompass a minimum of three academic years of full time graduate study. In addition to instruction in scientific and professional ETHICS AND STANDARDS, RESEARCH DESIGN and METHODOLOGY STATISTICS and PSYCHOMETRICS, the core program shall require each student to demonstrate competencies in each of the following substantive content areas. This typically will be met by including a minimum of three or more graduate semester hours (5 or more graduate quarter hours) in each of these four substantive content areas:

   a. Biological Bases of Behavior: physiological psychology, comparative psychology, neuropsychology, sensation and perception, psychopharmacology.

   b. Cognitive-Affective Bases of Behavior: learning, thinking, motivation, emotion.

   c. Social Bases of Behavior: social psychology, group processes, organizational and systems theory.

   d. Individual Differences: personality therapy, human development, abnormal psychology.

NOTE: Item 10 identifies the core psychology curriculum. In addition to these criteria, all professional education programs in psychology will include course requirements in specialty areas. The above curriculum requirements then, represent the necessary core but not the sufficient number of graduate hours for a degree in professional psychology.

Such information gives a state licensure board help in defining what doctoral programs qualify as being bona fide psychology programs or "are primarily psychological in nature." As suggested in the guidelines, American Psychological Association accredited doctoral programs, wherever they are housed, are considered to be psychology programs.

While an extended discussion is available in Theme Two describing the education and training similarities and differences among the helping professions and the controversies they engender, suffice it to say here that the content of such programs cannot be separated in importance from issues of credentialing.

With respect to credentialing per se, what has not been said here with particular regard to psychology or, by implication, for the other helping professions, is that the content of training or experience is not the whole of qualifying for licensure. It only defines who will be eligible to sit for a licensure examination. In other words, in many states, the *credentialing issue is not who passes the licensure examination but who will be permitted to take the licensure examination.* Thus, the concerns expressed by Bennett vis á vis the Ph.D. or Ed.D. degrees or programs in psychology versus those in education has nothing explicitly to do with whether these persons can pass the licensure examination but rather who, by definition of where they received their training, should be given permission to "sit for the examination." Thus, permission to be a candidate for licensure—in other words, to be allowed to take the examination—becomes a major gatekeeping process restricting access to the professional livelihood available if one is permitted to and is successful in passing the licensure examination. Such a matter becomes a major source of controversy.

Education, Competence, Both?

The uses of both education and training and the licensure examination as credentialing mechanisms have been major sources of controversy across the helping professions.

The first issue of controversy is whether the use of academic credentials is an appropriate reflection of individual competence to deliver psychological services. The second issue is whether a paper and pencil examination, usually multiple choice, covering some knowledge domain is an adequate test of one's ability to deliver psychological services. While these two matters are interactive, since, as we have just shown, the first largely determines who is permitted to take the second, they separately raise several controversial issues.

A number of observers (e.g., Ivey, 1982) have unequivocally stated that "education does not equal competence" (p. 132). Therefore, the major issue in the helping professions may not be what is the most appropriate training for psychologists, counselors, or other related specialists. The issue is what is competent and ethical performance, how can it be measured, and how can it be effectively communicated to the public? Ivey contended that "credentialism is only relevant insofar as it pertains to effective service delivery" (p. 132)... Thus, basing credentialing mechanisms solely on education, training, and test-taking ability, tends to mystify or obscure the actual practice of counseling and therapy" and places the emphasis of credentialing on what knowledge one has rather than what one can do.

Ivey cited some of the available research data which suggest that doctoral level psychologists or counselors are not the only persons who can make a positive difference in the lives of clients. Among such research data are reviews by Alley and Blanton (1976), Anthony and Carkhuff (1977), and Rappaport (1977), among others, who conclude that nonprofessionals are effective in delivering counseling and other mental health services. Berman and Norton (1985) have recently affirmed such a finding in comparing professional and para-professional therapists. The problem, of course, is that under most of the existing credentialing procedures, such persons would not be able to gain access to licensure or certification because they did not gain their education and training from an acceptably accredited institution or in the training pattern expected.

Narrow pathways to licensure through rigid education and training models and test-taking have been particularly challenged by minority populations who claim to be unfairly denied the opportunity to work in the helping professions by such means. Such claims seem justified on many grounds but, perhaps, the foremost one is that the poor and minorities are significantly underserved by existing mental health systems. Such systems tend to be dominated by white, middle-class individuals working out of white-middle-class theories and structures. As a result, up to 50% of non-white clients drop out of psychotherapy and, undoubtedly many others seek help from non-credentialed caregivers in their local neighborhoods (Sue & McKinney, 1975; Sue, 1977; Berzins, 1977). Likely, then, only alternative systems of credentialing or different views of what constitutes competence will address such concerns.

Competence

An implied corollary of licensure is the screening out of incompetent practitioners or, indeed, the provision of testimony to the individual competence of the practitioner who successfully receives a credential. However, a group of observers in the helping professions question that assumption. Gross (1978), for example, argued that "there is no evidence of any relationship between licensing and the quality of care" (p. 1013). Obviously, the quality of care could be considered a proxy for competence. He further stated, "The link between licensing and competence is the basis for societal support for licensing arrangements. I have questioned that link" (p. 1014). Gross's contentions are based primarily on the medical profession since in his view, medical licensure is the model that other professions aspire to.

Koocher (1979) put the matter somewhat differently when he said,

> the construct of competence as applied to psychological practitioners is obviously relative but if a credential is to certify that a given individual is qualified to practice, it should be founded on a clear notion of what is meant thereby. Does licensure, certification or any credential in question indicate a superior level of competence, a minimum level, or simply that a practitioner is not likely to harm anyone seriously? ...Within any of these levels a given credential may indicate competence to help all potential clients, only a small fraction of them, or it may simply assure that only a very small number will come to harm as a result of the practitioner's efforts on their behalf... The point to be made is simply that the construct of competence varies as a function of the type of professional service or particular credential. Furthermore, it is evident that those practitioners competent within certain spheres may have no talents or abilities within certain other areas, and also, they may fail to take cognizance of this limitation. (p. 697)

Koocher's views are instructive in several different ways. One, he suggests that the relationship between affirmations of competence and various types of credential differ. Two, because one is credentialed in a particular generic area (e.g., as a psychologist), that does not mean the practitioner is competent to deal with all populations and all types of problems. This is particularly a problem when, as in the case of a psychologist, a professional is licensed in most states on the basis of a generic examination of knowledge, not on the basis of the specializations (e.g., clinical psychology, school psychology, counseling psychology, industrial/organizational psychology) to which training was directed.

Koocher concluded his analysis by suggesting that

> whatever existing credentials in psychology do measure, they are clearly not highly valid measures of professional competence... By the same token, we must recognize that there are many skilled and competent mental health professionals who will not have the usual credentials, and we must seek to reduce unnecessarily rigid barriers to preclude members of the public from access to their services. Current credentials in psychology may provide some helpful information to the consuming public, but two Latin words may be inappropriately absent from most of these diplomas: *Caveat emptor.* (p. 702)

Assessment of Competence. Implicit in the foregoing discussion of the relationship or the lack of relationship between licensing or other forms of credentialing and the competence of those who are credentialed, are problems with the assessment of competence itself.

As we have seen thus far, the essential pattern leading to licensure or certification is completion of a prescribed education and training program including matriculation in some set of core courses in a particular discipline and, perhaps, supervised practicum or internship. Completion of these requisites permit one to have access to the examination which is the culmination of the credentialing process.

While some question the assumption that a prescribed set of educational experiences is equivalent to competency, others find difficulty in equating the results of an examination, particularly a multiple-choice examination covering generic knowledge, with competence. The problem at base seems to reside with an acceptable answer to what is meant by competence. Until competence is defined with reasonable precision, the ability to measure it with accuracy is suspect (Shimberg, 1982). In this regard, Shimberg quoted the work of Senior (1976) who has differentiated among the terms *knowledge, competence,* and *performance.* Citing medicine as the example, Senior suggested that competence is distinct from medical knowledge as measured, for instance, by multiple-choice exams as well as from performance in practice as assessed by the medical audit. Performance, according to Senior, "is always viewed in retrospect, after the fact, while competence pertains to the future—before the fact. It is the capability of carrying out an act when the time comes" (Shimberg, 1982, p. 20).

If credentialing mechanisms are to be related to competence, they need to be predictive of how a practitioner will perform within the scope of practice for which he/she will be granted the autonomy to engage. One way to do so is to rely on direct observation of performance. Such procedures are used in such fields as dentistry where a person seeking licensure is still required to carry out some set of tasks on actual patients considered to be representative of the scope of practice for which the person is being credentialed. In such cases, how the work is done and the finished work are evaluated against some set of predetermined criteria.

Because of the difficulty of reliable ratings of performance, the cost of such processes, and the problems of standardization and representativeness of the performance samples used, most licensing and certification boards in the helping professions do not now use performance assessments. Rather, they are likely to use written and oral questions designed to probe one's knowledge and problem-solving skills using simulated cases or vignettes. According to Shimberg (1982), the underlying assumption of such approaches is that while possession of knowledge and skills does not guarantee that they will be used, the lack of them virtually assures that they will not be used when the occupation arises (p. 22).

Viewed in such a context, current credentialing examinations may be the most parsimonious, valid, and reliable methods available given the various constraints under which they operate. But saying this assumes that they are related quite directly to job performance or the components of competence which the practitioner will have to demonstrate when in private practice. In the helping professions, this is a big *if* and the crux of considerable controversy.

Scope of Practice

Licensure, as stated previously, is assumed not only to reflect competence but to do so within the scope of practice by which the occupation is defined. Both of these areas are controversial among the helping professions.

Let us use psychology as the example. Most state licensure boards credential, license, or certify psychologists, not clinical, counseling, school, or industrial/organizational psychologists. The perspective is that any psychologist is a psychologist first and these skills are applied and used in some specialization second (Wellner, 1977). Such a rationale encourages the use of a generic examination for licensure of psychologists, not a separate examination for psychologists intending to practice with different populations and in different settings. Even so, the resulting credential places no restriction on what the successful applicant can do. Such a circumstance virtually assures that the examination will be academically oriented and focused on content dealing with limited domains of psychological knowledge rather than that reflected in the scope of practice which psychology attributes to itself. Such a generic examination puts those candidates for licensure who have been out of graduate school for some years more at risk of failure than those recently graduating. It, in general, puts poor test takers at risk of failure and makes the claims of validity for the test questionable since most of the candidates for licensure are not planning academic careers but rather plan to provide direct service in applied settings.

The lack of relationship between the psychologist licensure examination and the full dimensions of the scope of practice attributed to psychology is one issue. The other issue has to do with the comprehensiveness of the scope of practice and its virtual assurance that it will overlap with the domains in which other helping professions claim competence. For example, in 1967, the APA Commission on Legislation defined the practice of psychology as:

> rendering to individuals, groups, organizations, or the public any psychological service involving the application of principles, methods, and procedures of understanding, predicting, and influencing behavior such as the principles pertaining to learning, perception, motivation, thinking, emotions and interpersonal relationships; the methods and procedures of interviewing, counseling, and psychotherapy, of constructing, administering, and interpreting tests of mental abilities, aptitudes, interests, attitudes, personality characteristics, emotion, and motivation; and of assessing public opinion.
>
> The application of said principles and methods includes, but is not restricted to: diagnosis, prevention, and amelioration of adjustment problems and emotional and mental disorders of individuals and groups; hypnosis; educational and vocational counseling, personnel selection and management; the evaluation and planning for effective work and learning situations; advertising and market research and the resolution of interpersonal and social conflict.
>
> Psychotherapy within the meaning of this act means the use of learning, conditioning methods, and emotional reactions, in a professional relationship, to assist a person or persons to modify feelings, attitudes and behaviors which are intellectually, socially, or emotionally maladjustive or ineffectual. (American Psychological Association, 1967, pp. 1098-1099)

Although the 1967 definition has been an important influence during the rise of credentialing for psychologists and other mental health providers, it needs to be noted that the 1967 definition of practice was approved in a revised form in June 1985, by the Board of Professional Affairs of the American Psychological Association. The revised definition is as follows:

> Practice of Psychology is defined as the observation, description, evaluation, interpretation, and modification of human behavior by the application of psychological principles, methods and procedures, for the purpose of eliminating symptomatic, maladaptive, or undesired behavior, and of improving interpersonal relationships, work, and life adjustment, personal effectiveness and mental health. The practice of psychology includes but is not limited to, psychological testing and evaluation of intelligence, personality, abilities, interests and aptitudes; counseling, psychoanalysis, psychotherapy, hypnosis, biofeedback training and behavior therapy; diagnosis and treatment of mental and emotional disorder or disability, alcoholism and substance abuse, and the psychological aspects of physical illness, injury, or disability; psychoeducational evaluation, therapy, remediation and consultation. Psychological services may be rendered to individuals, families, groups, and the public. The practice of

psychology does not include the teaching of psychology, the conduct of psychological research, or the provision of psychological consultation to organizations, provided such teaching, research or consultation does not involve the delivery or supervision of direct services to individuals or groups of individuals. (American Psychological Association, 1985)

To the degree that the language of 1967 or 1985 is incorporated into state statutes defining the practice of psychology for purposes of licensure, virtually all activities of counselors, social workers, psychiatric nurses and other helping professionals are fundamentally illegal unless these professionals are supervised by licensed psychologists. This is true even though state licensing statutes defining a generic psychologist licenses persons without restriction of the practice of psychology and without regard to their training and experience in the various areas defined by the scope of practice. This is true even though other professional groups may have more specific training and supervision in some areas (e.g., group counseling, primary prevention, educational and vocational counseling) than do many psychologists.

As discussed in Chapter 1, the claim, for example, to competence in psychotherapy or to the prevention and amelioration of adjustment problems and emotional and mental disorders of individuals and groups has been made by psychiatric nurses, clinical social workers, and by mental health counselors. One of the ways that the ownership of psychotherapy was wrested from psychiatrists by psychologists was through arguing that it was not medically based and was a generic therapeutic process which laymen can provide. That argument continues to be used by other groups of helping professionals seeking professionalization and independent practice opportunities for their constituencies. Here again lay the seeds of major controversy.

Inevitable, given the breadth of the definition of psychology promulgated in 1967 by the American Psychological Association and recommended to state licensure boards in psychology, licensure statutes covering other mental health providers are likely to be in conflict. Some examples will illustrate the point.

As quoted in Sporakowski and Staniszewski (1980), the definition of marriage counseling in the 1971 New Jersey statute regulating marriage and family therapy in that state offers the following:

> The rendering of professional marriage and counseling services to individuals and marital pairs, singly or in groups, whether in the general public or in

organizations, either public or private, for a fee, monetary or otherwise. "Marriage counseling" is a specialized field of counseling which centers largely upon the relationship between husband and wife. It also includes premarital counseling, pre- and post-divorce counseling, and family counseling which emphasizes the spousal relationship as a key to successful family living. The practice of marriage counseling consists of the application of principles, methods, and techniques of counseling and psychotherapy for the purpose of resolving psychological conflict, modifying perception and behavior, altering old attitudes and establishing new ones in the area of marriage and family life. In its concern with the antecendents of marriage, with the vicissitudes of marriage, and with the consequences of the failure of marriage, marriage counseling keeps in sight its enabling marital partners and their children to achieve the optimal adjustment consistent with their welfare as individuals, as members of a family, and as citizens in society.

The State of Georgia defines the practice of marriage and family counseling in its 1976 licensure statute in the following manner:

"Marriage and family counseling" is a specialized field of counseling which centers largely upon the family relationship and the relationship between husband and wife. It also includes premarital counseling, predivorce and postdivorce counseling and family counseling. "Marriage and family counseling" consists of the application of principles, methods, and techniques of counseling and psychotherapeutic techniques for the purposes of resolving psychological conflict, modifying perception and behavior, altering old attitudes and establishing new ones in the area of marriage and family life. (Sporakowski & Staniszewski, 1980)

Depending upon the exact language of the psychologist's statutes in New Jersey and Georgia, the likelihood is that language overlap occurs with it in the Marriage and Family Counseling/Therapy statutes in those states. Similar examples could be identified for statutes dealing with social workers or professional and mental health counselors as well as other groups in the helping professions.

Information is not available about which groups may have attempted to keep the other from seeking a licensure statute in particular states; nor is extensive information available about court cases dealing with conflicts among such statutes. What is clear is that in some states, individual practitioners have been arrested and brought to trial for allegedly violating licensure statutes, either because they were not licensed at all or because the license they held did not encompass the specific technique or practice they were using. For example, a duly licensed professional counselor in Florida was arrested on the complaints of a third party insurance carrier because he was providing clients with biofeedback, a technique not covered by licensure for counselors. At this writing the case is still in litigation. In Ohio, an individual was conducting a part-time practice involving mental assessments of children but was not licensed as a psychologist. At the time of the incident, Ohio did not have a state licensure statute for professional counselors although it does have such legislation now. Having training in guidance and counseling, not in psychology, this individual had written to the Ohio Board of Psychologist Examiners to inquire if his work would result in problems with that Board. After receiving no response, he subsequently wrote to the Board again to inquire about their position on this matter. A short time later he was arrested for practicing psychology without a license although he had not previously heard anything from the Board. In this instance, the judge heard in favor of the defendant (State of Ohio vs. Cook) (Smith, 1978).

The potential for litigation among different licensure boards in a particular state or between a particular board and a practitioner whose credential is from another board but who has allegedly violated some standard of the first board is wide and deep. As such things occur they cause adversarial relations to be generated among different occupations in the helping professions and the climate for controversy to be an enduring one.

CREDENTIALING FOR CONSUMER PROTECTION

The primary rationale for most forms of occupational regulation and licensing is consumer protection. However, as we have seen earlier in this chapter, usually consumers are not the ones who clamor for the licensing of occupational groups but rather persons in the groups themselves. For the most part, research is very minimal to assess the significance between licensure and the quality of care provided consumers. Indeed, as we have seen, some observers see occupational regulation as a form of self-protection or monopolistic practice which restricts service delivery to specific groups of practitioners. To the degree that such views are valid, questions can be raised about the restraint of trade which occurs for some groups of practitioners not eligible for licensure or certification, the increased or decreased costs to the consumer which arise from occupational licensing, and the restrictions on freedom of choice of consumers in deciding from whom they want to receive services.

Licensing in the helping professions is directly tied to third-party reimbursement (discussed in Chapter 9) and to the independent provision of psychological counseling and related services (Danish & Smyer, 1981). Drawing from the work of Swagler and Harris (1977), Danish and Smyer observed that:

> In the past, most psychological services were delivered by providers in public agencies. When services are delivered in the public sector, the consumer receives the service through the agency, not from the individual psychologist. Agencies are administered by professionals who are in a position to evaluate the providers' backgrounds and assess their competence to perform in this situation. The agency is considered an 'expert buyer.' The agency then becomes accountable for the quality of service, and the consumer is protected.... In private practice such protection cannot be assumed. The provider loses the 'certification' the agency provides. (p. 18)

As a result of the shift from public psychological service delivery to private or independent practice, the potential consumer loses, in many instances, the evaluative system within which public agencies receiving either governmental funds or insurance payments must operate. In most instances, independent practitioners do not have the type and intensity of scrutiny that agencies do. Once licensed, the practitioner has almost unrestrained access to providing services for fees or insurance reimbursement to anyone and for any problem which falls within the scope of practice under which he/she was licensed. Given such circumstances, the naive consumer may actually have little freedom of choice to gain information about or understand the differences between existing independent mental health professionals.

Danish and Smyer (1981) raised a further important point with regard to consumers acquiring services from licensed "helping professionals" who obtain reimbursement from insurance. In many states and in many insurance or health maintenance plans, reimbursement can be claimed only if a psychiatric diagnosis or a diagnosis which fits the *DSM-III* classification structure is assigned to the client. Such diagnosis is then required to be supported by a treatment plan. In some cases, a provider and client may decide together what diagnosis to place upon the insurance forms to obtain reimbursement. In other circumstances, the provider decides upon the treatment to be used. Whichever case prevails, the question occurs as to consumer self-definition and its attendant implications for self-esteem, feelings of personal power to change one's circumstances or, indeed, the amount and type of support one is likely to receive from one's family and friends. Various studies (Farina, Fisher, Getter, & Fischer, 1978; McKnight, 1977; Abramson, Seligman, &

Teasdale, 1978) have demonstrated that negative self-definition and the attributions to oneself of mental illness lead to disempowerment, learned helplessness, social breakdown, and other results. Such issues caused Danish and Smyer (1981) to conclude: "The benefits to the provider of receiving third-party payments may be at the expense of the recipient's self-esteem and welfare" (p. 19).

Another major issue pertinent to consumers is how licensing and occupational regulation affect the costs of acquiring mental health or psychological services. Danish and Smyer (1981) also have made some important observations here. They contend that regulating the delivery of psychological services has three distinct costs: "The increased economic cost of the services, the disadvantages of uneven public accessibility, and the potential for 'benign neglect' of innovative services under reimbursement plans" (p. 16). Such costs are also applicable to other helping professions which are licensable.

Among the reasons for increased costs to consumers of regulating the delivery of psychological services, Danish and Smyer suggested such matters as the following: licensing restrictions diminish the number of eligible providers and increase prices such providers charge for their services; the demand that both public and private providers of psychological services be licensed and trained at the doctoral level raises the costs to the providers in obtaining training and in deferring income while engaging in extended preparation and these costs are ultimately passed on to the consumers; where nondoctoral level psychologists or other helping professionals deliver services, but under the supervision of doctoral level psychologists, the added cost of supervision increases fees.

More subtle but perhaps more important costs to consumers from the regulation of deliveries of psychological or other "helping" services is the availability of such services. Psychiatrists, professional psychologists, and other licensed service providers are not evenly distributed geographically. Rather such professionals are concentrated in affluent urban locations (Gottfredson & Dyer, 1978), not in rural areas or inner cities. Independent practice in the helping professions is market driven, just as are other entrepreneurial businesses. Independent service providers tend to cluster where a critical mass of clients are who can pay the fees involved. As a result, rural areas and inner cities tend to be underserved and some potential consumers are unable to gain access to, do not know about, or choose not to try to gain access to licensed providers because of high fee structures or problems of getting to where the services are available.

Danish and Smyer (1981) suggested that these conditions do not argue for training more doctoral-level licensed psychologists but rather for such alternative solutions as:

> (a) allowing nondoctoral level psychologists and providers from other professions who demonstrate competence to deliver services; (b) changing the manner in which services are delivered from individual therapy to more cost-effective procedures; (c) emphasizing preventive interventions; (d) encouraging self-help and natural helping intervention; and (e) developing better linkages with health care settings to increase accessibility to mental health services. (p. 18)

Ivey (1982) would likely agree with Danish and Smyer (1981) about the cost and accessibility issues for consumers which are present under the current system of regulation of mental health service providers. For example, he indicated that,

> Given the need for innovative new modes of mental health delivery, it is especially critical that special populations of varying race, age, and sex be given specific and special consideration in each community (p. 136)... There is real danger in any reassessment of delivery services that those most in need will again turn out to be those that receive the smallest amount of service. (p.137)

Ivey went on to say that,

> It is critical to note that mental health professionals are not necessarily the most qualified persons to work with special populations. Data are clear that clients stay in counseling and feel more satisfied with results when they are counseled by people whose background closely resembles their own. We can no longer assume that degree-oriented professionals are the "people of choice" for all mental health concerns. (p. 137).

Arguing against the current models of credentialing based upon specific approved programs of training, Ivey, like other observers noted in the Chapter, saw the need to provide new ways for individual practitioners, those representing culturally different populations and others, to demonstrate their competency to be licensed and to provide services to those who are underserved by the existing system. He made several recommendations for federal and state policy changes in occupational regulation which relate to such matters. They include the following:

> Given the diversity of the U.S. population, it is necessary to provide an array of distinct and diversified mental health delivery alternatives that are of demonstrated quality. Those who provide these alternatives must be screened for competence. These alternatives may or may not have traditionally certified practitioners on their staffs. Further, alternative service providers need not necessarily follow traditional routes of academic training and licensure.

...It is recommended that *alternative human* service agencies such as street clinics, volunteer alcohol prevention agencies, programs for battered women, and other innovative groups who do *not* have traditionally certified psychiatrists, social workers, and psychologists on their staffs be accredited for third-party payments (e.g., by insurance agencies, by state departments of social welfare, etc.) and for full access to all federal and state funds.

Research data are clear that these nontraditional agencies, operating at desired levels, can often serve the diversified U.S. population more effectively (and at less cost) than mental health professionals certified by traditional routes. A free marketplace thrives on competition. At present, psychiatrists, social workers, and psychologists have a monopoly on services, thus promoting an artificially scarce supply.

...It is recommended that individual certification for third-party payments be extended to new professional groups such as rehabilitation counselors, guidance workers, marriage and family counselors. Therapy and counseling are generic skills much as less expensive generic drugs are suitable alternatives to expensive "name drugs" from pharmaceutical concerns. Research again has demonstrated that a wide array of individuals can perform at the same level or at higher levels than many present psychologists, psychiatrists, and social workers. (pp. 133-134)

Many of the controversies which are associated with licensure and, indeed, with state licensure boards tend to *mix* professional and legal considerations. In a lengthy and insightful treatment of the legal context in which the regulation of professional psychology is embedded, Herbsleb, Sales, and Overcast (1985) have examined many of the legal issues and court cases which relate to licensure and certification. They suggest that the courts are firmly committed to the view that the goals of protecting the public welfare fully justifies the regulation of professions and occupations which may effect such welfare. Therefore, "the general question of whether licensure is the most appropriate regulatory vehicle is political—that is, a question of policy making that is remitted to the judgment of elected representatives" (p. 1166). Obviously, any political process can be a source of controversy and that which focuses on licensure is no exception.

Herbsleb, Sales, and Overcast went on to contend that the major legal principle which involves professional credentialing is that of due process. In this context, the due process clause imposes three essential requirements on which court challenges may be initiated: specificity, rationality, and fairness. Thus, professional standards for credentialing must be clear and intelligible, reasonably related to the practice which is being regulated, and fair as to how the processes of applying standards occurs. The due process clauses are the basis on which most of the legal challenges within States have been mounted whether they pertain to educational requirements, experience, examination content, and/or procedure. In addition to due process, a number of challenges to the credentialing of professionals has come in regard to federal antitrust legislation. Regardless of which challenge has been mounted, court findings have been mixed depending upon the substance of the issue. Nevertheless, credentialing in its multiple forms has survived across the nation. While this outcome may itself be controversial, it causes challenges of substance to be both professional and, ultimately, legal and to rest on empirical data rather than opinion.

SUMMARY

In Chapter 6 we have examined the role which credentialing mechanisms play in stimulating controversy among the helping professions. While several forms of individual or program credentialing are available in the helping professions, licensure, which controls both the use of title and the practice of service delivery, is the most powerful and the most controversial of these mechanisms.

Among the major foci of controversy are the direct linkage between education and training patterns, access to licensure examinations, and eligibility for third-party payments available to those who are licensed for independent practice. Such patterns are seen by many observers as exclusionary in their procedures of admitting persons to candidacy for licensure and livelihoods in their chosen fields. Thus, they unfairly deprive otherwise competent people from pursuing such livelihoods.

Also at issue in credentialing is the matter of competence assessment. Some observers contend that educational credentials and multiple-choice examinations, the standard requisites for licensure, do not equate with competence; that alternative ways to measure competence should be available to permit persons with nontraditional patterns of training or experience to demonstrate their skills in those states where different groups of helping professionals are licensed.

A further source of controversy attending licensure is the increased cost to consumers which now exists because of the practitioner levels of training or supervision required. Perhaps the important issue of controversy, however, is whether credentialing protects the practitioner or the consumer. The discussion in Chapter 6 concluded by examining several of the issues which are not now addressed in credentialing processes: the fact that licensed mental health practitioners are not adequately distributed geographically or by socioeconomic or cultural need—therefore, many of the culturally different, poor, and those in rural areas are underserved by the existing mental health delivery system; the need to provide credentialing capability and access to reimbursement for those non-traditional practitioners and agencies who do serve populations with special needs; the importance of recognizing that most of the mental health service delivery in the nation is provided by master's level practitioners from groups of practitioners not ordinarily defined as core providers or as eligible for licensure and third-party payment in most states.

Credentialing is frequently both the symbol and the crucible through which special interests, power, economic motives, territoriality, are played out. As a stimulus to controversy in the helping professions, credentialing is not a benign process.

THEME FOUR:
ETHICAL AND LEGAL STANDARDS

CHAPTER 7

LEGAL AND ETHICAL ISSUES IN THE HELPING PROFESSIONS

As we discussed in Chapter 6, among controversies in the mental health professions are those which are legal challenges and those which are primarily professional issues. While the two interrelate they are not the same.

A similar case can be made in the implementation of mental health services by individual providers. Both legal and ethical issues or controversies can be identified. While legal and ethical issues interact, they are ultimately different and need to be so considered if the controversies they engender are to be understood.

In Chapter 7, a number of the most timely of legal and ethical controversies are examined. While not exhaustive of all possible issues in this arena, they do include those which have considerable public interest and those which are somewhat more abstract, philosophical, or contextual in their content. In any case, such topics can have legal or ethical controversy or both associated with them.

Among the major areas of controversy to be examined are those of the right to treatment or habilitation; informed consent; research use of clients; sexual misconduct; duty to warn or inform; confidentiality; value conflicts; and, training in legal and ethical aspects of helping. These analyses will, however briefly, serve to condition the reader's thinking to how controversy can be conceived in the areas of legal and ethical practice.

TERMINOLOGY

In most discussions of the standards which should or must govern the conduct of helping professionals, a distinction is made between ethical and legal issues. *Ethical issues* usually refer to moral imperatives—the shoulds and oughts directed toward protecting the welfare of those who require the services of helping professionals. They are largely attempts at self-regulation by the professions. *Legal issues,* on the other hand, refer to the efforts of governmental administrative agencies, legislatures, and the courts to create rules of law which govern the practice of psychology, psychiatry, social work, and counseling.

While some aspects of the law reflect professional ethical standards, the law—except peripherally—is not determined by these standards. Ethical statements promulgated by the various helping professions are clear and straight forward (American Psychological Association, 1979; NASW, 1980; American Psychological Association, 1981; APGA, 1981). Each, in one way or another, addresses the practitioner's ethical responsibility to the client, to the profession, and to society (including an employer if one exists).

The ultimate consequence of legally unclear practice, incompetent practice, or blatant disregard of clear legal mandates, is a malpractice suit. Knapp (1980) defined malpractice as "an act of omission...that is inconsistent with reasonable care and skill used by other reputable (mental health care providers) of the same system and results in injury to the client" (p. 606). The lack of reasonable standards of care must lead to the injury. Examples of typical court cases include, but are not limited to, such problems as the following: failure to predict and take action on suicide risks, potentially violent clients who would do harm to a third party, improper treatment, breach of confidentiality, improper or unnecessary commitment, abandonment, failure to warn of possible adverse effects of treatment, sexual misconduct, undue restraints, inadequate care, misdiagnosis, and a variety of issues related to professional "policing," such as denial of access to a licensing or certification examination, ethical censure, improper job evaluation, and so forth.

In medicine, most of these client-psychiatrist harmful situations would be termed *iatrogenic* (from the Greek *iatros,* meaning physician). An iatrogenic state in medicine (hence, psychiatry) is an undesirable condition in a patient, induced or aggravated by the physician in the course of treatment. A patient comes in for elective surgery; the anesthesiologist botches the anesthesia; the patient is deprived of oxygen for too long a period; and the patient becomes a "vegetable." The cause is iatrogenic. No similar term relates to non-medical therapeutic interventions. Obviously, no ancient Greek word exists for counselor or therapist as we now understand the term, since none existed in those times. We might suggest that we take the Greek stem, *bouleuo,* to give counsel, or *boule,* meaning counsel, and create the word *boulegenic,* meaning an undesirable condition in a client, induced or aggravated by the therapist or mental health professional in the course of treatment. Thus, most law suits filed by clients against therapists are done so on a boulegenic basis.

In fact, however, we should remember that relatively few law suits are filed by clients against therapists. The reasons for this are not entirely clear. One reason may be that clients must prove "emotional damage," and this construct is difficult to determine. Another reason may be that the therapist-client relationship is such that the client does not easily consciously engage in assertively aggressive acts against the therapist. A third reason may be the fear of exposing oneself to the perceived stigma of society's recognizing that one is in treatment. Whatever the reasons, the number of actual cases are few, and the majority of those settled are for less than $5,000. Relatively few settlements of claims are for over $10,000.

We concentrate in this chapter on some of the more visible legal and ethical issues affecting practice in the helping professions. The fundamental issue addressed both legally and ethically is basically that of the rights of individuals versus the rights of society. The law is constantly changing, and many legal issues remain unresolved. With that *caveat* in mind, we turn to a brief delineation of the following areas about which legal and/or ethical controversies exist: the right of clients to treatment or habilitation; informed consent; research use of clients; sexual misconduct; duty to warn or inform; confidentiality; standard treatment modalities; professional disclosure; value conflicts; and training in legal and ethical issues. A number of issues are not addressed because of space limitations but are, nevertheless, important. Examples include issues such as fee splitting, failure to terminate clients who are not improving, outright fraud, advertising, and advice dispensed via the mass media.

RIGHT TO TREATMENT OR HABILITATION

Helping professionals who work within institutional structures are faced with the question of clients' rights to treatment or habilitation. Issues involved in this concept are most commonly those of placement in the least restrictive environment, rights within institutions, and involuntary treatment.

Placement in the least restrictive environment is a concept that has emerged recently. The Supreme Court has held that a person in a state institution has a right to reasonable care and safety, to reasonably nonrestrictive confinement conditions, and to such training as may be required by these interests. This mandate to ensure humane care and treatment without undue restraint has led to increased efforts at "deinstitutionalization" in the form of community-based care. Ironically, a major issue now appears to be that community placements are often so inadequate that currently a number of legal cases are filed in which individuals seek to return to institutional care. Some regard the release of mental patient to be a massive failure. Professionals may have overpromised what they could deliver to the politicians, thus leading to controversy. A delicate balance must exist between economics and science, as we shall see shortly.

Consent decrees, essentially contracts between the state and patients in state facilities in which terms of "adequate" or "active" treatment are addressed, are often the mode of enforcement of legal mandates. However, a legislative body often is unable (or unwilling) to provide the financial wherewithal necessary to implement the consent decree. Further, no accepted federal standards for consent decrees exist, thus leading to differences among states as to what constitutes acceptable staff/client ratios, per patient expenditures, necessary equipment, and the like.

Gutheil (1980) has pointed out the "conceptual misalignment" between the law and the helping professions. He argued that lawyers are concerned mainly with rights or limitations on the civil liberties of individuals. Helping professionals, on the other hand, while conscious of these rights, are concerned primarily with the effectiveness of a therapeutic intervention. Often the two foci are in conflict, as in the case of the use of medication in treatment. One faction regards it as mind-altering and, therefore, inappropriate; the other faction regards it as "mind-normalizing" (Mills & Gutheil, 1982) and, therefore, appropriate. The basic issue is whether treatments should be determined legally or clinically.

The obverse of the right to treatment or habilitation is the issue of involuntary treatment or institutionalization. Again, the conflict is between civil liberties and professionals' perceived needs for specific therapeutic interventions. Chodoff (1984) described this disagreement in philosophical terms as one of a utilitarian approach versus a deontological approach. In the utilitarian view, morality is defined by the extent to which any act serves the good of the individual or the society. In the deontological view, good consequences must be moderated by principles such as liberty, fairness, and justice. According to Cahn (1982), the major issue is basically a *quid pro quo* of exchanging effective treatment for loss of freedom. This view, of course, presumes that our treatments are indeed effective.

School psychologists are daily faced with another issue that is allied to the least restrictive environment and rights within institutions concept. That is the issue of placement of handicapped children. As a member of the Committee on the Handicapped (COH), the school psychologist must evaluate pupils and recommend placement in a least restrictive environment to provide for the special education needed and assure the education of the pupil to the maximum extent appropriate with other pupils who are not handicapped. In doing so, the psychologist frequently may be torn between the desire to "mainstream" the education of a handicapped child and the desire to provide the specialized services that appear to be required.

The fundamental conflict involved in issues of the right to treatment or habilitation is thus an individual's civil liberties versus the right of a duly certified or licensed professional to provide the treatment necessary to ameliorate or to control a given condition. It is a conflict between means and ends, between a type of benevolent paternalism and autonomy. In terms of involuntary commitment, state laws are reasonably clear (Beis, 1983). Most states agree that when individuals require protection for themselves or for others, institutionalization is appropriate. The conflict comes in determining when, indeed, an individual represents a substantial threat or risk to self and/or to others. Some states, for example, include drug dependency and alcohol in their criteria of a "mentally ill person," while others specifically exclude such categories of persons. When some do and some don't, the basis for controversy exists. Finally, a critical issue is the right of legislative bodies and courts to order conditions of treatment beyond the power of the treatment providers to deliver because of financial or personal constraints.

INFORMED CONSENT

In the late 1950s, the concept of "informed consent" began to appear in the professional literature. Continuing from our previous discussion of involuntary commitment, an interesting speculation is whether an individual so committed has the right to refuse treatment. In the mid 1970s, a group of involuntarily committed patients in Massachusetts and New Jersey sued not to be required to have psychiatric treatment without their consent. A number of lower court cases since that time have failed to provide a clear definition of the right of a patient to receive treatment.

Generally, the idea of informed consent exists in order that individuals have the freedom to accept or to reject a particular treatment. To do so, they need to have accurate information and the ability to process that information rationally in making a decision. Mills, Cummins, and Gracey (1983) described the three components that comprise informed consent as "capacity (competence, voluntariness of consent, and information (knowledge of risks)" (p. 50). In some states, when a person is adjudged to lack competence or is a minor and commitment is not voluntary, a surrogate, such as a guardian, may make consent decisions (called *substitute consent*). Unfortunately, such guardians are not themselves protected by law (Gutheil et al., 1980) and may consequently be sued.

Informed consent in relation to voluntary treatment is both an ethical and a legal issue. Altmaier (1979) suggested that all clients should be informed of the nature of the treatment and the possible risks (in non-technical language) and of the training and experience of the professional helper. A Presidential Commission has issued a report, "Making Health Care Decisions: The Ethical and Legal Implications of Informed Consent in the Patient-Practitioner Relationship." In this document are provided recommendations. The conclusion reached is that informed consent is a moral imperative, ideally based on mutual respect of practitioner and client and on shared decision-making. Clearly informed consent requires the helping professional to describe to the client the nature of the client's difficulty and the proposed treatment; to give some probability of success; to catalog possible alternative treatments; and to apprise the client of any potential risks.

What is not clear is to what extent the helper must conform to these ethical mandates and legal requirements. For example, how much information is sufficient to give an individual? How much must a client be told about side effects of treatment? Medication cases are one matter; non-medication cases are another. What are the criteria of competence or capacity? Halleck (1980) has noted, "Whenever a patient has a serious mental illness which interferes with his cognitive functioning, his perception, or his capacity to behavior in a self-serving manner, the question of his competency to accept or refuse treatment is always at issue" (pp. 84-85). Is a minor, *per se,* incompetent to consent to treatment? What is voluntary? If a client agrees to treatment in order to avoid a negative consequence (e.g., job loss, loss of child custody, revocation of parole, etc.), is this act voluntary or coercive? Should informed consent in mental health be restricted primarily to somatic treatment modalities (e.g., psychosurgery, electroconvulsive therapy, psychotropic medications), or should it include all possible treatment modalities, including psychotherapy? How far must the professional go in warning the client that psychotherapy involves risks? For example, Everstine et al. (1980) recommended providing clients with a written statement.

> Psychotherapy may involve the risk of remembering unpleasant events and can arouse intense emotions of fear and anger. Intense feelings of anxiety, depression, frustration, loneliness, or helplessness may also be aroused. (p. 833)

In addition, some recommend that the client be told that therapy may not work and, in fact, could make matters worse; that the cost may be substantial; and that consent to therapy may be rescinded at any time during the process.

RESEARCH USE OF CLIENTS

Ethical and legal issues are raised whenever clients or non-clients are utilized in research. This condition is especially pertinent when a potential risk exists to the research subjects. The reason research is carried out is, presumably, to provide advances in our knowledge in order that we may more effectively help people. The major critical issue is, therefore, whether the monetary and health costs of research are such that they justify the advances? Some use the medically oriented doctrine of "limiting harm" (Eichelman, Wikler, & Hartwig, 1984) to justify research as well as the more common argument of developing benefits—i.e., stopping people from committing harm while they are trying to do good.

Research, in general, contains many of the ethical and legal issues previously addressed: the rights of subjects, informed consent (both as a precondition and as an ongoing condition), and competency. Most institutions have a review board, a third-party safeguard of the client's autonomy, which determines if risks to the subjects are minimal and reasonable, if informed consent is appropriate, if data collection does not harm the subjects, if privacy and confidentiality are assured, and if no undue influence or coercion was or will be used in securing subjects. The Department of Health and Human Services requires (with the exception of certain types of research on educational instruction, tests, surveys, or public observations) that informed consent involves giving subjects a clear explanation of the purposes and procedures of the research. This description must include any notation of the risks or discomforts involved. Clearly participation must be voluntary.

Thus, the issues of subject autonomy (what can be done with the subject's body and mind), undue risk, and truth-telling are the major critical aspects of research, especially with populations "at disadvantage" (usually defined as psychiatric patients). Risk is not necessarily only physical or psychiatric but also extends to a subject's suffering indignity, deceit, or use as an object.

Compounding all of this is the fact that the non-invasive psychotherapies have not been completely proven as yet to have great effectiveness in the treatment of many mental disorders. Because "standard" treatments cannot be proven to have great effectiveness, to argue against the legitimacy of almost any type of non-traditional therapy being applied experimentally is difficult. Hence, some rather esoteric therapy modes have been effected and justified on the basis of research experimentation.

Research with human subjects has been viewed historically as different from inquiry into non-human phenomena. In one sense, many make a distinction between mind and matter, so to speak, and argue that human beings are so special, so unique, that the license given for inquiry into other segments of nature should not pertain to humankind. At the very least, the argument goes, techniques and conditions should be consistent with the higher nature and status of Man.

SEXUAL MISCONDUCT

No ethical issue receives more attention in the mass media than does sexual activity in therapy. This ethical issue is often changed into a legal issue as clients argue that they have suffered psychological damage as a result of sexual relations with a therapist. To be sure, data are available to suggest that few client-therapist sexual interactions ever reach the stage of legal action. Results of surveys indicate that as many as four to seven percent of clinicians have had sexual relations with their clients (Sadoff & Showell, 1981). Most workers in the helping professions are strong in their condemnation of sexual involvement with clients. Some base this view on the perceived vulnerability of the client who is presumed to be experiencing classic Freudian transference. Too, the therapist is thought to experience countertransference. The notions of transference and countertransference, however, are virtually untestable constructs. More helping professionals simply subscribe to the idea promulgated in every code of ethics that sexual intercourse between client and therapist is ethically reprehensible because it is thought to be countertherapeutic and exploitative and, therefore, that it is also likely to be illegal. Such is not necessarily the case.

Serban (1981) has summarized the justification of some of the newer therapy modalities which seem to encourage or at least condone sexually oriented interaction between client and therapist. He stated:

> If in classical therapy the emphasis was on interpretation, in the modern one it has shifted to closeness, empathy, warmth, love, expression of mutual feelings, and bodily contact. With the loose conceptualization of authentic human interaction, the boundary between the professional involvement and a personal one becomes increasingly blurred. (p. 77)

Sexual activity is usually thought to include but not be limited to intercourse, touching, fondling, caressing, petting, and/or kissing; oral-genital contact; masturbation; talking about intercourse; attempting intercourse; exhibition; or group sex. Some feel that the therapist has an obligation to end therapy as soon as a sexual relationship begins to develop; others feel that the therapeutic relationship can be resumed when the sexual relationship ceases.

The major study which demonstrates the harmful effects on therapy of sexual intimacy between therapist and client is that conducted by Bouhoutsos et al. (1983). They analyzed responses from California-based therapists who described 559 current clients who had returned to therapy after becoming involved in sexually intimate behavior with a former therapist. Their conclusion was, basically, that "When sexual intercourse begins, therapy ends." Approximately 90% of the clients were described by their current therapists as having suffered some ill effects from sexual involvement with their previous therapists. These negative effects included those on the client (personality adversely affected; negative feelings about the experience; a worsening of sexual, marital, intimate relationships), those on the therapeutic relationship (ended or interfered with therapy), and those on future therapeutic relationships (more difficult to recommence therapy with another therapist).

At the worst, sexual activity between client and therapist is seen by some as a form of abuse of the client, a violation of the intimacy sought in the client-therapist relationship. It allegedly betrays the client's trust, heightens his/her vulnerability, and, therefore, impedes effective treatment.

The consequences to the therapist of this activity can range from professional censure, to loss of license, to civil liability for money damages. Clearly a legal risk exists for therapists who engage in sexual relations with their clients. Parenthetically, Ewing (1984) has noted accurately that actual sexual relations are not the only type of exploitation of client vulnerability. He cited court cases involving a therapist who induced a client to turn over savings to him, and who caused a client to divorce her husband on the supposition that the therapist would do likewise with his spouse but did not, and another who lost a suit based on the allegation that he met with his client in public places and proposed a possible romantic rendezvous even through no findings of sexual relations were made.

DUTY TO WARN OR INFORM

The duty to warn or inform third parties of potential harm or danger always has been a critical issue in the helping professions and especially has been a "hot" issue since the famous *Tarasoff v. Regents of the University of California* (1976). A brief review of the case is necessary. In August of 1969, an outpatient in the U Cal/Berkeley Counseling Center confided to a psychologist his intent to murder a former girlfriend, Titiana Tarasoff. He asserted that he would do so when she returned to campus in the Fall. The psychologist, Dr. Lawrence Moore, informed campus police of the threat and recommended that the outpatient, Prosenjit Poddar, be involuntarily committed. The campus police talked with Poddar, determined that he seemed rational, and believed his denial that he intended harm to Ms. Tarasoff. Dr. Moore's superior, Dr. Harvey Powelson, a psychiatrist, also directed that Poddar not be detained. As might be expected, Poddar refused to continue treatment with Dr. Moore or to get any other assistance. In October, when Ms. Tarasoff returned to school from summer hiatus in Brazil, Poddar killed her.

The parents of Ms. Tarasoff filed suit, claiming that the police and the therapist had failed to warn them of the danger posed by Poddar. Although no law in America requires any individual to warn another about possible endangerment by a third party, the California Supreme Court noted that exceptions are created by a "special relationship" with either the person endangering or the possible victim and that the patient-therapist dyad constitutes such a special relationship. The court stated:

> When a therapist determines, or persuant to the standards of his profession should determine that his patient presents a serious danger of violence to another, he incurs an obligation to use reasonable care to protect the intended victim against such danger. The discharge of this duty may require the therapist to take one or more various steps, depending on the nature of the case. Thus it may call for him to warn the intended victim or others, to apprise the victim of the danger, to notify the police, or to take whatever steps are reasonably necessary under the circumstances.

Oldham (1978) believed the heart of the decision to be that where a therapist

> *actually* concludes that the patient presents a serious danger of violence to another, the therapist has a duty to warn the third person. In a case where the therapist did not actually believe that the patient committed a violent act, before

liability could result, the plaintiff would have to establish that the therapist should have foreseen this likelihood of violence. (p. 188)

The early upshot of Tarasoff appeared to be that therapists were indeed required to protect third parties from potentially violent clients, even at the cost of breaching confidentiality. Subsequent cases, however, make that conclusion less strong. Knapp and Vandecreek (1982) cited several cases in which courts have ruled that while therapists are statutorily allowed to breach confidentiality, they are not required to do so. The dilemma created by the desire to safeguard the confidential relationship on the one hand and the legal duty (or moral obligation) to warn of a potentially violent client on the other, has led to many suggestions for therapist self-protection. Among these are greater use of outside consultants and ethics committees of professional associations, routine attempts to assess likelihood of potential violence, and simply the exercise of better clinical judgment.

Many of the same issues are entailed with clients who threaten harm to themselves rather than to others. Failure to provide appropriate care for an obvious suicide risk could have legal implications. Therapists may reasonably be expected to assess the degree of suicide risk, especially when dealing with high risk clients (e.g., young women and recently widowed older persons). Most clinicians will recommend hospitalization if the risk is clear and apparent and, further, that once the client is hospitalized, suicidal precautions be taken in the management of the patient. Waltzer (1980) concluded that the likelihood of a malpractice finding is very small "if there was cognizance of the suicidal potential, and the treatment and management plans were considered therapeutic and in keeping with the needs of the patient" (p. 98).

A third major type of duty to warn or inform which also involves a breach of confidentiality is the case of child abuse. Swoboda et al. (1978) pointed out that much of the difficulty in these types of cases emanates from a lack of understanding of the distinction between *privileged communication* and *confidentiality*. Privileged communication "refers to a rule in evidence law that provides a litigant with the right to withhold evidence in a legal proceeding that was originally communicated in confidence" (p. 449). Depending on the state, privileged communication may exist between client-attorney, husband-wife, priest-penitent, doctor-patient, and therapist-client, among others. In other words, a relationship which requires mutual trust is legally protected. Confidentiality is different. The concept is based on an ethical rather than a legal standard and is meant to reassure clients that they have no fear of disclosure. More about this distinction later.

Despite the so-called children's rights movement of recent years (i.e., the recognition of children as independent individuals with legal and civil rights), the courts have essentially implied that setting up an adversarial procedure between parent and child should be avoided, since it undermines the family relationship, and that wide discretion is still permitted parents in child rearing. All states have child abuse and neglect laws. Mandatory reporting laws, however, are sometimes not so clear as they appear. What is abuse? Who must report abuse? How does privileged communication affect the decision to report? Physicians and social workers are usually specified in state laws. Other helping professionals are sometimes not. Would *not* reporting abuse lead to more good than harm (e.g., no adverse publicity) and thus justify defying the law? Professionals are often urged to be advocates for both policy matters affecting children and for individual children. In fact, Mearig (1982) suggested that "professionals go beyond traditional ethical guidelines and take personal risks to serve children's best interests" (p. 526). A professional, however, cannot and should not promise complete confidentiality to a minor, since a parent can force a therapist to breach confidentiality. One study (Swoboda et al., 1978) found that psychologists were more ignorant of child abuse laws in relation to privileged communication than were psychiatrists and social workers, but that a relatively low proportion of practitioners in any of these disciplines were familiar with the law. In fact, the language of the typical mandatory reporting statute is assertively *against* preserving confidentiality. We also should remember that privileged communication is a right of the *client,* not a right of the mental health worker.

CONFIDENTIALITY

The matter of confidentiality pervades many of the legal and ethical issues in the helping professions. We have previously indicated a distinction between confidentiality and privileged communication. Siegel (1979) related both ideas to the concept of *privacy,* "the freedom of individuals to choose for themselves the time and the circumstances under which and the extent to which their beliefs, behavior, and opinions are to be shared or withheld from others" (p. 251). Presumably, confidentiality must be assured for clients if they are to choose to waive their right to privacy and engage in complete disclosure, for the latter status has been through to be a necessary condition for effective therapeutic intervention. Yet, counselors and social workers, to cite just two types of workers in the helping professions, have long operated without a legal protection for confidentiality. Additional justification for confidentiality have come from arguments related to protecting clients from social stigma and promoting clients' rights (Denkowski & Denkowski, 1982).

Some issues in confidentiality are particularly nettlesome. One of these is related to third-party insurers, private or government, who require detailed information about clients and who store these data for retrieval in electronic data banks. The Medicaid audit is one such example. Obviously, confidentiality is destroyed in this situation. Requests for information from employers, schools, public agencies, and other health care professionals also are often honored because they are presumed to be of benefit to the individual. Another issue arises when a therapist has confidential information extracted from a third party with whom he/she had a professional association in the past. How is this confidential information used with a present client? Dulchin and Segal (1982), for example, cited the problematic nature of confidential information gathered in analyzing students from a psychoanalytic institute in one generation and then analyzing subsequent generations of relatives, friends, or colleagues.

When does writing about a client in order to advance knowledge for professional colleagues abuse confidentiality? When should or must confidentiality be breached? Some states require that confidentiality *must* be breached by the therapist under certain circumstances. We have previously observed the case of child abuse. In addition, in some states, matters of criminal action, certain court actions, expert report to an attorney, litigation between client and clinician (Popiel, 1980), when the therapist is court appointed, and when danger is perceived of client harm to self or others, are just a few examples of circumstances that must be reported. Group psychotherapy sessions further attentuate the idea of confidentiality. All in all, confidentiality is under so many legal assaults and is so difficult to maintain completely, that a committee of the California State Psychological Association (Everstine et al., 1980) concluded that little confidentiality exists.

VALUE CONFLICTS

A number of ethical issues are encountered when the implicit or explicit values of a therapist come into conflict with the values of a client. One such situation is that in which the religious values of an individual are thought by the therapist to be counter-therapeutic. Religiosity as an aspect of individual behavior has been extensively researched, but few definitive findings have emerged. On the face of it, potential conflict would appear to exist between therapist and client. Sevensky (1984) reviewed the data on what percentages of mental health professionals believe in certain religious principles (e.g., contact with the dead, life after death, personal immortality, etc.) and the existence of God, compared with the general population, and concluded that the two groups have different views of the world. He asserted:

> In short, many people hold beliefs which most doctors and scientists (and presumably most psychiatrists, psychologists, and other mental health workers) regard as impossible; they organize and make sense of their lives around meanings and goals which a majority of the scientific-medical establishment considers mistaken. And unless these differences are recognized, the possibilities of professional bias, misinterpretation or error in the psychotherapeutic process remain quite real. (p. 75)

Whether certain religious practices are regarded as pathological or as healthful often, then, depends on the orientation of the therapist. Studies which compare the mental health of religious versus non-religious individuals tend in meta-analysis to indicate that, in general, no decided group positive or negative mental health effects can be linked to religiosity (Bergin, 1983). Clearly, religiosity can be good (healthy) or bad (unhealthy) in individual cases. And even in clearly unhealthy cases, some believe that any attempt to alter the religious beliefs of clients is an affront to civil liberties (McLemore & Court, 1977).

McNeely and Oates (1978) have cited a number of religious symptom patterns that may distort the therapeutic process. These include the client's feeling that his/her emotional illness is the result of a lack of faith; that the therapist must be of the same faith; or that clients regard therapists as anti-religious or evil because the therapist is thought to evoke magic or sorcery, both of which are condemned in the Bible. More obviously, some schizophrenic clients and others may identify themselves with religious figures, such as Jesus, the Virgin Mary, etc., and other clients may believe that demons have possessed them. Other potentially distorted aspects of religiosity may include the client's feeling so unworthy that he/she is beyond God's forgiveness or that he/she has been abandoned by God.

When, then, is religiosity healthy and when is it unhealthy? As we have said, much will depend on the values of the mental health professional or on what some schools of therapy would describe as the therapists's countertransference reactions. A useful procedure may be to remember that the holiest, most respected and revered figures in most religions—the saints and the prophets—engaged in behavior that psychohistorians could easily describe as psychotic, asocial, neurotic, or, at the very best, bizarre.

Another type of value conflict emerges in cases when a mental health professional believes that a professional colleague or the employing institution is acting in less than a professional manner. The British Psychological Society's (1983) *Guidelines for a Code of Conduct for Psychologists* states that psychologists shall

> where they become aware of misconduct by a professional colleague that cannot be resolved after discussion with the colleague concerned, take steps to bring that misconduct to the attention of those charged with the responsibility to investigate it, doing so without malice and with no breaches of confidentiality other than those necessary to the proper investigatory process. (p. 244)

A number of articles in the professional literature address employer-client conflicts. At times the welfare of the client and the rights and reputation of an employing institution are at odds. In the abstract, one would surely aver that the client's welfare is paramount; in the diurnal material world we live in, however, well-meaning professionals may be constrained by prospects of economic loss, disapprobation of one's peers, and other potential retaliatory actions. Simon (1978) suggested that one way to avoid any ambiguous feelings that a professional may have about "whistle-blowing" is to include explicitly in a document such as the *Guidelines for the Employment of Psychologists* (1972) a statement such as the following:

> The primary responsibility of the psychologist is to the client. The psychologist must resolve conflicts of interest between the employer agency and the client on the basis of this responsibility. (p. 334)

Still another series of potential value dilemmas emanate from issues surrounding psychological assessment. Beauchamp and Childress (1979) have delineated two ways to examine ethical issues. *Beneficence* is the duty to act positively in the interest of others. *Nonmaleficence* is the duty not to act negatively in relation to clients (as in a boulegenic occurrence). In looking at the potential abuses and misuse of assessment and labeling procedures. Adelman and Taylor (1984) suggested that concerns regarding false negative and false positive identifications, stigmatizing effects, self-fulfilling prophesies, and the like might also be viewed in relation to the idea of utility—achieving the greatest number of positive results (and the least number of negative outcomes) for all people involved in an action. In other words," does the potential good help outweigh potential harm, or, more generally, are the costs likely to be less than the possible benefits" (p. 17).

Some evidence exists that those who engage in psychological assessment are often casual about the manner in which the results are used and safeguarded (Berndt, 1983). Newer computerized technology opens the opportunity for potential abuses in assessment procedures. Goodyear and Sinnett (1984) argued that the ready availability of automated interpretation services has led to their use by untrained personnel (e.g., technicians, physicians, etc.) and to overtesting because of the potential profit stressed in promotional materials. To guard against these possible abuses, they suggested that consumers be advised to raise the following questions:

1. Is this test necessary?

2. Will the interpretations be valid for me?

3. Is there a certified psychologist associated with the program who is responsible and can be consulted freely about automated findings?

4. What guarantees are there of accuracy in scoring?

5. What safeguards are there for confidentiality of data and results?

6. Are the savings of computerized testing passed on to me?

In an effort to provide helping professions workers with assistance in evaluating ethical problems, Van Hoose and Paradise (1979) suggested the application of five elements of analysis: (1) identify the problem or dilemma according to source (e.g., client versus institution); (2) identify any rules or guiding principles to help resolve the dilemma (e.g., published standards of the insitution or the profession); (3) generate possible and probable courses of action; (4) consider potential consequences for each course of action; and (5) select the best course of action.

Any person who has ever taken a basic philosophy course knows full well that values can be categorized as either absolute or relative. The former are considered to be universal and unchanging and equally applicable regardless of culture, history, form of government, or the like. The latter are values that may vary from situation to situation or from time to time, depending on a variety of conditions at a particular time and place. Obviously no attempt has been made at a system of codifying conduct that is universally accepted by every helping professional. Each sorts through notions of "right" and "wrong" in a search for personal relevance. Van Hoose and Paradise (1979) offer an interesting guideline when they state:

> The counselor or psychotherapist is *probably* acting in an ethically responsible way concerning a client if (1) he or she has maintained personal and professional honesty, coupled with (2) the best interests of the client, (3) without malice or personal gain, and (4) can justify his or her actions as the best judgment of what should be done based upon the current state of the profession. (p. 58)

TRAINING IN LEGAL AND ETHICAL ASPECTS OF HELPING

When a Watergate occurs and involves so many attorneys, schools of law are subject to pressures to increase the intensity of the preparation they give to their graduates in dealing with ethical issues. Similarly, Medicaid fraud invariably produces demands for medical schools to enhance the ethical preparation of their students. In the helping professions, no such stimulation is needed, because a constant agitation has been for formal preparation to help practitioners cope with ethical dilemmas and understand legal requirements. Welfel and Lipsitz (1984) concluded that general agreement exists for requiring some form of ethics training in graduate education in psychology. The situation appears to be the same in the other helping professions. Yet, no formal studies have assessed the effects of such training on practitioners in their actual practice.

Several writers have suggested that formal ethical training for mental health professionals include direct instruction in moral philosophy, values clarification designed to help trainees to discover and to assess more accurately their own values, and an understanding of the ethical principles of the specific profession (Abeles, 1980; Corey, Corey, & Callahan, 1984; Losito, 1980).

ADDITIONAL RESOURCES

Because this chapter covers so wide a range of legal and ethical concerns, we can do little more than simply raise some major critical issues. A number of recent books offer excellent discussions in more depth than space considerations here allow. Among these are the following:

Corey, G., Corey, M.S., & Callanan, P. (1984). *Issues and ethics in the helping professions.* Monterey, CA: Brooks/Cole.

Ewing, C.P. (Ed.). (1985). *Psychology, psychiatry and the law: A clinical and forensic handbook.* Sarasota, FL: Professional Resource Exchange.

Fischer, L., & Sorenson, G.P. (1985). *School law for counselors, psychologists, and social workers.* New York: Longman.

Grisso, T., & Sales, B.D. (1978). Law and professional psychology. Special issue of *Professional Psychology, 9*(5).

Hopkins, B.R., & Anderson, B.S. (1985). *The counselor and the law.* Alexandria, VA: American Association for Counseling and Development.

Hummel, D.L., Talbutt, L.C., & Alexander, M.D. (1985). *Law and ethics in counseling.* New York: Van Nostrand Reinhold.

Keith-Spiegel, P., & Koocher, G.P. (1985). *Ethics in psychology.* New York: Random House.

THEME FIVE: TECHNIQUES, STRATEGIES, AND PROCEDURES

CHAPTER 8

CONTROVERSIES IN TECHNIQUES, STRATEGIES, AND PROCEDURES OF THE HELPING PROFESSIONS

The tools of the mental health professions are theories of behavior, assessments, classifications of behavior, and interventions in behavior—for example, counseling, psychotherapy, group work. Within each of these domains are sets of assumptions; social science paradigms; differential weightings of biological, social, and psychological factors which have been incorporated in varying forms within the various mental health professions. As these emanate from dissimilar disciplinary origins—e.g., differential psychology, psychodynamic-social learning-cognitive psychology, medicine, sociology, cultural anthropology—they open or shut different "windows" on behavior and how it should be altered. These "windows" or lenses are in turn translated into procedures by which to classify and act on the behaviors of interest. Obviously, science, art, politics, and culture get intertwined in such matters and different groups of mental health professional espouse various combinations of explanations and interventions as their own. Such differences breed controversy.

In Chapter 8 are examined some of the major controversies related to theories and techniques used in the mental health professions. Particularly at issue are classifications of behavior, testing and assessment, and the biases inherent in such mechanisms from the standpoint of their relevance and sensitivity to cultural variation among clients. The controversies discussed here vary in their intensity and in their likelihood of resolution. They are for the most part continuing problems which create tensions among professional groups and, in a larger sense, for the total mental health enterprise.

Other sections of the book have focused on major issues which have divided the helping professions: identity, credentialing, training, legal and ethical issues, economics. In this part, we take a somewhat different tack and examine several of the major techniques and strategies which, in some cases, may be controversial because of the nature of their conceptual foundations or outcomes sought between professional groups and in other instances controversial within a professional group. Testing and classification of behavior are examples of the latter. In some form or another, all of the "helping professions" use techniques by which to classify and assess behavior and while cross-professional controversies may exist about their use, also arguments and controversies exist about the techniques per se.

In this chapter the techniques or strategies visited—e.g., classification of behavior, cross-cultural techniques—may better be described as revisited. They already have been viewed in other parts of the book through different lenses than will be used here. The basic intent of this chapter is to examine techniques and procedures which are used by all of the helping professions or which are emerging as issues for the helping professions separately or collectively. In either of these conditions, they represent the "stuff" of controversy.

SOCIAL SCIENCE PARADIGM

In considering controversy in techniques and strategies, one first needs to consider the conceptual paradigms and theoretical systems which guide such techniques. What are the behavioral assumptions about growth, learning, normality which are at the core of classification and intervention? What are the epistemological bases on which the mental health professions rest? Although these questions are raised here for purposes of context, neither the purpose of this book nor the space available permit a reconstruction of the assumptions and theories which give form and substance to each of the helping professions.

Suffice to say here is that different views on the nature of scientific knowledge and how it is best obtained, the interaction between epistemology and substantive theory, and the methodological commitments of scientists in the helping professions frequently underlie debates within and between professional groups and public policy makers. For example, Amundson (1985) has provided a historical analysis of the "place versus response" controversy in psychology, a controversy which matched a group of cognitive psychologists against a group of S-R behaviorists, in which he argued that the great difficulty in resolving the issue was due to unacknowledged differences in epistemology between the parties.

Amundson further contended that the importance of epistemology to psychology is due to the special relations between the tasks of epistemology and the tasks of psychology. He outlined three major epistemological topics: "the nature of knowledge, the conditions under which it is most likely to be achieved, and the capacities possessed by humans which make them potential knowers" (p. 128). While the first two topics have relevance to any science, the third one, "the human abilities which makes knowing possible," is the special domain of psychology and by extrapolation of the other members of the helping professions as we have come to deal with them in this book. Thus, much of the task of psychology and its related sub-disciplines or applied subsystems "is empirically to discover precisely what knowledge-gaining abilities the psychological subject possesses" (p. 128). But at this junction is where the controversy begins as these opposing theories, for example, operationalism, cognitivism, neobehaviorism become elements of debate, shapers of scientific methodology, and possibly, constraints upon the questions asked and the models of behavior which are ultimately constructed. Thus, in Amundson's view epistemology and theory need to be paired in a form of logical ground/figure combination which confirms the principle of *epistemological parity: Accept only those theory/epistemology pairs in which the epistemology would be appropriate to a psychological subject being truly described by the theory.*

Such a principle provides a test of competing theories and continues to draw controversies about techniques and strategies back to their basic assumptions about and representations of either observable or unobservable behavioral phenomena.

Such a perspective is extended by Kilmann (1982) who argued that the major contributions and break throughs in the history of a social science paradigm occur because at each stage of development a prior assumption was challenged and then rejected. Kilmann contended that one can characterize the progress of social science theories as a decade by decade process of questioning and refining the underlying assumptions that scientists make concerning the nature of human behavior, social environments, and the interactions among them. Kilmann further argued that social scientists

> should not assume that all assumptions if made explicit would be considered valid, obvious, or even reasonable. Rather, we should surface and examine the most critical assumptions in any scientific pursuit (if not all the assumptions), since these assumptions get at the heart of whether one's theories or (tentative) conclusions are reasonable and valid for the time being.

He concluded that there are really three stages of analysis by which assumptions might be uncovered: stakeholder analysis—generation of a list of all or most assumptions affecting a conclusion; belief-assessment analysis—evaluation of those assumptions according to some criteria of importance or centrality; and, conclusion analysis, the re-examination and perhaps modification of the initial conclusion once the critical assumptions have been exposed, then validated or altered (p. 4). Such a process permits the development of a matrix of assumptions which compare those which are less-important, most-important, certain, and uncertain. This in turn can lead to a determination of the unlikely truth of a conclusion or to a specific design and action steps by which assumptions can be tested. Since theories can be competing explanations for similar observed phenomenon, and because it is unlikely that single research studies will fully support or reject a complex theory, the expeditious procedure is to add to whatever other method of science is involved an analysis of the assumptions on which a particular theory is based.

With respect to the underlying rationale for psychotherapy, Howard and Orlinsky (1972) contended that implied in such a process is "some conception of *human nature* or personality (the material to be worked with), *human fulfillment* (the ideal to be sought), *human vulnerability* (psychopathology), of *therapeutics,* and of the *therapeutic profession.*

Taken together, they comprise...the Therapeutic Belief-Value Complex" (p. 617).

That some members of the mental health profession tend to skip over underlying assumptions about human behavior and make inferences with no behavioral references or engage in negative labeling has been empirically demonstrated (Case & Lingerfelt, 1974; Gingerich, Kleczewski, & Kirk, 1982). Where this occurs it can lead to selective attention to client behaviors which disconfirm the label or to client self-fulfilling of a label. Again, what is often at issue in such "professional" behavior is an insensitivity to the assumptions which underlie any set of labels and a need to test the epistemological validity of the label as it is demonstrated in the particular client's behavior. The inaccuracy or accuracy of such superficial labeling and its potential for negative consequences to clients is another focus for controversy among mental health professionals of different levels of training and theoretical perspective as well as between such professionals and members of the public.

A final brief example of the importance of the underlying assumptions of social science paradigms as sources of controversy has to do with the multiple disciplines which feed into the conceptualizations used by the "helping professions." For example, while the term "mental health" tends to be treated in many research studies and descriptive pieces as a unitary concept having an absolute meaning, in fact many conceptualizations of mental health have different meanings and implications for practice. Four such classifications and their conceptual roots have been described by George and Brooker (1984). They include the following:

1. "Mental health as freedom from illness" which derives from a medical perspective, biological origins, and a homeostatic notion of the equivalence of a lack of symptoms and mental health. Thus, mental health is the antonym to mental illness.

2. "Mental health as an ideal personality type," has its roots in a utopian and psychoanalytic perspective which measures mental health against some mythical total harmony or balance of forces.

3. "Mental health as transactional systems" suggests that healthy behavior changes over time and space in interaction with situational elements.

4. "Mental health as multiple perspectives" suggests that mental health is relative and must be considered in terms of multiple criteria as they appear in the individual case.

Obviously, each of these models of mental health holds different implications for interventions with clients, for the formulation of models of appropriate or inappropriate client behavior, and, indeed, for the development of theory. The point, is, however, that each of these definitions of mental health is different, rests upon different assumptions, and implies different intervention techniques. Until each is empirically tested against the others, the usefulness of each is unclear and uncertainty exists as to whether or not the four classifications can be integrated. The overarching point is that if one group of helping professionals adheres to one definition of mental health and another group of helping professionals uses a second definition, the outcome is likely to be controversy, debate, or perceived need to isolate one's group from the other. This may occur in spite of some overlap in assumptions between the two definitions or a possibility that if the basic assumptions of a definition were clarified, the group holding a particular definition would no longer do so.

All of these prefatory remarks are by way of background to the consideration of areas of controversy in techniques or strategy and acknowledgement that the roots of such controversy frequently lie with differences in meaning, language, or epistemological assumptions by which groups of helping professionals can be differentiated.

METHODS OF STUDYING PERSONS

Perhaps the most controversial of the techniques commonly used in some way or another by all of the helping professions is that of testing, assessment, and the classification of persons' behavior. Sometimes the controversy has to do with when testing should be done; or, what should be tested, by what means, and by whom. Some professional groups are primarily committed to individual psychological evaluations; others use group assessments. Some professionals value information on aptitudes, interests, achievements; others are mostly concerned about psychological traits or states; some professional persons test every client with a standard battery; others customize or tailor their test usage.

Such preferences for assessment usage by different professional groups tend to be less complex or difficult to resolve than do the underlying questions of the validity of tests of different types; the reliability of diagnoses under different conditions; clinical versus statistical assessment; the characteristics of the entity being measured (e.g., depression); when and how physiological measures should be combined with behavioral measures; and, particularly cultural issues in testing.

Clinical Assessment

Like most other elements comprising the cultures of the differing groups of "helping professions," assessments, testing, behavioral classification each have their own language systems and multiple definitions of related processes. Professional groups differ in whether they refer to the information collection processes describing clients as diagnosis, appraisal, assessment, or history-taking. Different mental health occupations describe their assessments and classification procedures from vantage points which give more or less credence to the need for certain kinds of information, at different points in the therapeutic process, for various purposes.

Even within such a context, however, considerable difference of opinion occurs about whether classifications of behavior or assessment are really necessary. For example, Hertz (1970) has observed that

> the predominant behavioristic trends in our field contend that there is no need to explain human behavior at all. All that is required is ability to modify it. Hence we should have no concern either with the dynamic aspects of disordered behavior or with its etiology. From such reasoning the conclusion follows that there is not need for our diagnostic tools. Furthermore, the emergence and rapid development of community psychology with its focus on community social systems and community institutions, make it unnecessary to be concerned with the understanding of intrapsychic systems.

Again, it is argued that there is no need for the traditional clinical skills or diagnostic techniques.

Within the language of assessment and behavioral classifications, the term "clinical assessment" is frequently used. Clinical assessment has been described as "the process by which clinicians gain understanding of the patient necessary for making informed decisions (Korchin, 1976, p. 124). Korchin and Schuldberg (1981) contended that the intent of clinical assessment

> is description of prediction toward the ends of planning, executing, and evaluating therapeutic interventions and predicting future behavior. Any of

numerous techniques can be used, singly, or in combination, depending on the orientation of the clinician and the specific questions for which answers are sought. Thus, interviews with the client or with others; observation in natural or contrived situations; or the use of tests of different functions, varying in length, objectivity, psychometric refinements, and inference might all be included. The immediate goal may be the relatively precise measurement of a particular psychological function or the construction of a working image or model of the person. (p. 1147)

Woody (1980) indicated that

clinical assessment is a set of processes and procedures for human services professionals. It is inherent to all professional functions, be it reaction in the initial contact with a prospective patient, the decision to accept or reject a patient, the services to be offered and the techniques to be used, the decision to terminate treatment, or the impression of the treatment's efficiency and relevance to treatment, or the impression of the treatment's efficiency and relevance to treating other patients. (p. xxxxi)

In Woody's view clinical assessment is a professional service encompassing much more than the use of psychological tests. Further, from this perspective are four critical points in clinical assessment. One, the procedures are not restricted to being objective, standardized, or quantifiable. Much of the data comes from interviews or observations. Two, clinical assessment is principally individually focused—idiographic rather than nomathetic—intended to construct a profile of the strengths, weaknesses, problems, behaviors by which this person can be more accurately and intimately known by the clinician. Three, it is problem oriented. Four, the clinician, diagnostician, the assessor has the responsibility of "applying and maintaining astute clinical acumen" (p. xxxi).

Within such perspectives, four dimensions tend to intersect and become elements of potential controversy: psychodiagnosis, psychometrics, and clinical versus statistical prediction. According to Korchin and Schuldberg (1981, p. 1147), in paraphrased form, psychodiagnosis uses a number of procedures, projective as well as more objective and standardized tests with interpretation including symbolic signs and directly scorable responses, in order to tap into and describe various areas of psychological functioning at both conscious and unconscious levels with the goal of describing individuals in personological (idiographic) rather than normative terms.

The psychodiagnostic orientation puts the clinician rather than the test at the center of the assessment process. The clinician has to organize and conceptualize the questions to be answered, the techniques to use, and finally integrate diverse findings in to a coherent whole. At all points, clinical judgment and inference are required, and the value of the assessment findings ultimately depends heavily on the skill and knowledge of the interpreting clinician. (Korchin & Schuldberg, 1981, p. 1148)

Psychometric versus Psychodiagnostic Tradition

The psychometric tradition differs from the psychodiagnostic tradition on several counts. For one, the former is typically concerned with normative or comparative perspectives rather than primarily idiographic perspectives. The central question is how the client or patient compares with others who have been tested and defined as falling within a normal range of behavior, or as evidencing specific types of emotional or behavioral disorders, or as manifesting certain types of psychological traits, performance potential, motivational preference or other characteristics which can be demonstrated empirically to exist and to be predictive of some set of behaviors. The psychometric tradition, frequently labeled a trait and factor or actuarial approach, emphasizes objectivity throughout the measurement sequence engaged in by the examiner and by the person being assessed as well as in the outcomes achieved. The intent of the process is to reduce inference, judgment, and subjectivity by the examiner and as a characteristic of the assessment process. Issues of test reliability and validity, the precision of test items, the forms and standardization of the test, and its administration are central to the psychometric orientation. The fluid stimuli of projective testing, psychiatric diagnosis and similar psychodynamic assessment processes are not compatible with a psychometric approach to assessment.

At this juncture of psychodiagnostic and psychometric views of assessment, one encounters the controversy engendered by the issues of clinical versus statistical prediction (Meehl, 1954). In essence, *assessment of individual behavior, however it is done, is concerned with predicting future behavior on the basis of past or present behavior and determining whether what is predicted supports the need for mental health intervention and, if so, the type of treatment plan which should ensue.* The actual process of making a prediction on the basis of assessment data can take one of two forms or combine elements of both.

The first of these methods is the clinical or case study method, what we have called clinical assessment previously. Here the mental health specialist operates as a clinician who, on the basis of interview data, test scores, or other observations, formulates some hypotheses about the counselee's behavior. Such an approach tends to be intuitive and subjective.

The second method of prediction is the actuarial or statistical method. Here the client's test data are classified into categories representing performance. The mental health specialist then uses a special computer program, actuarial table or other device providing statistical frequencies of behavior of other persons classified in the same way to compare the individual client to such normative tables. These data are thus mechanically combined (for example by means of a regression equation or expectancy table), and a probability figure or other predictive weight results.

Meehl's early work (1954) in comparing the efficacy of clinical versus statistical predictions has shaped many of the controversies between such methods. He investigated 19 studies having unambiguous results which predicted success in some kind of training or schooling, recidivism and/or recovery from a major psychosis. Ten of these studies failed to find a difference between the clinical and statistical method of assessment; nine found differences in favor of the statistical method of prediction; none produced a difference in favor of the clinical approach. Watley and Vance (1964), among other researchers, have found similar results as those of Meehl.

To argue that all of the issues of assessment among the helping professions can be captured in the dichotomy of clinical versus statistical prediction would be overly simplistic and obviously untrue. Many dimensions of the therapeutic process or the assessment or information collecting aspects of such processes do not now lend themselves to as much precision or statistical analysis as some observers would desire. Thus, mental health specialists must rely to a greater or smaller extent on their own intuition and training to formulate appropriate questions, to collect relevant information, to interpret available data accurately, and to help clients (patients, counselees) formulate treatment plans or action goals which are realistic and credible.

However, each of these aspects of the therapeutic process and its interaction with assessment and classification of individual behavior become potential points of controversy. They include:

1. The relative degree to which one group of mental health professionals is imbued with a clinical assessment versus a statistical prediction mentality? This obviously relates to the therapeutic purposes, the clinical training, and the epistemology of each group. For example, psychiatrists are

much more likely to use clinical judgment and projective techniques than are psychologists or professional counselors. Part of the explanation for this disparity is the historical reliance of psychiatrists on clinical psychologists to conduct assessments for them; psychiatric disappointment with the results of assessment; and psychologists' dismay over the lack of appreciation of their efforts (Berg, 1984). Psychologists and professional counselors are much more likely to be trained in statistical techniques and in standardized psychological measures than are psychiatrists or psychiatric nurses. Professional counselors are much more likely than other groups of helping professionals to be trained in and use aptitudes, career information, and interest or values assessments. Psychologists are more likely to use trait/state psychological assessments and other standardized psychological instruments. In a study of attitudes towards clinical assessment by members of the Association for the Advancement of Behavior Therapy, the finding was that in terms of future emphasis it appeared that both behavioral and objective personality assessment were expected to continue in popularity, projective techniques were viewed as having little future utility (Piotrowski & Keller, 1984).

To extend this point is not really necessary except to say that how helping professionals are trained to view and use assessment as a clinical or statistical tool becomes a major ingredient of controversy among them.

2. The language system by which the recipient of testing or assessment is known is also an issue among many groups of the helping professions. How one labels the person to receive some form of therapeutic intervention has a lot to do with how that person's needs are conceived. Is this person a patient, a client, a counselee? These terms obviously have different value loadings with regard to the likely diagnostic entities involved. Is the person to receive help a person who is sick, mentally ill, experiencing problems of living, or coping with unresolved developmental tasks? How the therapist addresses each of these perspectives tends to affect how he/she conceives the field of likely questions, problems, or treatments to be engaged. The matter of controversy here has

to do with not only the validity of the labels but that different helping professional groups use them differently. Again to be overly simplistic psychiatrists, some clinical psychologists, and psychiatric nurses are likely to refer to patients. Counselors, counseling psychologists, social workers, marriage and family therapists are much more likely to refer to clients or even counselees.

3. A major, perhaps *the* major, issue in assessment is the validity of whatever classification structure is used as the model from which symptoms will be interpreted, diagnoses will be derived, and treatments are conceived. In this scenario, diagnosis is the critical lynchpin to the rest of the process. It typically involves clinical judgment as well as a cognitive map of how the particular mental health specialist views the behavioral domains of concern to him/her.

Woody (1969, p. 77) offered three requirements for diagnosis. They include "the present functioning or characteristics should be evaluated and described; possible causative factors of etiology should be posited; and a prognosis should be made and a treatment approach recommended" (p. 77). Arbuckle (1965) stated it a bit differently: "Diagnosis may be considered as the analysis of one's difficulties and the causes that have produced them. More clinically, it may be thought of as the determination of the nature, origin, precipitation, and maintenance of ineffective abnormal modes of behavior" (p. 220). Finally, and perhaps most directly to the point is the observation by Shevrin and Shectman (1973) that "In the diagnosis of mental disorders the diagnostician elicits and observes a range of psychological functioning which he(she) considers relevant on some theoretical grounds for understanding the disorder..." (p. 451).

Thus, the issue is how an individual therapist conceives of the interplay of emotional, behavioral, intrapsychic, and environmental factors in causing an individual distress. What theoretical notions do they use to construct such models? In such instances the question of interest is how does the science of classification interact with the art of diagnosis?

Clearly, different therapists using different theoretical models do not behave in the same way with regard to assessment, diagnosis, or classification. For example, various psychologists object to what they see as an overemphasis on intrapsychic processes as the major etiological factors in emotional difficulty. Behaviorists, for example, would weigh situational determinants as much more important than intrapsychic processes; community psychologists view social factors as more important in causing mental health problems than are internal individual processes; humanistic psychologists or those who embrace a Rogerian conception of client-centered therapy dismiss testing and assessment as major tools and argue that understanding the individual's interpretation of his/her phenomenological world is much more relevant than interpreting or labeling behavioral patterns using some external classification systems. Family therapists and social workers would likely want to know more about family dynamics, communication and relationship patterns, and related processes than about individual symptoms.

Therefore, given such contradictory perspectives on the appropriateness and substance of classification systems, it is not difficult to understand that virtually any labeling of behavior or classification system can be the center for controversy. Whether its focus is "nosology," the classification of diseases, as is inherent in the various systems of major mental disorders or other forms of classification such as taxonomies of vocational or work adjustment problems, mental health practitioners trained in various clinical specialties and using different theoretical perspectives are likely to value and conceive the integrity of such classification structures differently.

Blashfield and Draguns (1976) have contended that any classification system should meet at least four evaluative criteria.

> First, the systems should be able to be applied in a reliable fashion. In other words, different diagnosticians should be able to apply the system in essentially the same manner and replicate the judgment of another diagnostician.
>
> Second, the classification system should cover those behavioral areas relevant to some domain of patients or clients.
>
> Third, the system should have descriptive validity; categories which are relatively homogeneous in their content.
>
> Fourth, the system should have predictive validity; it should lead to treatment decisions which are appropriate to the category of disorder described.

These four evaluative criteria are formidable goals for any classification system to meet. Clearly, some observers do not believe that existing classification systems or, indeed, psychiatric diagnoses based upon them do or can meet such criteria (e.g., Frank, 1975).

DSM-III

As has been discussed in other parts of this book, *DSM-III* as the major classification system used for emotional and behavioral disorders among virtually all persons in the mental health profession has not received universal endorsement in its coverage or in its conceptualization. Part of this reaction may be because of its origins in psychiatry and part of the reaction may stem from other more substantive reasons. For example, in 1977, the American Psychological Association's Task Force on Descriptive Behavioral Classification reported that

> the proposed DSM-III fails to provide a satisfactory method of classification for the following reasons: (1) it is a disease-based model inappropriately used to describe problems of living; (2) it has consistently shown high levels of unreliability of the specific categories; (3) it is a mixed model, the groupings variously based on symptom clusters, antisocial behaviors, theoretical considerations, or developmental influences; (4) categories have been created or deleted based on committee vote rather than on hard data; (5) the labels have assumed strong judgmental qualities, frequently resulting in bias and social injustice; (6) it offers low capability for indication of treatment modality, prediction of outcome, or determination of required duration of interventions, characteristics both desirable clinically and of major importance to third party payers. (1977, p. 1; quoted in Woody, 1980, p. xxxvi)

In some ways the criticism of *DSM-III* by the American Psychological Association's Task Force on Descriptive Behavioral Classification is mild compared to the debate that has ensued within the ranks of the American Psychiatric Association itself. In one such debate which took place at the American Psychiatric Association Convention in Toronto, in May of 1982, four distinguished psychiatrists, one of whom chaired the working group which developed the *DSM-III,* discussed in comprehensive fashion the advantages and the disadvantages of this classification system (Klerman, Vaillant, Spitzer, & Michels, 1984). To summarize as succinctly as possible the elements of this debate, the advantages and disadvantages are tabulated in Table 8.1.

This debate affirms a point which was really implied in the beginning of this chapter. Classifications of behavior or of nosology, major disorders, are constructions, inventions if you will, of the multiprobabilistic nature of behavioral ingredients; classifications or

TABLE 8.1

CONTROVERSIAL PERSPECTIVES ON *DSM-III* AMONG PSYCHIATRISTS

Advantages	Disadvantages
1. Represents a reaffirmation on the part of American psychiatry of its medical identity and its commitment to scientific medicine (p. 439).	1. It ignores other cultures, lacks adequate sensitivity to value judgment and to cross-cultural and cross-generational moves (p. 542-543). It is parochial (p. 542).
2. It embodies the concept of medical disorders, reaffirming psychiatry's acceptance of the modern medical model of disease that was crystallized in the late nineteenth century (p. 540).	2. Ignores the fact that most diagnoses reflect dimensions and continuums not absolutes. It is reductionist (p. 543), it does not discuss broad, unifying patterns.
3. For the first time an official nomenclature has incorporated operational criteria with exclusion and inclusion criteria...these criteria are based on manifest descriptive psychopathology rather than on presumed etiology—psychodynamic, social or biological (p. 540).	3. It confuses state and trait. Pays too much attention to transient surface phenomena and too little attention to clinical course and human development. Even the best defined disease can have very different symptoms in the same patient at different ages (p. 543).
	4. It is dynamic. Pays too little attention to pathogenesis.

TABLE 8.1. CONTINUED.

Advantages	Disadvantages
4. *DSM-III* underwent field testing reliability (p. 540).	Because the etiology of many psychiatric disorders is uncertain, it is ignored (p. 544).
5. A multiaxial system was introduced to accommodate the diverse aspects of patient's existence.	5. It sacrifices validity for reliability (p. 545).
6. Implicit in the creation of *DSM-III* and the mode of its formation is the necessity for change—the push for DSM-IV.	6. The task force that forged *DSM-III* was not representative of the interests, the values, the diversity of the profession (p. 549).
	7. Does not recognize that there are multiple enriching paradigms in American psychiatry (p. 550).

diagnostic categories are hypotheses, not empirical facts applicable to all clients or patients.

Certainly if systems of classification are flawed or do not meet the tests of evaluative criteria previously described, diagnoses and treatments provided by those groups of helping professionals who use such systems can themselves be flawed and lead to controversy between the helping profession and the public or policy-makers. Also questions are raised of how useful systems of diagnosis are under emergency conditions or settings which are less than ideal. For example, Lieberman and Baker (1985) compared the diagnoses made for 50 patients in an emergency room with those made during a subsequent inpatient hospitalization. They found an acceptable level of reliability for broad diagnostic categories, such as psychosis, depression, and alcoholism. However, the diagnosis of more specific subtypes of mental illness, such as schizophrenia and bipolar disorder were not made reliably in the emergency room nor was nonalcoholic substance abuse. Such findings about diagnostic precision suggest problems with the reliability or structure of classification models as well as with the training of those who apply them. In either case, they add to the body of controversy which surrounds classification of behavior as a process, a technique, and a conceptual model.

Psychobiological Assessment

One of the issues, if not controversies, which is now on the threshold of significant impact in both the diagnosis and the treatment of affective disorders has to do with the psychobiology of depression, mania, and anxiety and the effects of drugs as treatment modalities. Preliminary evidence shows that different types of affective disorders reflect differential sensitivity to the effects of tricyclic drugs. In addition, recent research in biological psychiatry has not yet been reflected in the measurement of biological variables in combination with the most reliable and sensitive clinical outcome and behavioral measures (Katz et al., 1984). As the relationship of specific components of depressive, manic, or other affectively disordered persons are dismantled into those affect, expressive and activity characteristics presumably closely tied to central nervous system functioning and to the differential impact of psychotropic drugs on these functions, they may ultimately alter both classification systems and the use of certain traditional treatment approaches (e.g., the "talking cure").

The continuing and as yet unclear opposite side of the psychobiological assessment issue is that even though psychotropic drugs or other medications provide relief or long term stabilization of certain behaviors, where do concerns for drug-dependence and habituation become major concerns and, beyond such an issue, what combination of, for example, cognitive interventions and physiological procedures are appropriate for some disorders, e.g., Generalized Anxiety Disorder (GAD), even if such combinations of interventions are not necessary or not feasible for other disorders? (Last, Barlow, & O'Brien, 1983). The degree to which such a question is a research question or a controversy is itself unclear. It is probably both. Research is certainly indicated. But, the matter becomes an issue when different professional groups line up to advocate a biological and, therefore, a chemical treatment only versus those who advocate only a psychological approach.

Psychiatry is diligently pursuing ways to deal with some of the compartmentalizing of mental health treatment of divisiveness among practitioners which can be stimulated by successes in the psychotherapies. For example, Abroms (1983) suggested that one of the major tasks facing contemporary psychiatry

> Is finding a paradigm that retains the valuable contribution of psychoanalysis but that places it in the context of a more comprehensive account of mental illness. Such a paradigm must make sense of multiple etiologies and treatments, particularly the combined use of psychoactive drugs, individual dynamic therapy, behavior modification, and family, group, and milieu approaches. ...The leading candidate for the job is biopsychosocial eclecticism. This position maintains that psychiatric disorders have biological, psychological, and social determinants, and that optimal treatment involves a combination of biological, psychological and social intervention... It provides a model in which, for example, a biochemical explanation of depression need not conflict with a psychoanalytic or a family systems account. Each of these modes of explanations would in fact occupy a different level of hierarchy in which the family systems or social level would represent the most comprehensive, holistic account, subsuming the more elemental biochemical and psychoanalytic accounts. ...Conflicts would arise only when parochial proponents of one of the levels maintained that their account provided the whole truth rather than only part of it. (p. 740)

Perhaps a sub-issue which flows from the biological nature of some of the affective disorders is the preliminary data which suggests that the pharmacokinetic effects of some drugs differ in elderly versus younger patients. The clear evidence that elderly patients are being treated more often with psychotropic drugs then are younger patients and particularly in major depressive disorders becomes an important element in the search for interactive effects between biological and psychological correlates of affective disorders, and for classifications of comprehensive treatment regimens (Feighner & Cohn, 1985).

Another view of emerging insight into the interaction between physiological and psychological or psychiatric disorders has been reported by Schiffer (1983). In this study the author assessed 241 inpatients and outpatients on a neurology service to determine the presence of emotional disorders as a primary, secondary, or nonexistent diagnosis. Of the 241 patients evaluated, 101 (41.9%) had sufficient symptoms to justify a *DSM-III* diagnosis. Ten of 57 inpatients were admitted to neurology with a chief complaint that could be classified as primarily psychiatric; 5 of these 10 patients were found to have no neurologic illness. Of the 184 outpatients, 32 were primarily psychiatric and 30 of these had no neurologic illness. Thus, 17.5% of both the inpatients and outpatients on this neurology service had a primary psychiatric diagnosis which most frequently could be described as a conversion disorder, anxiety disorder, or somatoform disorder. The majority of these 42 patients had no neurologic illness.

In addition to those neurology patients who had a primarily psychiatric problem, Schiffer also found a large group of persons who had a primarily neurologic illness and in addition a secondary psychiatric disorder: the most common included alcohol abuse, depression, and anxiety syndromes. In some instances the psychiatric disorder preceded the neurologic disease and in others the reverse was found to be true.

These data when combined with data from primary care physicians confirm the high incidence of those with diagnosible mental disorders among those who seek care from other than mental health professionals. Between 15% and 40% of primary care patients have diagnosable mental disorders. Further, most patients with mental disorders are seen only in the primary care section of the medical care system even though general physicians who see these persons do not record a psychiatric reason for the visit. While, for example, general physicians record a psychiatric diagnosis for about 4.4% of primary care visits, they record a mental health reason for visits or provide psychotherapeutic drugs or psychotherapy or therapeutic listening much more often. The National Ambulatory Medical Care Survey (Jencks, 1985) has shown that in 58% of visits in which a psychotropic drug was prescribed and in 57.6% of visits in which psychotherapy/therapeutic listening was provided, no mental diagnosis was recorded.

These conclusions have several controversial elements which include the following:

1. Given the high incidence of mental disorder which occurs under the guise of physical complaints is sufficient reason available for increasing the degree of psychobiological assessments in routine evaluations of mental disorder?

2. Why do general physicians continue to dispense psychotropic and psychotherapeutic treatment without either making a psychiatric diagnosis or referral of the patient to a mental

health specialist in the community, e.g., psychiatrists, counselor, psychologist, social worker?

3. Is there a major problem of a lack of sensitivity by general care physicians to mental disorders? Are they untrained to recognize and intervene in or refer such cases even through they dispense psychotropic mediations or other mental health treatments, perhaps in an undifferentiated way.

4. How should pharmacologic agents such as anti-anxiety drugs, anti-depressants, and anti-psychotic drugs be used to manage behavior or produce arousal levels that facilitate psychotherapy or other cognitive interventions? If a client or patient is taking such psychotropic agents to what do they attribute the outcomes of psychotherapy? If they attribute satisfactory outcomes entirely to pharmacologic or other external agents, that may result in an indefinite dependence on drugs that may be unnecessary, expensive, dangerous, or useful only episodically, or a lowered likelihood that the gains made in psychotherapy will be maintained without indefinitely long psychotherapy (Brooker, Bechel, & Mareth, 1984).

5. If many affective disorders are primarily biological or chemical in origin, are therapeutic interventions which use only verbal interactions between counselor and client ineffective and/or misrepresented to the public? What are the ethical or legal implications of such circumstances for the therapist of for the client?

Test Bias and Cross-Cultural Assessment

While psychobiological assessment and treatment may be relatively recent or, indeed, emergent controversies in the mental health professions, issues of test-bias and cross-cultural assessment are ongoing issues whose visibility tends to ebb and flow in concert with other issues of social justice and pluralism among American sub-populations. At the heart of such controversies are social concerns over standardized testing.

An important issue to acknowledge is that many critics object to the influence which virtually any form of testing exerts in this society. They observe that tests are major factors colleges and universities use in making decisions about admissions. Schools use them to decide upon which track a student will occupy. They are also major factors in the decisions of employers about who should be hired, trained, or promoted. Tests play important roles in clinics, in agencies, and in mental health facilities in evaluating the achievement, intelligence, and personality of many people. Such results are frequently used to identify those whose behavior is retarded, arrested, abnormal, or deficient. In so doing many test users attribute an inappropriate amount of confidence to the results of testing as "objective" markers from which decisions can be made. By the content included and the criteria of success established test makers tend to shape goals for individuals and structure the characteristics of social institutions dependent upon test results. These are formidable influences upon a society, the potential roots of bias against subpopulations in a culture, and a matrix in which many different forms of controversy can arise and be sustained.

Haney (1981), among others, has traced the history of social concern over standardized tests and testing. Much of the recent controversy has been focused on the appropriateness, if any, of using standardized tests and test content conceived by and validated on predominantly middle class White populations with Black populations or other minority groups whose developmental and educational experiences, economic conditions, and language systems have been different from those groups on whom the test was originally developed. But, the controversies surrounding test bias really do not begin here. As Haney has demonstrated, social concern about testing began with the development of the Stanford-Binet scales by Terman and the Army Alpha test of World War I. The social debate about testing also has encompassed such issues as the meaning of intelligence, its genetic inheritability, the social functions that tests serve, the appropriate use of personality tests, the genetic-developmental content of the "IQ" score, test disclosure, test bias, and truth-in-testing (p. 1021).

Haney suggested, in line with the earlier comments about epistemology and assumptions as important ingredients of controversy in the helping professions, that social concerns over standardized testing tend to be as much matters of social and political philosophy as they are technical matters of scientific measurement. Thus, the perennial controversy on standardized testing can be dismantled into such issues on the one hand as the construct or predictive validity of tests and on the other hand such issues as the utility of test information, or, if one prefers, the social functions of standardized tests.

One of the seeds of the controversy among the mental health professions with regard to testing is captured in the notion of the social functions of standardized tests. Haney made the point that such functions do not depend on the scientific measurement qualities of such instruments. For example, he reported that the two instruments which have by far the most references in the professional testing literature are the Rorschach and the Minnesota Multiphasic Personality Inventory (MMPI). He asked why such tests are so widely used and, then responded, that surely the reason is not because of their proven validity and reliability as measurement instruments (p. 1020). He cited reviewers who had suggested that the Rorschach had played an important role within the psychodynamic approach to psychopathology because it provides data rich with hypothetical dynamic associations which can be used to formulate complex personality structures and complex dynamic interactions as the cause of the observed behavior. As Haney, observed, then, "the Rorschach is popular not because it provides vital answers to specific questions, but because it multiplies the questions," and, thereby, yields information which "can be interpreted in numerous different ways" (p. 1030).

In this respect, other mental health groups who do not embrace a psychodynamic construct of behavior would find the utility of the Rorschach to be nil and, indeed, would likely impugn, either overtly or covertly, the empiricism or the professional competency of the mental health specialists who use such an instrument. This point can be extended to the perceptions of virtually any mental health group of the validity of another professional group's use of assessment, classification, or intervention techniques.

Indeed, given the assaults on the validity of projective techniques from many professional quarters, Hertz (1970) has observed that even those who employ projective techniques are asking with growing frequency such questions as: Is our theoretical position sound? Have our preparations been adequate? Is our research worthwhile? Are our services relevant and effective? In her view these are questions which reveal a sense of inadequacy, tension, restlessness, and dissatisfaction within the ranks of clinical psychology and other users of projective techniques.

Lewandowski and Saccuzzo (1976) and Cleveland (1976) also have outlined the decline of psychodiagnostics in clinical psychology and particularly the use of projective techniques. They have cited a variety of factors which contribute to the steady erosion of the use of such tests:

cost of administration, negative connotations surrounding psychological tests, poor university preparation of clinical psychologists in testing, the outdatedness of Thematic Apperception Test (TAT) pictures and of items in such individual intelligence tests as the WAIS, society's wish to blur all individual differences be they sexual, racial or cultural, and newer forms of psychotherapy that minimize testing.

Test Bias

As suggested earlier, the issue of test bias is perhaps the most significant of the controversies between mental health professionals and the public at large and between groups of mental health professionals representing majority and minority group views of test utility and validity.

Some observers contend that test bias is not a singular matter, but one with many aspects: e.g., over-interpretation, sexism, content, differential validity, the selection model, the wrong criterion, and the testing atmosphere (Flaugher, 1978).

Other observers argue that the main features of test bias lie in their content, modality, and structure as well as in application and interpretation. Therefore, standardized tests are inappropriate for use with populations whose cultural, linguistic, economic, or social background differs from those in the majority culture for whom the test was designed and validated (Garcia, 1981). Others assert that in the case of sex bias in testing the evidence points to society as the prime culprit (Diamond, 1976) even though test content and biased use of test results are clearly implicated. Essentially the same factors have been found (Tittle, 1974) in studies of sex bias in educational measurements and in vocational interest inventories. Other observers contend that in many instances the question, Is this test biased? is the wrong question. A test is designed to reflect a certain ability or trait, in a given cultural context. These observers believe that tests accomplish their purposes well (Clarizio, 1978; Sedlacek, 1977). Therefore, the pertinent question is, "Is our society biased?" or as a subset of such an issue "Is our educational curriculum biased?" In such a view, the controversy is not whether or not a particular test has predictive validity, but rather whether the criterion being predicted is appropriate to Black children, or women, or whoever is put at risk by such a procedure. In the view of Williams (1975) no need exists to pursue further the mythological "culture fair, 'culture common,' or 'culture free' tests unless they all relate to a culturally fair curriculum and most importantly a culturally fair society" (p. 87).

Cole (1981) has suggested that a large gap occurs between public concerns and social policy issues regarding testing and those concerns which are primarily technical and reside principally among mental health professionals.

Cole (1981), Cronbach (1980), and other scholars of testing have differentiated between the technical aspects of test bias and the questions of proposed use of tests which are really ethical or policy questions of bias. For example, such scholars are concerned about whether or not a test accurately measures what it purports to measure. This is a scientific and technical question involving assessments of criterion-related or predictive, construct, or content validity, or, indeed, the more recent efforts to combine these three measures of validity into a broader understanding of the meaning of a particular score (Cronbach, 1980). In the latter view, the different types of information reflected in the various approaches to validating a test's accuracy are simply types of evidence which singly or in combination attempt to reduce the technical bias, the lack of accuracy in what is measured, the inappropriate interpretation of test scores, and the misranking of persons on the construct or content measured.

But the public issue of concern in test bias is not a technical question. For the most part, it is a question of ethics or values. Simply stated, the questions are, regardless of the technical validity, the accuracy, of the test, should it be used for the proposed purposes? What are the potential consequences of testing or the affects upon social values which inhere in a particular type of test?

To make the point clearer, a test can be designed which accurately predicts performance in some educational or occupational set of tasks. Indeed, it may accurately indicate that White students or males are more likely to be successful than Black students or females on these tasks. Thus, in its predictive validity it is unbiased in its technical or psychometric qualities, but the social and ethical questions begin where questions of technical bias stop. The question arises in this example, Should the test be used for selection purposes? If it is, White or males will continue to gain in access to opportunities and Blacks or women will continue to be impeded in access to opportunity. Is such a result ethical, does it represent an appropriate social policy? Does the test accurately reflect the social history of the groups? For example, even though the test accurately differentiates the groups on the basis of their potential performance, it is not able to factor in the fact that Blacks and women have been penalized in their current performance on the basis of previous inferior educational opportunities, limited developmental experience, or lack of encouragement. What part should the causes of different types of test performance play in using the test results? These are not issues of test validity per se but rather of policy and ethics and values. They raise policy questions about "differently weighting" the characteristics of applicants to attempt to compensate for past social wrongs or the use of quotas in selection of applicants. They also raise other questions of ethics or policy. Should tests be used to select or facilitate access to opportunity? These are the issues which are the legal and ethical questions which arise in the public forum.

Gordon and Terrell (1981) also put the criticisms of testing into a social context. They contended that the,

> Critics of testing argue from a sociopolitical context, and thus challenge the very purpose, as well as the developed technology of standardized testing. Defenders of testing argue from a traditional psychometric context, with little or no concern for political or social issues. The arguments of the two parties cannot be understood and appreciated without reference to those contexts. (p. 1167)

Gordon and Terrell argued that the reasons for testing at the beginning of this century and for several decades afterward have changed and so must the purposes of testing. In their view, a meritocratic approach to testing designed to identify those few scarce human resources who deserve special attention is no longer viable in a period when the availability of human resources has increased and the meritocratic selection of a few as a goal has given way to a shift in the approach to allocation of opportunities that has evolved from changes in the social and political environment. The assertions of group superiority on the basis of test scores and the subsequent control of the opportunity and reward structure to retain low-status groups in some socially assigned position, has given way to an attempt to democratize access to opportunity, thus the use of tests also should change. As understanding grows about the pluralism in and diversity of the affects of ethnicity, gender, race, and social class upon cognitive and affective structures, learning styles, motivation, and related matters, these should be reflected in purposes for assessment. They contended that,

> The proper course of assessment in the present age is not merely to categorize an individual in terms of current functioning, but also to describe the processes by

> which learning facility and disability proceed in a given individual so that it is possible to prescribe developmental treatment if necessary. ....the equalization of opportunity may require that intervention be responsive to the functional characteristics of the person to whom the opportunity is being made available. It must be determined where the examinee is in terms of function, how he or she got there, and how growth within the examinee's particular social and cultural environment can be enhanced. (p. 1170)

Another element of the test bias issue has to do with whether the conventional tests used to screen persons in or out of opportunities appropriately measure factors related to success in particular environments. The use of the Scholastic Aptitude Test (SAT) for college admission has been a rallying point for such an issue, particularly in regard to factors it does not measure which are found to be important to success by Blacks. The point is made that what the SAT actually does is assess the degree to which a student "has been exposed to a particular type of material" (Hixson & Epps, 1975). Such tests include virtually no information relating to "learning ability, motivation, extra-academic knowledge (often useful in college), quality of high school instruction, achievement orientation, career aspirations, and a host of other factors which in the final analysis determines who succeeds and who does not" (p. 119). This perspective is also typically supported by the fairly widely accepted statistic that the correlation between SAT scores is high school and college grades is about .50, although the band of correlations found in most studies tends to range between .40 and about .60. The essential point is that a correlation of .50 would account for approximately 25% of the variability in college grades. Therefore, the 75% of the variance which is unexplained by scores on the SAT leaves much room for Blacks and Whites to differ on factors making for success including the weighting of the motivational factors mentioned previously. Put even more succinctly, "for so-called marginal students (defined by SAT test results) the SAT score has *no* relationship to their future performance whatsoever" (p. 122). Such findings have led various observers to urge that separate prediction equations be developed for race-sex groupings (Pfeiffer & Sedlacek, 1971) or that highly valid specific academic predictions be developed for Blacks and Chicanos although not necessarily for Whites or Orientals (Goldman & Hewitt, 1976).

In a technical sense, the roots of controversy between psychometric properties or qualities of specific tests and the social purposes for which they are used is an acknowledgement that any assessment, testing or other type of measurement procedure, has many validities not just one. In this sense, then, we can not accurately speak of the validities of the measure themselves when the reality is that we are actually referring to the validities of the inferences from the measures. "The kind of validity statement we seek in any given measurement situation depends on the kinds of inferences we wish to make. This fundamentally is a value judgment" (Guion, 1974, p. 290). Assuming that a test has an absolute, unidimensional, or single validity frequently is at the heart of the controversy about testing which arises among professional groups and in relation to public comment. Thus, however scientific or empirical the development of any measurement instrument may be, its probable multiple validities and the inferences which can be made from it, bring it into the realm of values and social contexts. From such perspectives, many of those who argue about tests are, in fact, talking about different validities or inferences which can be assigned to the same test than are those with whom they argue. In the process, they miss the context of the other's statements thereby making a potentially resolvable debate an acrimonious and unresolved one.

Anastasi's analysis of trends in psychological measurement over a fifty year period (1985) has added another element to the growing chorus of voices describing the interaction between the individual and his/her social context. She, too, argued that implications for testing must be examined both in terms of the contexts in which test takers developed and the contexts in which they are to perform. Perhaps, more importantly, she contended that the knowledge base of the past fifty years has shown an increasing appreciation of the modifiability of human behavior rather than its fixed effects. In this sense, affective variables may be seen as intervening variables in behavior and they in turn may change in response to societal change.

Anastasi has discussed the social context of testing with respect to cross-cultural content. In essence, different cultures provide different opportunities or reinforcements to learn or to implement different cognitive skills, form particular concepts, participate in logical analysis or engage in abstract thinking. Thus, behavior is linked to specific contexts. One way of trying to respond to such realities has been the search for culture-free or culture-fair tests. These technologies have been disappointing in their utility because in the last analysis human behavior is not culture free it is loaded with characteristic patterns of aptitudes or other forms of behavioral expectation which come from social institutions and other cultural artifacts.

To pursue the point a bit further, the problem of test bias in sociopolitical terms is one of responding to cultural difference which in practice becomes cultural disadvantage. Since each culture or sub-culture defines and reinforces behaviors, values, cognitive structures which are adapted to its needs and values, being exposed to a test based upon a different set of cultural norms is to experience test bias and cultural disadvantagement. The issue is not whether the behavior measure is inherently better or worse than some set of norms but how it is different, the implications that such difference holds for adaptation and performance, and how the dominant culture can respond to implications of such difference. In large measure, this is the view Gordon and Terrell (1981) take of how assessment might be used to facilitate opportunity rather than to select people out of opportunity and to assign them to a fixed pool of persons in some inferior status. Obviously, mental health professionals who take an "absolutist" view of how people differ and who therefore believe that differences within or across cultures are "fixed" will view as controversial those discussions of the social context of testing and how such realities need to alter the purposes of testing. So, too, will those persons whose only perspective on testing is a psychometric one. Clearly, the need to consider the environmental context of behavior in all psychological measurement raises questions about the experiential background and learning history of individual test takers, norm groups, the assessment of learning disabilities, cultural differences, and cross-cultural comparisons. Each of these is a challenge and a seed-bed for controversy.

CROSS-CULTURAL COUNSELING AND THERAPY

While systematic consideration of the social context of testing has emerged as a potential antidote to test bias, the issues related to the cultural differences of persons receiving psychotherapy and counseling are likely to grow in their importance in the immediate future. Regardless of whether one is a psychiatrist, a psychologist, social worker, a mental health counselor, a marriage and family therapist, or a psychiatric nurse a principal mental health intervention used is psychotherapy or counseling. However, just as tests and classifications of behavior are not culture free, indeed they measure content which reflects cultural material, neither counseling nor psychotherapy are culture free nor without values assumptions.

Several decades ago, the advocates of psychotherapy and counseling argued that these processes were value-free and provided a relationship climate which was scientifically detached from the values of clients (Walters, 1958). That rather naive era has now passed and the mental health professions are in a more realistic period in which the realization is clear that any intervention in the life-space or life-style of people carries with it values implications or, indeed, actively promotes values (London, 1964). Bergin (1985) has recently suggested that "values are orienting beliefs about what is good for clients and how that good should be delivered" (p. 99). Thus, values influence, if not permeate, counseling and psychotherapy, theories of personality and pathology, the design of change methods, the goals of treatment, and the assessment of outcomes (p. 99). Other observers have similarly suggested that client's values make up much of the "content" of counseling, and that the values of the counselor enter into the "process" of counseling (Pietrofesa, Hoffman, Splete, & Pinto, 1978, p. 55).

Speaking directly to the values of the individual mental health practitioner, May (1963) has contended that

> Values are presupposed in every step the counselor makes in his [sic] own integration, but not in the sense that the counselor's values or even society's values are handed over or subtly implied as the only possible ones or the preferred ones. The counselor can best help the counselee arrive at his [sic] own values by admitting (though it need not necessarily be verbalized) that he [sic], the counselor has his [sic] own values and has no stake in hiding the fact, but that there is no reason at all that they will be the most meaningful or fitting values for the counselee. (p. 95)

As the observations of Bergin (1985), London (1964), Pietrofesa et al. (1978), and May (1963) attest, values inherent in counseling and psychotherapy are powerful influences in how interventions are conceived and carried out. The question of controversy arises when one examines the assumptions of counseling and psychotherapy about appropriate therapeutic outcomes. Are they appropriate to all clients? Are they transportable across cultures?

Cross-Cultural Implications of Counseling and Psychotherapy Models

Many authors have noted that the counseling profession and other mental health specialists have historically been grounded in assumptions that emanate from a white, Anglo-Saxon Protestant would view (Sue,

1981; Wrenn, 1962). Other authors have asserted that counselors functioning with this "world view" tend to prefer clients who are young, attractive, verbal, intelligent, and successful (YAVIS) (Schofield, 1964). Controversy arises when clients not in possession of these attributes receive treatment which is inappropriate and results in disillusionment with and premature termination of the therapy process (Padilla, Ruiz, & Alvarez, 1975). Part of the stimulus to such disillusionment lies in unexamined values within the counseling and psychotherapy models used and whether such values are compatible with the client's cultural history.

Rather than considering that the counselor's values and the intervention strategy used may run counter to the client's value system, therapists sometimes label the client as being "abnormal" or "unresponsive to treatment" (Buss, 1966). Such a counselor mind-set can be demonstrated by examining the topic of self disclosure within the therapeutic relationship.

Many western counseling approaches focus on client-therapist verbal interchange as the principal vehicle by which successful therapy occurs. Often, the degree to which the client engages in self-disclosure determines how that client is perceived by the therapist. Clients who are willing to self-disclose are usually viewed in a positive light by the therapist. Clients who are not as willing to self-disclose are often labeled "resistant" by the counselor. The client's reluctance is perceived by the therapist to be an indication of underlying individual pathology (Jourard, 1964) when the alternative and more defensible explanation for the client's behavior is likely to be a cultural one.

In such a context, often the case is that the therapist does not understand or give sufficient weight to the cultural antecedents of a client's behavior and thus the result is inappropriate labeling of behavior rather than a sensitive and perceptive differential diagnosis. Perhaps, equally important, a core condition of any therapeutic relationship, that of accurate empathy, has been grossly violated by the therapist (Rogers, 1951).

Such an example illustrates the nub of much of the controversy which attends criticisms of counseling and psychology as a cross-culturally insensitive. Many counselors fail to acknowledge the diversity which exists in cultural conditions. For instance, Yiu's research (1978) indicated that Chinese-American college students disclose less than their Caucasian counterparts regardless of their degree of assimilation to the

United States. Saner-Yiu and Saner (1985) also noted that the Taiwanese-Chinese culture prizes interpersonal relations, group identification, and family bonds but deemphasizes the natural expression of feelings. Such a frame of reference obviously conflicts with middle-class American tendencies toward self-disclosure.

Ridley (1984) pointed out that, in many instances, the client's reluctance to engage in self-disclosure is a healthy response to the cultural conditioning to which the client has been exposed. For minority populations, Grier and Cobbs (1968) have referred to this reluctance as a "healthy cultural paranoia" on the part of minorities as they interact with individuals and systems that are frequently racist in nature. Thus, seemingly counselor insensitivity to client values and cultural mores often leads to inappropriate counseling interventions which, in turn, results in the exacerbation of the client's issues of concern rather than his/her alleviation.

Certainly the issue of the cultural implications of counseling or psychotherapy is not confined to the matter of self-disclosure or only to White-Black issues. The potential pool of issues and controversies which arise within the application of cross-cultural concepts to counseling and psychotherapy is wide and deep.

Culture-Bound Theories and Techniques in a Land of Immigrants

For most of the history of the mental health professions in the United States, the theories of counseling and psychotherapy and the techniques and the assumptions about behavior change which flow from them have been primarily *intra*cultural, not *inter*cultural in their focus. Theories and practices have tended to take a universalistic or "etic" (Sue, 1978) view of human behavior rather than one which acknowledged the cultural distinctiveness of most persons in the United States, a primarily "emic" view. Such a homogenized view of cultural assumptions belies the historical reality that the United States is a land of immigrants who have brought with them, regardless of when they arrived and under what conditions, assumptions, traditions, world views, and cultural constructions which carry their residual effects upon perceptual priorities and formulations of space and time from the nations, societies, or tribes which are their ancestral legacies. Even the only non-immigrant population in this country, the native American Indian, was not and is not monolithic in cultural background. The Indian tribes and nations which have been in place in this country since before the foreign settlements began to occur more than four centuries ago differed than as they do now in their religious orientation, languages, sex roles, methods of economic and physical survival, and other behavioral norms (Benedict, 1934).

When one adds the cultural diversity of wave after wave of immigration to this nation from Europe, Africa, Latin America, Asia, and the Middle East, one can recognize that approaches to psychotherapy or counseling which are intracultural only or, indeed, which treat cultural heritage as benign have limited applicability in a pluralistic nation such as the United States.

The significance of cultural diversity to therapy has been emphasized by McGoldrick, Pearce, and Giordano (1982) in their book *Family Therapy and Ethnicity*. In it these authors have pointed up the continuing intergenerational effects which family background transmits or reinforces through values formation; orientation to the past, present, and future; how one views and interacts with strangers and persons beyond the family boundaries; how one interprets one's obligations and responsibilities to others; how one views work or marriage or childbearing; what one defines as a problem and as an appropriate array of solutions; or how one copes with cultural identity. Such ethic traditions and their roots in the family of origin as a national or international phenomenon persist for long periods of time in individual concepts of who they are and the behavioral norms to which they subscribe. Such factors shape behavior and lay a base for the interactions which are likely to occur in therapy and the likelihood of it yielding successful outcomes.

Within the broad parameters of cultural diversity and its accommodation with models of psychotherapy and counseling is the need to acknowledge the potential tensions which arise from a socioeconomically middle-class therapist and a client of a different socioeconomic perspective. The argument can be made that such conflict can occur when the counselor limits himself/herself to viewing client behavior through a psychological lens which assumes individual action to be the prime determinant of success or happiness. In such a view, individual initiative, planfulness, deferred gratification, and achievement orientation may be values, consciously or unconsciously, imposed on the client by the counselor. In such situations, clients for whom such values are neither prized nor socially inculated are often assigned attributions of "unmotivated" or some other label when they are, in fact, acting out a personal script or value set to which they have been culturally conditioned.

In one sense, the counseling perspective just described is a unidimensional psychological view. The values it prizes assume that unfettered individual action is available to all clients and that competition, achievement, and activity are goals and processes which signal maturity and positive mental health. But such a view does not reflect sociological perspectives. Sociological views tend to argue less that persons can choose behavior unrestrained by environmental constraints and more that one's values are largely situationally determined (Roberts, 1981).

Sociological views also emphasize that the social structure represents the context in which each person negotiates his/her identity, belief systems, and life course. The social structure is the seed bed from which values emerge. Depending upon the social structure of which one is a part and to which values one has been conditioned, values of the client and the mental health professional may be quite similar or dramatically different. The point of course is not that value sets are in themselves normal or abnormal, they simply "are."

As entities which shape and motivate individual behavior, value sets are a complex mix of individual psychology about the types of initiative and action which are appropriate and the sociological or contextual limits which define, permit, and reinforce or constrain such individual behavior. Unless such individual-environmental interaction is understood by mental health professionals, differential value sets and their relationships to cultural diversity are not likely to be fully appreciated as ways by which clients organize their personal realities.

Cultural diversity in client populations have other implications as well. As was suggested in the previous section on test bias, since psychological tests examine samples of individual behavior, the cultural milieu of the individual will be reflected in his/her test performance. In this regard Anastasi (1982) has noted the following:

> Each culture fosters and encourages the development of behavior that is adapted to its values and demands. When an individual must adjust to and compete within a culture or subculture other than that in which he or she was reared then cultural difference is likely to become cultural disadvantage. (p. 286)

Therefore, what is considered to be an objective assessment instrument within a majority culture, may not be so within a minority culture or for persons from a cultural orientation different from that on which the instrument was standardized.

Such perspectives remind us that decision-making, the development of self-identity, and life chances do not only occur within political, economic, and social conditions that influence the achievement images and belief systems on which individuals base their actions. They occur within different cultural constructions which reinforce certain types of behavior and try to extinguish others. They occur within different provisions of mechanisms by which to assist the individual to deal with questions of cultural identity, achievement, illness.

Instances of Cultural Diversity

If one assumes that the pluralism of the United States is reflected in the continuing immigration which it permits, the arranging of many of its citizens into culturally defined neighborhoods however they are described—e.g., ghetto, barrio, etc.—or the residual effects across generations of family roots which originated in other nations, then the controversial question becomes, Does the equalitarian premise of the American creed, "All men are created equal" mean that "All people are pretty much alike?" Or, do psychological characteristics actually differ across groups and have behavioral implications which have some predictability?

Peabody (1985) has recently studied national psychological characteristics. His research has compared psychological characteristics among the English, Germans, French, Italians, Russians, the American, Northern and Southern Europeans, Swiss, Irish, Finns, Dutch, Southern and Eastern Europeans, Austrians, Greeks, Turks, Czechs, Hungarian, Spanish, and Phillipinos. He also has summarized other major works concerned with the examination of intercultural diversity across national groups. On balance, this work suggests that when national psychological characteristics are compared, partial differences rather than complete differences occur among groups. Some behavioral manifestations tend to overlap across nations while others are quite different. Another tenet of his study is that national characteristics are due to historical developments and therefore they can and do change over time. Some national psychological characteristics change rapidly under the onslaught of technology, for example, or occupation by foreign troops, while other national character changes are much more subtle and slow.

Peabody and his research colleagues in the several nations with which his study was concerned used scales composed of trait-adjectives to differentiate national groups on the basis of such major behavioral sets as tight vs. loose control over impulse-expression and self-assertiveness vs. unassertiveness. The varieties of trait-adjectives comprising the 14 scales used in his study assessed both descriptive and evaluative dimensions of national character. Pairs of adjectives such as thrifty-extravagant, inflexible-flexible, inhibited-spontaneous, cooperative-uncooperative, cautious-rash, opportunistic-idealistic, peaceful-aggressive are exemplars of the substance which alternately went into factor loadings and studies of variance among native and out-of-country observers.

Perhaps the most striking result of the Peabody study is the finding that psychological characteristics of the national groups which were targets of the investigation are distinguishable and consistent (p. 57). Time and space does not permit an analysis of the specific psychological characteristics found to characterize each of the national groups or their similarities or contrasts with other groups. In summary the national groups tended to have comparative differences on the basis of (1) social relationships, (2) social rules, (3) control of hostility, (4) impulse control, and (5) authority and hierarchial relations. Clearly the variations in how each of these differences is reinforced and portrayed in a particular nation are internalized by many, if not most, of the individuals in that national group. Thus, modal behavior for one national group is likely to be different from that for other groups. Indeed, the rules for interaction or action in a situation are largely cultural with respect to private and public relationships, the formality of communications, and the intimacy of spontaneity by which such relationships are conducted (p. 31).

Roots of Intercultural Diversity

Obviously, the historical influences on international cultural diversity have diverse origins and timing. The Protestant ethic and the Calvinist traditions with regard to work and achievement have been similar for Americans and English as compared with the lack of effects of such influences on the Russians or French or Italians. On the other hand, the latter two groups have been influenced by the Catholic and Latin traditions much more than the English or Americans or Germans. The Russians and Germans have been imbued differently with supra-individual goals, communal feelings, and solidarity. This is true of many other groups. The latter can be conceived as relating to the contrasts between Gemeinschaft relationships and Gesellschaft relationships and the transitions between these relationship clusters as nations have evolved from primary, peasant, tribal, small community social orders to more complex, impersonal, secondary, socially differentiated, interaction patterns (Parsons, 1951; Lipsett, 1963). *Gemeinschaft* relationships are likely to be particularistic, ascriptive, and broad. In such a model, family and friends are treated much differently than other people, standards of treatment of people are differently applied, people are related to in terms of their birth and ascribed status not their actual performance, and their relationships tend to be broad and communal. On the other hand, *Gesellschaft* relationships are likely to be more characterized by universalism in standards applied to people regardless of background, people are more likely to be treated in relation to achievement or performance than their ascribed status, and relationships are more likely to be limited than broad.

When one turns away from European and Christian traditions to the East, to the Chinese and to the Japanese, one finds the major influences of Confucism, Zen Buddhism, and the Code of Bushido. Here we find family fidelity, self-discipline, social bonding, and public and private virtues which are different in behavioral manifestation from those found in the national character of European nations.

Research across national psychological groupings demonstrates that national groupings are not just political units but psychocultural shapers and reinforcers of behaviors culturally distinctive, at least in part, from other national groupings. Vaizey and Clarke (1976) have suggested that nations create social metaphors as the bases for personality characteristics, child-rearing practices, education, and other social organizations. Concepts such as the "socialist personality" used in a nation such as East Germany to define those behavioral traits which youth and adults should try to emulate are not simply slogans, they are filters of information, sanctions of conduct, psychological boundaries, and seedbeds for value formulation. As Gestalt Psychology and, more recently, the work of the cognitive therapists has demonstrated, human perception and judgment are determined by the organization and, indeed, the availability of information from the outside world. As Snygg and Combs (1949) stated many years ago, one behaves as one perceives. The fact is that one is taught what to perceive and how to behave and such teachings are different across societies. "These differential schedules of reinforcement result in cultural differences in perceptual selectivity, information-processing strategies, cognitive structures, and habits" (Triandis, 1985, p. 22). According to Triandis (1972), cognitive structures may best be summarized by different elements of subjective culture such as categorizations of experience, associations among the categories, attitudes, beliefs, behavioral intentions (self-instructions about how to behave), norms, roles, and values.

Also other types of confirmation of international cultural diversity exists in terms that matter to cross-cultural counseling and therapy. One such form of evidence of cultural diversity lies with the way in which psychological disorders are viewed across national groups or cultures. For example, Draguns (1985) has reported that "while large-scale multicultural investigations have demonstrated that the same major disorders occur in a variety of very different cultures, ...a wealth of research reports have documented the operations of cultural influences upon the manifestations, course, and outcome of psychological disorder" (p. 55). For example, experiences of personal guilt in depressions are predominant in countries with a Judeo-Christian heritage but infrequent or atypical in settings with other religious traditions. In schizophrenia, ideational and paranoid symptomatology is characteristic of countries at a higher level of economic development and high rates of literacy. Catatonic manifestations are prevalent in many traditional, rural, and non-industrialized settings (p. 56). Similarly, among American ethnic groups class-related, culturally, and religiously based differences in psychiatric symptoms have also been observed (Dohrenwend & Dohrenwend, 1974).

Kleinman (1980), a psychiatrist trained in Anthropology, has done extensive cross-cultural studies on medicine and psychiatry, particularly in Taiwan. His work focuses on three major elements: illness experiences, practitioner-patient transactions, and the healing process. One of his major conclusions is that,

> in the same sense in which we speak of religion or kinship as cultural systems, we can view medicine as a cultural systems, a system of symbolic meanings anchored in particular arrangements of social institutions and patterns of interpersonal interactions. In every culture, illness, the responses to it, individuals experiencing it and treating it, and the social relationships relating to it are all systematically interconnected... These include patterns of belief about the causes of illness, norms governing choice and evaluation of treatment; socially-legitimated statuses, roles, power relationships, interactions settings, and institutions... (p. 24)

> Patients and healers are basic components of such systems and thus are embedded in specific configurations of cultural meanings and social relationships. They cannot be understood apart from this context. (p. 25)

Further, beliefs about sickness, the behaviors exhibited by sick persons, including their treatment expectations, and the ways in which sick people are responded to by family and practitioners are all aspects of "social reality" in a particular culture; in this sense, clinical practice, the range of clinical phenomena in a particular culture, and conceptions of illness are cultural constructions, systems of symbolic reality not entities with absolute, unequivocal reality across all people and cultures. These culturally-mediated symbolic realities enable individuals to make sense out of their inner experiences. These realities help shape personal identity in accordance with social and cultural norms. In this view, symbolic meanings influence basic psychological processes, such as attention, state of consciousness, perception, cognition, affect, memory, and motivation (p. 42).

Transportability of Models of Counseling and Therapy Across Cultures

In pluralistic societies such as our own, a mix may exist of social and individual expectations for the outcomes of counseling services, particularly as they are provided to different population sub-groups. Beyond that point, however, the provisions of counseling services can be stated fairly as significantly affected by the characteristics of the society in which they are found. In this sense, in every nation, counseling, social work, marriage and family therapy, career guidance, psychotherapy, and other mental health services are sociopolitical processes which reflect the values which individual nations attribute to helping its citizens with various types of personal, career, or psychological problems. But, such provisions also vary because, in essence, every counseling approach is a form of environmental modification which carries political overtones through the assumptions and value sets inherent in it.

If the cultural characteristics of a nation and the value sets inherent in a particular counseling approach do not match, such a counseling approach is not likely to have adherents and is not likely to be successful in that particular action. As Reynolds (1980), among others, has reported, western psychotherapists have a particular way of looking at and processing human behavior; eastern psychotherapies have a different way of defining behavioral norms and intervening in them. One set of therapies is not necessarily a substitute for the other because cultural value sets and assumptions make some forms of counseling and psychotherapy ineffective or unacceptable in nations or cultures different from those in which such interventions were formulated. For example, psychoanalytic therapy has not acquired much clinical popularity in Japan despite its rather wide acceptance in Europe and less but substantial support in the United States. The explanation seems to lie with the fact that psychoanalytic theory values such behavior as individualization, self-consciousness, and independence from parents as prized therapeutic outcomes. These are not the behavioral norms of Japan. Confucianism the code of Bushido, Zen Buddhism, and related philosophical guides to Japanese behavior values family unity and respect, loyalty to others, subjugation of individualism to group identity, self-discipline, and gratitude to others.

Speaking to the transportability of counseling theories, Saner-Yiu & Saner (1985) contended in their research that the value assumptions embedded in counseling approaches derived from an individualist culture (e.g., the U.S.A.) are in conflict in their adoption in a collectivist nation (e.g., Taiwan). Others addressing counseling in African and in Middle eastern nations have indicated that many assumptions taken for granted in some cultures are simply not shared across cultures: e.g., "I" consciousness, rights to private life and opinion, individual initiative and achievement, the forms and content of interpersonal relationship (Shanhirzadi, 1983; Okon, 1983).

Against the type of cross-cultural perspectives just described, Sue (1983) urged the helping profession to acknowledge the shortcomings of attempting to resolve ethnic minority issues or cross-cultural controversies relating to the uses of counseling and psychotherapy by utilizing convergent reasoning in an attempt to arrive at "the solution." Sue argued for the incorporation of divergent reasoning in attempts to gain cultural sensitivity. Rather than forcing a dichotomy between etic and emic perspectives as we described them at the beginning of this section, Sue advocated a synthesis of the two, emphasizing their complementarity in the attempt to understand human nature. This viewpoint is a departure from past tendencies to opt for singular definitions of culture and values with regard to the goals of counseling and psychotherapy. Such an approach is itself controversial because it can result in discomfort on the part of the counselor who must accept a certain degree of ambiguity required to acknowledge the need for cultural pluralism rather than assuming the validity of generalizing a specific value system and world view to all clients.

CONCLUSION

Every technique used in the mental health profession and each model of behavior which guides the application of interventions carries within itself, the potential to elicit controversy. The reasons for such a conclusion vary. In some instances, the assumptions about why techniques are to be used or their intended outcomes are not clear or are insufficiently based on empirical information. In some circumstances, the fundamental explanations for the emergence of or changes in behavior are interpreted quite differently by varying groups of mental health professionals. The theoretical systems which explain the etiology of different types of behavior, their course, and how they may be altered place greater or lesser emphases on biological, social, or psychological factors. Therefore, controversy ensues among and between professional groups who weight these factors in dissimilar ways.

Perhaps the most controversial element in either models of behavior and their classification or in the intervention techniques used is that dealing with the effects of cultural distinctiveness of clients. Can tests or psychotherapies, for example, developed in one cultural context be used in another? How do test and psychotherapies impose values on clients which are not shared across all cultures? These are the growing roots of controversies within the professional ranks of mental health service providers and between such providers and persons representing minority or other culturally distinct groups.

THEME SIX: ECONOMICS

CHAPTER 9

THE ECONOMICS OF MENTAL HEALTH PROFESSIONS

Mental health services use resources and reduce the cost of services. The question is what is the cost-benefit ratio of such services in relation to not providing such services at all and in relation to their impact on other aspects of the health care system. In a national climate of cost containment of social and health services, the cost-effectiveness of mental health services within institutions and among private providers has become both important and controversial.

Another major category of controversy is that of third-party payment. Federal legislation, insurance carriers, and other third-party payers are not consistent with regard to which mental health professions can be reimbursed for services provided. In many third-party payment situations, physicians are the dominant persons who must refer to or supervise other mental health care providers. This condition elicits interprofessional tensions, identity questions, and other issues of controversy.

As the provision of mental health care has moved from institutional settings increasingly to private practice settings, it has engendered increased concern about credentialing, education and training, supervision, regulation, and other matters which are ultimately translated into economic questions such as who can be paid for what, under what conditions, and from what sources?

Many of the controversies in the helping professions are economic in origin or economic in outcome. Typically, such economic issues are tied to issues of power, credentialing, training, identity, political actions, or history. These factors are frequently interactive, rather than divisible and independent. As has been indicated in other chapters each of these factors is at the heart of the controversies among mental health practitioners and between such professional groups and the public—defined as either clients, policy-makers, or insurance bodies.

Whether interactive with other factors or not, the economic dimensions of the helping professions are sufficiently important subjects of controversy to be considered in their own right. While many forms of controversy are at issue in the economic arena as it pertains to the helping professions, at least three broad categories of concern tend to be at the center of such discussions. One is the matter of fee-setting in private practice. The second has to do with the substance of third-party payment and who is eligible to receive it. The third concerns the costs/benefits of different forms of mental health delivery and the comparative status on such a criterion of different groups of mental health professionals.

Each of the three categories of economic controversy elicits differing levels of emotionality and complexity within the helping professions. The ensuing discussion will focus on the major issues which arise in each category and their effects upon the helping professions.

FEE SETTING IN PRIVATE PRACTICE

The delivery of mental health services in the United States has become increasingly a matter between a private practitioner or a group of mental health specialists in private practice and a client(s). As government support for mental health services at the institutional or community level erodes and larger proportions of the population become clients, under their own volition for personal enhancement or for remedial and therapeutic reasons or because they have been referred by employers to psychologists or counselors, the matter of fee-setting becomes an area of controversy among mental health practitioners in private practice, between practitioners and clients, and between practitioners and those groups in the community who might contract for their services.

Due to the differential availability of third party payments to different types of mental health providers, even though each charges the same amount per hour of service, patients may pay a larger proportion of fees in some situations than in others. For an example, in a study of the patients of psychiatrists and psychologists in independent, office-based practice, Taube, Burns, and Kessler (1984) found in a national study that

> psychologists' patients pay a higher percentage of their costs for ambulatory mental health care out of pocket, 55% of the annual costs for visits to psychologists, as opposed to 33% for visits to psychiatrists... The highest proportion of out-of-pocket expenditures 'for psychiatrists' patients is for those with under 4 visits (55%) which may be a function of deductibles for mental disorder coverage. (p. 1442)

This proportion drops to 28% after 4 visits for psychiatrists but remains at over 50% for psychologists. Another way to look at these differences also is provided by Taube, Burns, and Kessler who reported that in comparison of coverage under government programs, 43% of psychiatrists' charges are paid by government sources compared to 22% for psychologists' charges (p. 1443).

Contractors for mental health services are not always third-party payers in the traditional sense; they will be discussed in the next section. Rather a growing stratum of community organizations contract with mental health specialists in private practice to provide services to employees or others. For example, Employee Assistance Program are typically funded by business, educational, and industrial organizations to provide mental health services to "problem employees," persons with chemical dependency, emotional, or family problems which interfere with their work productivity. In order to preserve the privacy within the work place of those workers referred for treatment, many industrial organizations prefer not to provide mental health treatment themselves. Instead, they contract with private mental health practitioners outside of the organization to provide such treatment. In such cases, fees for service become a major issue. Another example of such contractual arrangements occurs with base service units charged with providing mental health/mental retardation services in a community. Frequently, such community MH/MR units do not have the funds to create the full-time staff necessary to meet the demands upon their services. Therefore, they hire part-time staff or contract with other mental health specialists on a fee-for-service basis to maximize the services their budgets will permit. Ordinarily, hiring a part-time staff or paying for the contractual time of specialists in private practice reduces overhead costs (e.g., fringe benefits for staff and housing) to the agency thus permitting a greater percentage of the mental health dollar to be spent on direct services to clients. Usually, however, such governmentally funded, community-based organizations have restrictions on how much they can pay for each therapist hour. Often this rate is substantially lower than that charged by mental health practitioners in private practice and causes controversy to ensue among those practitioners who accept such lower fees for service and those practitioners who believe that to accept such lower fees is to undercut the system of fees for service being charged in a community by private practitioners.

The controversy surrounding contractual fees for services as just described, while a raging controversy in some communities, is really benign in comparison with other issues in this economic area. The more important controversy applies to the use of a fee as a therapeutic issue in its own right.

Fee as a Therapeutic Issue

Professional literature often contains opinions or theories regarding the therapeutic value of charging fees for mental health services. Among those of interest are the views of such persons as Adams (1968), Dightmen (1970), Mintz (1971), and Pope, Weller, and Wildinson (1975).The problem is, however, that most of these views are speculative, not empirical in origin. Bugental (1968), Kades and Winich (1968), and Kanter and Kanter (1977) are among those who have called attention to the lack of research about the effects of financial transactions among providers and consumers of mental health services.

At least three primary issues surround the matter of fees for mental health services. One has to do with the prevailing view in the clinical and social work literature that fees in themselves are therapeutic to the client. For example, if the client pays for help, he/she is making an investment in getting well; the client is taking responsibility for his/her improvement and this is itself therapeutic (Dightman, 1970). A second issue is, Does fee paying generate sufficient revenues to make a significant contribution to the maintenance of services? The issue here is not only the therapeutic value of fee paying by the client but the more practical one of suggesting that with a combined contribution by the consumer and by government, the services provided will be of a better quality, more comprehensive, more available, and off-setting to the reduction of government subsidies. A third issue has to do with whether fees create a form of unintended economic discrimination by deterring certain clients from expressing their needs for services (Newkirk, 1983) or, indeed, from using the services available. In other places in this book, we have indicated controversies about the alleged middle or upper class biases which tend to be built into traditional forms of mental health delivery in private practice and in many governmentally supported delivery services. Particularly at risk in this regard are the inner city minority populations and the rural poor.

Newkirk's review (1983) of the systematic study of fees for mental health services indicated that the three issues cited previously have not been dealt with as outcome measures or, in the few cases where they have been addressed, the results have been contradictory.

Fee in the Counseling Relationship

Whether or not a substantial research literature is available for dealing with the fee-for-service, the matter of billing for services rendered or receiving money directly from clients is an important and controversial issue for both neophyte and experienced mental health specialists. A number of observers have decried the lack of training in psychiatry or social work about money matters. Undoubtedly, the training of other mental health specialists is equally devoid of attention to this issue.

Pasternack (1977) has written about the psychotherapy fee as an issue in psychiatric residency training. He described the range of behaviors of psychiatric residents in dealing with patients for whom a low fee sliding scale is based upon different income and insurance characteristics. In the institution he studied, residents were to assign fees during the intake and evaluation period and were supposed to supervise payment of fees to the clinic. In investigating why the clinic was receiving very little income even though a large volume of outpatient visits had occurred, the evidence was that resident behavior was quite variable with regard to fee setting. Some residents set fees below established clinic norms or engaged in other outlandish practices. Some simply ignored the matter and never mentioned the fees to their patients. Some colluded with the patients to undercut the fee schedule or to allow large outstanding bills to continue to be unpaid. Such behaviors were seen to affect the substance of the therapy and the therapeutic relationship in various ways.

Pasternack described a number of patterns of patient and resident behaviors which related to "fee misconduct." One common patient pattern was the request for a lower fee. These requests were most often more inappropriate than realistic and were frequently efforts by the patients to test the psychiatric residents' willingness "to abet dependency." Some residents easily succumbed to these patient wishes to be treated with "special indulgence" without considering the dependency issues implicit in the demands. Other patients were "patently sociopathic and manipulative" in their fee negotiations with the resident therapists. Some were overtly dishonest in falsifying the income information they provided to the clinic. In some instances, resident were successful in using such behavior as therapeutic material which reveals much about their socialization within the family, the engrained sociopathic traits inherent, guilt feelings about exploiting others, and the distrust of others with regard to monetary matters. In some instances the profound guilt which attended the dishonesty and falsification of monetary matters gave rise to severe psychosomatic problems which also provided important therapeutic material.

In other instances, particularly where a third party payer was involved, patients frequently tried to avoid direct responsibility for the services being provided to them. Again, coercing the resident into taking responsibility for obtaining such payment often revealed immaturity, dependency, and unwillingness to take responsibility for other aspects of their lives. Some patients would make a claim for insurance but did not want the clinic to provide accurate information to the payer.

On some occasions, residents encountered patients who simply refused to pay or to recognize the right of the clinic to charge a fee. Such cases also provided an opportunity to set limits and to cause such patients to live up to their part of the relationship.

Pasternack suggested that while in such instances the therapist might be tempted to focus on the non-payment of the fee as the primary issue, in fact non-payment may have more important implications: resistance to therapy, infantile adaptations, social pathological manipulation, dependency, and other therapeutic matters. Failure to look more deeply at such fee-paying behavior can corrupt the therapy if not actually destroy the therapeutic relationship. Pasternack strongly urged that residents be helped to deal realistically with the setting and collecting of fees just as residents are asked to help establish other boundaries in therapy. The recommendation is further that residents understand the many meanings attached to the fee and the complex emotional issues which patients act out via deviant fee behavior. The most effective stance seems to be the need for a firm policy about fees with an empathetic understanding that fee behavior is part of overall therapeutic work. Finally, also important is the understanding that fee setting remains controversial within therapy, particularly in regard to such issues as charging for missing scheduled appointments and the ambivalence which fee-setting and collection causes therapists themselves.

Beginner Anxiety. The controversial character of fee-setting and collection in mental health services is not confined to psychiatric residents in training. Randolph (1975) has described the problems of beginning a private practice in psychiatric nursing including the problems associated with fees. Adler and Gutheil (1977) have discussed the problems which accompany the establishment of fees in beginning private practice for psychiatrists and for social workers after the completion of a training or clinic experience. They discuss the issues of beginner anxiety: "giving," "getting," and fees; and fees and the transference-countertransference interface. These will be summarized in turn.

"Beginner anxiety" may appear in several forms with regard to fees and may involve issues of self-esteem, narcissism, entitlement, and competitive elements. Indeed, the beginner may react in an overall sensitive manner to just starting out. Such circumstances may manifest themselves in several ways. One may be to charge less than the going rate in a local area. While this procedure may reflect the practitioners' concerns about being new and relatively less experienced than other practitioners in the area, it may be seen by others as undervaluation of one's work or of undercutting others. Other manifestations of beginner anxiety take the form of obsessional behavior about the language and appearance of the billing form or how one announces one's fees, whether one identifies one's therapeutic sessions as hours, appointments, meetings, or something else, as well as an overemphasis/underemphasis on avoidance of the fee as an issue. In the latter case, the practitioner may allow the bill to accumulate excessively because of traumatic feelings about confronting the patient about the bill.

Giving and Getting. Part of the controversy which surrounds "beginner anxiety" is probably an extension of a lack of understanding of deviant fee behavior as a therapeutic issue previously described by Pasternack. But certainly another controversial element is practitioner identity with regard to "giving" and "getting." Some mental health professionals conceive their roles as altruistic, benevolent, and giving. Thus, they conceive of charging a fee or handing a patient a bill as an aggressive act toward the patient; as an act incompatible with their views of how counselors should act. They consciously or unconsciously feel guilty and sometimes expect transference problems associated with the fee for which they themselves create countertransference problems. In some instances, mental health practitioners become healers in order to get back what they give: caretaking, love, etc. Thus, fee charging is conflictual to them because they are afraid that it will interfere with the client responses which the healer is unconsciously seeking. Schonbar (1967) put it well when he stated:

> Some therapists feel guilt about "selling" a human relationship, seeing it as a kind of prostitution. Similarly, there are those who, despite Freud's admonition (in his 1913 paper "On Beginning the Treatment"), cannot admit of the crass businesslike aspects of the treatment situation in terms of satisfying their own needs for status and security.

Transference-countertransference. A further controversy identified by Adler and Gutheil is described as "fees and the transference-countertransference interface." In this view, fees for service can elicit from clients a wide range of transference behavior such as anger or comparative/competitive elements and counter-transference phenomena such as inhibition. At the heart of such transference-countertransference phenomena are client unwillingness to assume adult responsibility for payment, or feelings that a lower fee than is typical among practitioners means that the therapy is less good and in fact devalues the patient. The therapist's counter-transference behavior tends to symbolize an unwillingness to confront the patient about money matters or an inhibition to press the therapy in particular ways because of fear that it may increase anger or other resistances rather than seeking these as therapeutic material to be worked on.

Credit for Treatment. The problem of how much to charge the patient and how to present and collect the fee are continuing dilemmas even for experienced practitioners. Indeed, it is overlaid with another complication: Should one extend credit to patients in treatment? Hofling and

Rosenbaum (1980), two psychiatrists in private practice, have studied this question among some 157 psychoanalysts and psychotherapists. Hofling and Rosenbaum start from the premise, first advanced by Freud, that

> the classic stance of the analyst has been that he "leases his time" to the patient on a contractual basis. The patient is expected to pay promptly and regularly for his or her assigned four or five hours per week, regardless of whether or not there is any apparent benefit or even whether or not the patient appears for his appointed hours. (pp. 327-328)

Aside from these practical matters, Hofling and Rosenbaum also recognized the central significance of the transference-countertransference elements involved in the financial transaction.

Into this mix of practical and theoretical elements of the economics of patient-therapist negotiations about fees is that of extending credit to the patient and the effects of such a procedure on the course of therapy. In order to investigate this situation, Hofling and Rosenbaum distributed an extensive questionnaire to some 250 psychiatrists who were primarily engaged in intensive long-term therapy and were thoroughly trained in dynamic psychiatry so that they would recognize and attend to subtle changes in transference and countertransference phenomena associated with the extending of credit. They received 157 usable responses to their questionnaire.

Several findings are interesting. One is that most of the psychiatrists in the subject pool did extend credit to patients. The great majority of patients gave evidence that such a procedure had a favorable effect on them. However, also noted was that both transference and countertransference phenomena were observed in the majority of the cases showing unfavorable effects. This finding was seen by the researchers as suggesting that when patient and therapist fail to distinguish (emotionally) between realistic and subjective aspects of their relationship or transaction in an element such as the introduction of a credit extension, the procedure is likely to be associated with adverse effects. Another interesting experience is that some therapists always seemed to have favorable results with extending credit; other had almost uniformly unfavorable results. While the data available to speak to such a finding were limited, the finding does suggest that therapists differed in the emotional context or skill with which money matters with patients are handled and how such concerns are treated within the therapeutic situation itself.

**Medical-Nonmedical
Practitioner Fees**

Sax (1978), a clinical social worker in private practice, reviewed a number of the professional and psychosocial dynamics of fee setting from both rational and nonrational points of view. Many of these have been discussed previously in this chapter and will not be reiterated here. However, she made several additional observations that deserve consideration. One is that nonmedical practitioners—e.g., psychologists, social workers, counselors, marriage and family therapists—almost uniformly charge less than psychiatrists. Why? Is this a function of identity, of skill, of competence? It is probably a function of one's view of the social attribution, the identity hierarchy, ascribed to psychiatrists as medical doctors compared to other types of healers.

A second issue is what should determine the monetary yardstick applied to psychotherapy or counseling? Aside from supply and demand considerations, how much is psychotherapy worth? Depending upon its outcomes it may, in fact, be priceless or worthless. Aside from such a matter, the question is what does a fee represent? The therapist's time? The therapist's training or skills? Outcomes? The issue is not clear and, indeed, the philosophical potential of such questions may obscure the practical necessities of earning a sufficient income to warrant remaining in private practice. In the latter regard Sax suggested that as a mental health practitioner one has both a personal self and a professional self. In the first instance, it becomes necessary to bring into focus one's own individual and private relationship to money. In the second instance, it becomes important to examine the implications of money as a transference object. Each of these selves and each of these meanings of money become important aspects of the economics of mental health services and, indeed, of the controversy surrounding such economic issues.

THIRD-PARTY PAYMENT

Fee setting, the transference and countertransference implications of money, and the particulars of the mental health practitioner's personal and professional identities are each highly significant issues when economic matters are between the client and the practitioner. However, an equally important if not overarching matter in the economics of the mental health professions concerns "Third Party Payers." In such circumstances, the client or patient does not directly pay for services, an insurance company or other third party does.

Third-Party Payers

While the number of third party payers increases, a number of carriers tend to be frequently used as the source of funds for mental health services: governmental sources including Medicaid, Medicare, Social Security Act rehabilitation, Worker's Compensation, CHAMPUS; and insurance companies including Blue Cross/Blue Shield, Aetna, Metropolitan, Travelers, Prudential, and Occidental. As will be discussed later, these third-party sources differ in their reimbursement guidelines from state to state and with regard to who is an eligible provider. Indeed, except for psychiatrists, the opportunity for other mental health specialists to participate in fee for service, private practice and thereby seek third part reimbursement is a phenomenon which has emerged in significant magnitude only since 1970.

Even so, however, psychiatrists have not been without their own difficulties in securing reimbursement for their services. Fink (1978) has described in some detail the politics of funding as it has benefitted medical and surgical trainees and practitioners to the detriment of psychiatrists. He suggested that such circumstances have left the field 10,000 psychiatrists short in the United States, decreased the pool of available candidates for training in psychiatry, causing psychiatry to become seriously dependent on foreign medical graduates to fill positions in training programs as well as in community mental health centers and mental health clinics. Fink indicated, for example, that in 1975-76, on a nationwide basis, 50%, and in some states, as many as 90% of all psychiatrists in the *public sector* are foreign medical school graduates.

In Fink's view, the economic problems of training and practice in psychiatry have caused problems of identity internal to the field and brought it under "heavy pressure from the other mental health professions (psychology, social work, psychiatric nursing) for equal privileges, reimbursement, and their "piece of the action. The medical leadership of the team is attacked and disputed. Third party payers wish to exclude or severely limit the annual and lifetime payments for psychiatric services in future national health insurance and health maintenance organizations (p. 16). In this view psychiatry becomes unique among medical specialities, as the only one in which practice methods are dictated by funding sources.

Fink also argued that another bit of evidence, also economic in origin, which demonstrates psychiatry's diminished position in the community is the rash of anti-psychiatric, protect-the-patient, right-to-treatment laws. The latter essentially places the psychiatrist in competition with psychologists and other mental health specialists seeking third party reimbursement for mental health services.

As suggested elsewhere in this book, mental health counselors, clinical social workers, psychiatric nurses and marriage and family therapists are meeting with differing degrees of success in obtaining licensure to practice as an independent mental health specialist and less frequently to obtain third-party payment as well. Psychologists have been much more successful in achieving such opportunities although they are not always eligible for all possible third-party payment or for such reimbursement without referral or supervision by a physician.

At this time, all 50 states have psychologist licensure/certification statutes. By 1979, 29 states and the District of Columbia had legislation recognizing psychologists as qualified, independent health practitioners eligible for direct insurance reimbursement. In most instances, these states have what has come to be known as freedom-of-choice (FOC) laws in which consumers or third-party payers can choose psychiatrists or psychologists or sometimes other mental health specialists to provide specified types of mental health services. In addition, since 1974 or so, the U.S. Congress has passed a number of different laws in which the practice of psychology has been recognized as being eligible for various types of reimbursement from federal health plans or insurance sources. These include such early and prototypic pieces of legislation as PL 93-112, the Rehabilitation Act of 1973; PL 93-363, the Federal Employee Health Benefits Acts; PL 93-416, Federal Employee Compensation Act as amended; PL 93-222, the Health Maintenance Organization Act. Each of these acts recognized psychologists as eligible to receive health care benefits within various changes in independent insurance plans or state provisions by which psychologists as well as psychiatrists or other recognized providers could be eligible for third-party reimbursement (Dorken & Webb, 1980). A major third-party payer which has considerable potential to affect the payment for and delivery of mental health services is the long proposed and debated National Health Insurance Plan if it were to include mental health benefits.

Controversy surrounding third-party payment takes many forms. As suggested in earlier sections of the book, it raises questions about what kinds of mental health specialists are eligible for third-party payments. Should such reimbursement be confined to "core providers" as was discussed in Chapter 1? If not, who and on what basis? In most states, to have received a license or a certificate as a mental health specialists of some type does not automatically make one eligible for third-party payment. It depends upon state statutes and, indeed, the extant regulations of the individual third-party payers about what can be reimbursed and who can be reimbursed. Each of these issues and others leads to diverse forms of controversy.

Does Third-Party Payment Increase Consumption of Mental Health Services?

As discussed earlier in this chapter, fees can be potential deterrents to the use of mental health services or they can possibly lead to economic discrimination among consumers. Obviously, such a charge also can be levied at many forms of third-party payment. Whether an individual does or does not have health insurance or insurance riders which reimburse for mental health services is likely to be linked to his/her affluence or socioeconomic status. Unless one is covered by Social Security or other blanket coverage participation in insurance is likely to be voluntary, expensive, and not acquired by all individuals or families. Thus, reimbursements for mental health services are not available under insurance plans or other arrangements to many people who could use the benefits but cannot afford the premiums. This is one of the reasons why some observers argue for National Health Insurance, an issue we will come to a bit later. As we will note then, such insurance coverage is itself a source of controversy.

One of the sources of controversy surrounding third-party payment is the assumption held by some persons in the insurance industry that third-party payment actually increases the consumption of mental health services. Indeed, variations on this theme suggest the insurance industry's fear that (1) people would bring a mental illness on themselves or would use treatment for self-actualization and (2) they fear the risk of providing never-ending treatment for incurable illness (Sharfstein, 1978). Underlying such controversies is the reality that mental illness in the United States is not seen in the same way that physical illness is. In general, unlike the physically ill person, the mentally ill individual is frequently considered to be responsible for causing or bringing on an anxiety state, depression, or an alcohol problem. According to Sharfstein:

> Despite recent developments, many people feel that serious mental illness is incurable and drains public and private resources of society. The issues of public support for the lion's share of mental treatment is also related to the fact that different types of mental illness are related to social class. Studies associating the most severe pathologies with the lower social classes maintain the poorhouse image for treatment of the mentally ill.... Thus at the one extreme private insurance companies are wary of mental health coverage because of the "moral hazard" of people bringing a mental illness on themselves or seeking self-actualization or self-fulfillment through mental treatment, and at the other extreme they are wary of the thousands of the incurables who languish in custodial institutions. The insurers fear that either extreme will bring financial ruin to an insurance program. (p. 1186)

Is the Medical Model the Only One Reimbursable? While a number of studies refute the views of insurance companies about mental illness (see later sections of this chapter) and argue for greater education of third party payers by groups of mental health specialists and the professional associations which represent them, the concern here is the substance of the controversy which inhibits the extension or the comprehensiveness of third-party payments for mental health services. Sharfstein, speaking from a psychiatric view of third-party coverage, suggested that the rapid increases in health care coverage in general causes third-party payers to insist that the "provider of care demonstrate that every dollar spent is for medically necessary and appropriate care." He observed that while most in-patient psychiatric care can be reviewed on the basis of admission criteria and length of stay norms, out-patient psychiatric care becomes more problematic especially where intensive psychotherapy and psychoanalysis are involved.

Sharfstein indicated that in terms of mental health coverage by third-party payers the following accountability issues are frequently raised:

1. What is the validity of the diagnosable condition? Is it a medical condition?

2. Is the treatment offered the most cost effective? Would shorter term individual treatment or group treatments produce an equally good result?

3. What are the qualifications of the person who provides the treatment? Since there is no board certification for intensive psychotherapy, who is qualified to conduct this technically demanding treatment? Why is a medical degree necessary for talking treatments? Which nonphysicians are qualified?

4. To what degree does the communication of information from the person who provides the treatment to the insurance carrier compromise the privacy of the therapist-patient relationship? How much peer review should be expected for this treatment? What about prior authorization? When does providing the information interfere with the treatment itself?

5. Finally, in any open-ended benefit structure, the question remains: At what point can you say that treatment has gone far enough and should go no farther? With psychotherapy, however, it is unlikely that a predictable increment of health will be evident with each increment of treatment. The phenomena of resistance, regression, and negative transference lead to a wave curve of treatment progress. (p. 1187)

Chodoff (1978), also a psychiatrist, extends a number of Sharfstein's issues with regard to the effects of third-party payment upon the practice of psychiatry, particularly that of private practice or office-delivered psychiatry. He suggested that among other issues of considerable importance, third-party payment has again caused the medical model to be a problem. (The reader will note that later in this chapter the Derner-Albee debate addresses this issue in a somewhat different but equally important manner.) According to Chodoff, the "medical model" is a term that is employed widely and generally rather loosely.

> It has been equated solely with organicity—one is not sick unless he or she has a demonstrable organic lesion. In a broader and more inclusive definition, "sickness" describes a form of deviant behavior with the following characteristics: It is negatively valued by society, it is involuntary—the individual displaying it is not responsible for his or her "sick" behavior—and it falls under the professional purview of physicians. Any individual satisfying these criteria assumes what has been called the "sick role" and becomes a "patient." (p. 1141)

Chodoff went on to suggest that some psychiatric patients simply do not lend themselves very well to the medical diagnostic process.

> In general, psychiatric patients seen in various settings include a very wide continuum of troubled human beings. At the unequivocally "medical" end of this spectrum are individuals with various forms of organic brain disease. Next are the major psychotic disorders, followed successively by the symptomatic neuroses and the personality disorders included and described in DSM II. However, psychiatrists also treat some patients with more or less serious character deformations resulting in persistent maladaptive disturbances that do not conform specifically to the DSM II categories (this is also true, although possibly to a lesser extent, of the broader and more inclusive DSM III). Legitimate differences exist as to where along this continuum the division should be made, but it is clear that the patients at one end comprise a very different population from the "patients" at the other end and that the latter can be included under even an elastic definition of the medical model only with a good deal of Procrustean manipulation. (p. 1142)

Chodoff suggested that perhaps the most important question facing psychiatry as a profession is the medical model question—to what extent are psychiatrists, physicians, and the people they deal with professionally, patients? (p. 1142). This question obviously refers to the tension between those psychiatrists whose chief or only treatment modality is psychotherapy and those psychiatrists who identify more fully as physicians who offer a range of mental health treatments. For the former it also causes conflicts with nonmedically trained psychotherapists and other mental health specialists. He then went on to articulate the problems that third-party payers impose on the practice of psychiatry. One, of course, is that they want a definition, a diagnostic label, of the "illness" which the patient has. Thus, regardless of how a given psychiatrist feels about the validity of the medical model or how inappropriately or uncertain a previous diagnosis seems to fit a specific client, the psychiatrist must render one if the patient is to have his/her mental health treatment reimbursed by the third-party payer. This in turn brings up the significant issue of confidentiality. Does the patient want his/her diagnosis provided to the third-party payer? If not, how does this affect the therapeutic relationship or, indeed, the patient's continuation in therapy?

Beyond such issues, Chodoff also suggested that third-party payments are likely to increase both the supply of practitioners and of the patients who otherwise could not have afforded such treatment. It does some other things as well. Third-party reimbursement also influences the modalities, intensity, duration, and goals of treatment planning. The availability of such money may consciously or unconsciously make the difference in whether the client will receive long-term intensive psychotherapy or brief direct psychotherapy, whether the patient will be treated as an outpatient, in the office, or be hospitalized. It is also likely that the concerns for cost control by third-party payers will increase the likelihood of peer review and monitoring of the professional activities of their colleagues and the development of more rigid standards about when treatment of a particular kind, duration, or intensity is called for. The intent of third-party payers is to obtain direct and clear information which can be translated into payment criteria. Unfortunately, a major issue here is that a lack of outcome research in psychiatry makes it difficult to develop such third-party payment criteria.

DeMuth and Kamis (1980) examined the relationships between source of fee payment and volume of service utilization for 321 admissions to a county mental health system. What they found indicated that source of fee (e.g., public third-party sources including Medicaid, state welfare, county welfare, or self) was essentially unrelated to service utilization (e.g., in-patient day, partial hospitalization, individual or family therapy, crisis or group therapy, case management, medication check). The primary determinants of service utilization were clinical factors. Such findings provide information which helps to dispel fears that public third-party payments encourage overutilization of mental health services by needy, severely disabled clients. "The results also dispute the claims that clients utilize services more related to economic or provider variables than to characteristics of the client's mental disability" (p. 795). Of course, possibly different results would be achieved at a profit-making, proprietary institution.

Will the Poor Benefit from Third-Party Payments?

Implicit in the findings of DeMuth and Kamis and some of the earlier discussion in the section on fee-setting is whether the poor will benefit from such mental health provisions. Indeed, one of the major arguments against the provision of mental health benefits in National Health Insurance is that the poor and minority groups would not seek out psychotherapy under NHI (Albee, 1977). In essence, the contention has been that the NHI coverage for psychotherapy would represent a subsidy to the affluent by poorer citizens because the latter simply do not find available mental health services with their middle class bias to be appropriate for them.

Edwards, Greene, Abramowitz, and Davidson (1979) have suggested that the arguments in the professional literature about whether the disadvantaged would use psychotherapy fall into four categories of hypotheses. They include the following:

1. Attraction Hypothesis. Mental health professionals cannot create clinical settings that will attract the poor. Even if they could, the poor would not use them for help with mental or emotional problems.

2. Duration Hypothesis. Even if the poor sought treatment, they would receive fewer sessions than would more affluent groups.

3. Elitism Hypothesis if the poor were given treatment as extensive as that accorded the affluent, they would (a) receive second-class services such as medication clinics rather than elite services such as individual, group, or family psychotherapy; (b) be treated by nurses and social workers rather than by psychologists and psychiatrists; and (c) be treated by staff rather than by clinicians with faculty appointments.

4. Effectiveness Hypothesis. Even if the poor sought treatment and were offered the same quantity and quality of treatment as the more affluent, they would profit less. (p. 411-412)

These four hypotheses seem clearly to capture much of the conventional opinion and research dealing with the use of psychotherapy by poor and minority groups. However, Edwards, Greene, Abramowitz, and Davidson go on to refute each of these hypotheses. They did so first by reviewing the professional literature and suggesting that most of the bases for the conventional folklore about the lack of use of psychotherapy by the poor comes from research done before 1970. According to their analyses, more recent data, particularly that describing the impact of the National Community Mental Health Centers Program, describe programs that attract and are sought out by disadvantaged groups. In particular, they note the research from the nationwide community Mental Health Centers Program which indicated that the poor constitute the majority of admissions with 84% of persons provided treatment in 1973 having incomes under $10,000 (Sharfstein, Taube, & Goldberg, 1977). Edwards et al. also found mixed results in the literature regarding the relationship of socioeconomic status or education to length of treatment. No studies could be found which literally suggested a relationship between income level and quality or status of psychotherapeutic services delivery; certainly the data about Community Mental Health Centers Programs did not suggest such links. Finally, the literature about lower socioeconomic class individuals benefitting less from psychotherapy than did those from higher socioeconomic levels also was found to be equivocal. Lorion (1974), for example, found from his review of available studies that psychotherapeutic outcome did not differ according to class membership.

Based upon the literature dealing with the four hypotheses previously identified, Edwards et al. (1979) designed an experiment to directly test each of the hypotheses cited with different samples of adult and child outpatients served in a consortium of community mental health centers providing mental health services in Sacramento County, California. Their findings did not support many of the major reservations about including coverage for psychotherapy under NHI or, by extension, other third-party payment programs. Specifically, they found that the community mental health centers studied were attractive to the poor, they were used more by the poor than by higher income groups, and they better met the estimated psychiatric needs of the poor than those of other higher income groups. They found that duration of psychiatric treatment, as measured by number of medication clinic visits, individual psychotherapy sessions, and group psychotherapy sessions, was equivalent across income groups. They found no substantiation for the allegation that the poor received second-class treatment. Individual psychotherapy was the modal treatment for all income groups, not only the more affluent. Finally their clinical outcome data did not show differences by income level. Rather, the poor benefitted as much from psychotherapy as did the other income groups (p. 417).

Edwards et al. suggested that in spite of the clinical lore to the contrary, mental health professionals can and do provide mental health settings and treatments that attract and are effective for the poor. Such an observation does not mean that all mental health settings provide such outcomes but rather that where the poor receive effective mental health treatment likely such critical ingredients as the following are present: location of clinics are easily accessible to the poor, clinicians are committed to providing psychotherapeutic strategies that are particularly effective in treating the poor, and that fee structures are established that make psychotherapy financially feasible for both patients and taxpayers.

Who Pays?

Unfortunately or fortunately, depending upon one's point of view, the controversy about third-party payment is not simply a function of increased use of mental health services or the effectiveness of such services for particular groups although such concerns may be the ones which are stated by insurance carriers or other third-party payers. Implicit in such an argument are more complex issues of the nature of insurance and who really pays it. In *arguing for mandatory coverage* of psychotherapy in general medical insurance, McGuire cited three reasons which, in his view, support such a perspective: (1) some important benefits of psychotherapy reach beyond the patient and the patient's family; (2) people may generally underestimate the value of psychotherapy and need "encouragement" to seek care; and (3) in attempting to attract the "best risks" in an insurance pool, private insurers tend to offer too little coverage for mental conditions. Many mental health specialists, particularly those in private practice, would note agreement with these positions and wonder why third-party payers, public and private, do not come into the twentieth century and simply make such payments available for any kind of mental illness, for psychotherapy as treatment, and to evidence their full enlightenment by mandating such coverage for any person involved in their health plans. Other mental health specialists agree with McGuire's reasons.

Maher (1982), a clinical psychologist, took to task the pro-third-party payment for mental health services cited by McGuire. He reminded his fellow clinical psychologists of the essential wisdom of the old aphorism, "There is no such thing as a free lunch." Rather, in the public arena of national health insurance or other federally supported health care provision, mandation of support for mental health care is a tax upon all, those who use it and those who do not. In the private arena, the world of insurance carriers and health maintenance organizations, mandating mental health benefits rather than free choice of mental health service provision causes the good-risk subscriber to subsidize the bad-risk subscriber. This is also a form of taxation but not as vivid or recognizable as that which prevails in the public sector.

Maher reminded his colleagues that insurance carriers do not provide benefits to policyholders; policyholders provide benefits to each other. Insurance carriers simply act as middle people—at the added cost of administration, advertising, agent's commission, dividends to stockholders—in a process in which policyholders pay each other's bills, out of some common pool of funds contributed by each policyholder for losses sustained in the areas covered by the insurance.

In opposition to most current procedures in insurance coverage, the mandating of payment for mental health services in current arguments for third-party payment mixes the good-risk policyholder with the bad-risk policyholder. In the public arena, where free choice ordinarily prevails, insurance carriers must try to define risk pools as precisely as possible and adjust their premiums accordingly or they will lose business. In the case of federal or national health insurance where mental health coverage is mandated for all, incentives to define risk pools or offer different types of coverage is lessened. In any of these circumstances, as Maher argued,

> Coverage of psychotherapy by insurance presents unusual actuarial difficulties and that mandatory coverage represents a tax upon good-risk subscribers for the benefit of bad-risk subscribers and of the practitioners whose bills are paid from the insurance sources. It also benefits carriers who are thereby relieved of the problem of dealing with a predominantly bad-risk pool. (p. 10)

Maher continued his arguments against mandatory insurance coverage for psychotherapy on several other grounds in response to the three points cited by McGuire in support of such coverage. McGuire's first point essentially suggested that the social costs created by the mentally ill are a burden upon the taxpayer via the costs of hospitals, social services, etc., and that we all therefore have a stake in the provision of effective treatment—presumably because it will lead to fewer tax burdens. Maher's counter-argument is that such a viewpoint rests upon dubious assumptions because very little effective research evidence is available to support the alleged fact that psychotherapy deals effectively with mental illness or that it does so with regard to mental illness of the kind that creates large costs to the taxpayer. McGuire's second point is that because people undervalue the benefits of psychotherapy, they use too little service. National health insurance which mandates provision for treatment of mental illness would encourage us to use more care and thereby correct our mistakes. Maher again countered by adding that such a provision would directly or indirectly cost the policyholders for several reasons including the likelihood that people would make claims for preexisting conditions. Premiums, therefore, must inevitably rise. The possibility is likely that good-risk policyholders will use more psychotherapy or other mental health services because of the difficulty surrounding the definitions of who should or should not need such treatment.

Is Psychology a Health Profession?

The major differences expressed by McGuire and Maher about the need for or validity of third-party payment for mental health services, more specifically psychotherapy, in National Health Insurance or similar coverage are extended from a different vantage point by Derner and by

Albee. Derner (1977) took the position that clinical psychology is a health profession. According to him,

> It has been a health profession from the point where observation and practice were applied to diagnose and therapeutically intervene in helping persons who suffer from maladies of the mind. Some of these maladies consist of learning difficulties which are most evidenced in schoolroom/book learning disability. Some of these maladies consist of learning difficulties in which the exigencies of living have led to a variety of coping styles that are manifestations of the anxiety which sears the soul. Some of the maladies are destructive habits such as smoking which is learned under one set of motivations and becomes functionally autonomous under another set of motivations. (p. 3)

Derner went on to argue that psychology is a health profession because for more than three decades, university psychology departments and researchers in psychology have been actively competing for funds from the National Institute of Mental Health. He concluded his analysis of the matter by suggesting:

> The excellent results in reducing physical health problems through the effective use of even brief mental health treatment should encourage psychology to increase our efforts in rendering mental health services and extend ourselves to make such service more readily available for human welfare by the inclusion of psychology as an independent health profession reimbursable under national health insurance. (p. 6)

Albee (1977) totally disagreed with Derner's position about including psychology, or more specifically psychotherapy, in a program of National Health Insurance. He does so on several grounds. First, and perhaps most important, he contended that most of the problems that bring people to a psychotherapist's office are not illnesses but are social or interpersonal in origin. He further argues that to perpetuate acceptance of a medical, illness, or defect model of mental or emotional problems is to argue that mental illness is an illness like any other. Rather, he suggested that these people are not sick, but experiencing various types of problems in living; changing a person's habits and self-confidence does not belong in the health-illness arena as it is cast in a form such as National Health Insurance would necessarily do. Albee argued that National health Insurance should not cover psychotherapy as practiced by anyone: psychiatrists, social workers, psychologists. He does so on the basis of the monetary costs of such a blanket provision as well as because the insurance should not cover problems of living as he defined them. He argued that the best outcome in National Health Insurance would be for the Congress to exclude nearly all of the conditions presently considered under the general term mental or emotional illness. This would mean "that the services of neither psychiatrists nor psychologists would be covered except in those very clearly specified (and clinically unpopular) cases involving psychosomatic, neurological, and organic conditions, and perhaps a few specified patterns requiring intensive emergency intervention" (p. 6).

While Albee's stance against the inclusion of psychotherapy in National Health Insurance is predicated upon definitions of health, mental illness, or problems in living and upon the costs of such legislation, several other issues are raised which deserve note. One is that including mental illness as a reimbursable treatment area would require persons to be labeled or to label themselves in one of the categories of mental illness (e.g., those of the DSM-III) to be eligible to receive treatment. Since, in Albee's view, most of these categories are not really mental illness but behavioral or social problems, to label oneself as mentally ill casts a self-perpetuating stigma which is not helpful to resolving the problem. A second issue is that if psychotherapy were not included in a National Health Insurance plan it would likely cause a greater emphasis to be placed on primary prevention rather than on one-to-one therapy to resolve problems in living. Albee saw the latter as one-to-one patchwork of symptom reduction which really cannot be effective in controlling or preventing the mass disorders of social or interpersonal problems-in-living which now affect many people. Finally, Albee argued that the power of medicine is such that psychology would continue to be dominated by psychiatry. In such a scenario, coverage for psychologists' treating mental patients would need to occur under psychiatric supervision with all of the implied second-class stigmata for psychologists that such a circumstance would include.

The controversies inherent in the Derner-Albee debate and that of the McGuire-Maher counterarguments are fascinating because of the range of issues they embrace and because they represent conflicting viewpoints held among psychologists. If the debates just summarized were between psychiatrists and psychologists, additional nuances and controversies would no doubt emerge. Even so the debates unfolded suggest again that the economics of the mental health professions do not stand apart from issues of power, training, political savvy, definitions of mental illness, and other matters dealt with in other parts of this book. Relatively few of these matters have been scientifically or empirically tested; rather they are matters of politics within and between professional groups and third-party payers.

Probably many of the issues surrounding the inclusion of psychotherapy in proposed National Health Insurance plans find their parallel in existing third-party payment plans. Currently, third-party payment procedures are likely to differ from state to state and even within states. As a result, probably a provider group (e.g., psychologists, counselors, social workers) cannot resolve at the national level the conditions or procedures by which third-party reimbursement will be made by a payer (e.g., insurance group). Rather insurance companies differ by states or other jurisdictions in their coverage, in who will be reimbursed, and in similar pertinent matters. For example, Blue Cross/Blue Shield has approximately 100 separate plans or regional jurisdictions in the United States. While each of these plans has some basic similarity, differences in state freedom-of-choice statutes or other regulations cause the plans to differ in their coverage and guidelines.

Third-Party Recognitions of Psychological Services

An interesting study of third-party recognition of psychological services in one state, Missouri, is instructive about many of the controversial elements of third-party payment. Dujovne (1980) examined the reimbursement guidelines for psychological services which existed among 26 insurance companies in Missouri. At the time of the study the Missouri state licensure law for psychologists was not in effect and no freedom of choice legislation existed. Beyond that it was not possible to obtain the names of companies which sold health insurance from state sources or from the American Psychological Association. However, through a variety of other information, the researcher was able to identify and survey 26 sources of health insurance including several government plans [e.g., the Civilian Health and Medical Program of the Uniformed Services (CHAMPUS) and the health insurance plan for government employees].

The findings were that although the range of services varies from insurance plan to insurance plan, most insurers do offer coverage for selected psychological services. Specifically, companies were asked if coverage was available for seven different services when provided by psychologists: outpatient individual therapy, inpatient individual therapy, inpatient group therapy, outpatient family therapy, outpatient marriage counseling, vocational guidance, and biofeedback. The results were that vocational guidance was not covered by any plan. Marriage counseling was covered only by CHAMPUS. Three companies did not recognize psychologists as providers (probably because of the lack of licensure for psychologists or the lack of freedom of choice legislation in Missouri at the time).

Three companies recognized psychological testing only. Most of the remaining companies offered coverage for individual outpatient therapy and individual inpatient therapy although reimbursement for outpatient group psychotherapy and outpatient family therapy was inconsistent. Biofeedback was covered by only four companies. Blue Cross/Blue Shield, the only company surveyed in two locations within the state, covered a variety of psychological services in Kansas City but the St. Louis Branch recognized psychological testing only.

Thirty percent of the companies that recognized psychological services required physician supervision of psychologists. Forty-two percent of the companies that covered psychological services required a physician's referral. All of the companies that recognized psychologists as providers offered the same coverage to psychologists and physicians.

Psychiatrists as Referral Sources or Supervisors. The requirements for physician supervision of psychologists or referral from physicians to psychologists found by Dujovne in her study is obviously a festering concern among many psychologists. Albee's work alluded to this problem as discussed a few paragraphs ago. Burns (1978) as well as Julius and Handal (1980), among others, has suggested that while the autonomy of psychologists as independent practitioners has been established in many settings and statutes the basic issues of professional competence, roles, and status between psychiatry and psychology remain as controversial as ever. The only difference is that the context is now third-party payment.

Julius and Handal observed in 1980 that none of the National Health Insurance proposals before Congress at that time specifically designated clinical psychologists or other psychologists as an independent (i.e., not supervised by an M.D.) provider of mental health services. Much of this proposed legislation cites psychologists as Physician Consultants. What is even more interesting is that most of the legislation refers to physicians, not even to psychiatrists, without designation of any required psychological experience on behalf of the supervising physician. Thus, the assumption is that psychologists' services would not be considered reimbursable unless these services are authorized and/or supervised by an M.D. In this sense, psychological services would be utilized when deemed medically necessary. Supposedly such restrictions are intended through medical referral and supervision to control overutilization and contain costs (Bent, 1976). In fact, however, they fly in the face of the Freedom of Choice statutes now existing in many states, restrain trade, and reopen historically bitter conflicts between psychiatry, psychology, and other mental health providers in those states which do not yet have Freedom-of-Choice statutes making psychologists, clinical social workers, or other providers eligible for third-party payment.

Such findings as these in the reality of the therapeutic marketplace raise several issues. Why the inconsistency of coverage across insurance plans? Why the inconsistancy of acknowledging psychologists as providers. Why the requirement in so many plans to have psychiatrists as supervisors of psychologists or the source of referrals to them? It is likely that these questions would be extended if the other groups of mental health providers—counselors, social workers, psychiatric nurses, marriage and family therapists—had been the focus of questions of coverage or supervision. The fact seems to be that for the most part, these groups are not yet in the central vortex of issues surrounding third-party payment. This is not to suggest they should not be but rather that their time may not yet have come.

As Dorken (1980) has observed,

> As the frictions between psychology and psychiatry are resolved, the competitive conflict between the nurse specialist practitioner and the clinical social worker will become more broadly apparent... The economics of market competition and penetration and monopoly are not casual. Jurisdictional disputes have an economic conflict at their core.... Even without NHI, the growing economic presence of third-party intermediaries has created a health economy of enormous proportions. Efforts to exert economic control invite challenges of unfair competition and antitrust action. To the extent that one profession seeks to define its practice in a fashion to exclude all or some of the practice of another learned profession, there is an interference both with the advantageous relationships that the other professions has established and with its contractual relationship with clients or agencies. Such interference is damaging; it is a tort objectionable under common law. (p. 669)

In the case of psychiatric nurses or nurse practitioners, it is not simply that physicians define their practice to exclude others, it is also a function of the historical relationships which have evolved between physician and nurse. For example, many state laws presently restrict the practice of nursing by requiring nurses to act under the auspices of a doctor's order. Such dependent functions sometimes conflict with independent nursing assessments during ongoing nursing care which, therefore, requires joint planning (McCloskey & Grace, 1985). The historic development of nurses as "Doers" not "Thinkers," to the advantage of hospitals and doctors alike inhibits the development of private nursing practice. Other restrictions on extending the scope of practice of nurses include factors such as physician-control of insurance programs, a recent surplus in the supply of physicians (which decreases any willingness to delegate functions to nurses), and the problem of access to malpractice insurance.

Evidence is available to indicate that increased delegation of responsibilities by physicians to other providers leads to cost savings and extensions of care; however, this evidence also provides impetus to efforts for broadening direct payment coverage to nurses as independent practitioners (Siegel, 1984, p. 24).

As suggested previously, the basic issues concerning third-party reimbursement for nursing services....

> affect professional relationships as well as nursing roles, and add new emphasis to the concept of professional autonomy. In addition, they assault the traditional physician-dominated reimbursement system. For example, as a salaried employee in a joint practice setting, a nurse's services are seen as a cost or liability on the economic ledger rather than as a revenue-generating component of the system. Such a financial arrangement relegates nurses to a less than collegial relationship. When one professional signs for and claims reimbursement for services legally performed by another professional, it is...exploitation. Yet...this happens in private offices and clinics when physicians submit claims to insurers for services independently performed by nurses, or when the obstetrician signs the reimbursement forms and birth certificates for babies delivered by nurse midwives. Unfortunately, not only is the revenue credited to another professional, but the official records do not accurately reflect nurses' services, making it difficult to collect data needed to support a change in the system. (Griffin, 1982, p. 409).

These perspectives and their realities are the stuff of controversy.

HMOs, PPOs, and DRGs

Into the mix of controversies related to third-party payment for various groups of mental health professionals, particularly as related to the possibility of National Health Insurance, has come several additional structures which are relevant to the discussion. As indicated at other points in this book, whether or not mental illness really exists beyond those brain diseases or organic injuries which affect mental functioning or whether the majority of behaviors falling under such a label are really problems in living, and while it may be debatable whether or not psychologists and other mental health specialists should be considered part of the health care system, they are being swept up in the cost containment concerns now blanketing the nation.

Much of the energy which has made third-payment so important in the economics of the mental health professions comes from the dramatic shift in the 1970s of mental health care from institutional settings to private practice. As long as only a few mental health care providers were in independent practice, controversies about credentialing, power, and economics were more academic than real. Certainly, issues have been and are presently raised about how institutionalized mental health care provisions would be reimbursed and the degree to which private insurance might be involved but, within such a context, the issues are different than those which have been discussed here in relation to the independent practice of mental health services providers.

What seems to be happening is the insertion into the third party payment debate of a new set of controversial elements frequently known by the acronyms as HMOs, PPOs, and DRGs. Respectively, these sets of letters mean Health Maintenance Organizations, Preferred Provider Organizations, and Diagnosis Related Groups. While these organizations are not substitutes for National Health Insurance they have been stimulated by many of the same goals—e.g., to provide quality health care in cost effective ways—and they have inherited many of the controversies which attend third-party payment and the access of different mental health service providers to such payment.

Health Maintenance Organizations (HMOs) have existed in this nation since the turn of the century but they received their impetus to growth from passage of the Health Maintenance Organization Act of 1973 (PL 93-222) which was seen by the Nixon administration as a major building block of a true national health system, not just a sickness system (DeLeon, Uyeda, & Welch, 1985). By 1993, the expectation is that over 50 million Americans will be enrolled in HMO's. The Health Maintenance Organization agrees, in a sense like insurance, to provide specific health services to enrollees for a prepaid, fixed payment. Thus, the HMO profits if it can find ways to keep enrollees healthy rather than providing them the various health services to which their payments entitle them.

Several perspectives are worth noting here. One is that the HMO contracts with health care providers, including psychologists and other mental health care specialists, to deliver the services to plan enrollees as required. Usually such fees are lower than those which a provider might normally expect in private practice. In addition, the mental health specialist becomes an employer of the HMO. While such an arrangement may give greater stability to one's income it also reduces the autonomy of the provider by setting limits on fees and how many visits the provider is permitted to implement and charge for in different diagnosable categories. As enrollees in the Health Maintenance Organization grow in number, they inevitably also reduce the pool of clients available to those mental health professionals in private practice and may ultimately squeeze such persons out of practice because of insufficient client populations.

HMOs initiate several other issues related to the future of independent practice. One is that independent psychologists or other mental health care professionals eligible to receive payments under Medicare or Medicaid historically could only do so incidental to physician referral and supervision. The net effect was that psychologists and other non-medical mental health providers were seen as paraprofessionals under this legislation. On the other hand, as of 1982, nurse practitioners, and in 1984, psychologists were recognized as able to function autonomously within risk-sharing HMOs for purposes of Medicare reimbursement.

What is also interesting about the psychologist's role in an HMO is the growing view of such persons as behavioral medicine specialists rather than psychotherapists (DeLeon, Uyeda, & Welch, 1985). This emerging phenomenon is a function of the growing evidence that some 60% of visits to physicians are really for emotional treatment and the resultant reduction of medical costs. Such awareness of the psychologist's contribution to the cost reduction efforts of an HMO has led to other role changes as well. It has added insight into the need for psychologists in HMOs to participate in the treatment of various medical conditions that include behavioral change as a critical part of the recovery process: e.g., chronic pain, eating disorders, hypertension, many types of heart disease, and addictions (alcohol, drugs, nicotine), among others (Tulkin & Frank, 1985). Further, the involvement of the mental health provider, particularly the psychologist, in interdisciplinary teams in HMOs concerned with behavioral change, reductions in recidivism, and adherence to medical treatment as a way of increasing the cost effectiveness of the HMO, has also subtly but surely increased perceptions of psychologists and physicians as partners not superordinates and subordinates.

Controversies surrounding the potential effects of HMOs to reduce opportunities for private practice for non-medical mental health professionals and to alter their roles to providers of behavioral medicine, not psychotherapy, is exacerbated by two other emerging structures in health care. One is the Preferred Provider Organization and the other is the Diagnosis Related Group. In a major sense, PPOs are similar in their effects to those of HMOs. Specifically, PPOs are groups of specialists who attempt to obtain contracts to deliver health care and/or mental care services to the employees of a specific firm, university, school, or governmental agency. The assumption is again that the medical care costs for employees of the organization with whom a contract has been secured will be lower and the quality of care higher under a Preferred Provider organization than if these employees go to health care professionals on the open market to obtain service. The effects again are to cause psychologists and other mental health care providers to develop new skills in targeted brief therapy (Cummings, 1986), for example, and to shrink the client pool of the private practitioner whose livelihood rests on the availability of a large pool of clients with freedom of provider choice and access to third party payment. Under a PPO arrangement, employees must go for service to those practitioners who are members of the PPO. This obviously reduces client freedom of choice even though it may increase cost effectiveness.

The final acronym of concern in this section is the DRG, Diagnosis Related Groups. Also a cost containment device, DRGs fundamentally mean that hospitals treating Medicare patients receive payments based upon the predetermined rates assigned to the diagnostic groups assigned to the patient at discharge. A classification system developed at Yale University now has 467 DRGs based on disorders in different organ systems (e.g., gastrointestinal, respiratory, mental, and nervous diseases). Thus, payment is based on the average costs associated with the treatment regardless of what the actual treatment costs are (Uyeda & Moldawsky, 1986).

For the moment, certain settings are exempt from the DRG based payment systems if they meet certain requirements. These include psychiatric, rehabilitation, children's and alcohol/drug treatment hospital, and units in hospitals. Even though these institutions may be exempted from DRG provisions, they are still exposed to other cost constraints being levied by various federal reimbursement procedures.

Several potential controversies exist under the DRG approach. One is that the financial provisions make it essential for hospitals and other effected agencies to deliver services as inexpensively as possible. While such processes may ultimately reduce the quality of care, it may also cause mental health care to be seen as a "frill" or "luxury" rather than a necessity when it is not differentiated from other treatments in particular medical problems. As Uyeda and Moldawsky (1986) noted within the context shaped by DRG approaches,

> Professional autonomy is no longer unquestioned; groups throughout the entire range of health care professionals are being held accountable for the cost effects of their treatment decisions, a purpose that is considered by many to be diametrically opposed to professional training and orientation. (p. 62)

> Treating the DRG averages as norms can create a "self-fulfilling process" which may not consider the patient's well-being and ability to function as the treatment criteria. Finally, the DRG system relies on "an acute care model of disease and cure. DRGs are based on treatment that focuses on a specific incident. Mental and nervous disorders do not easily fit such a model; chronic disability often means multiple incidents that require treatment in multiple settings. (p. 62)

The impact of DRG's and other emerging aspects of health economics have been examined by Biegel (1986) with respect to Psychiatry's future. He identified 10 trends that seem not to be confined in their impact to psychiatry but are likely to also affect other mental health care providers. They include, in modified form, the following:

1. *Prospective payment will become the predominant method of reimbursement.* What this basically means is that whether for psychiatrists or others the DRG notion of paying only so much for treatment provided in a particular diagnostic category is likely to expand in mental health payment systems. The open-ended, cost-based systems of the past are increasingly vulnerable.

2. *There will be changes in the current DRG-based method of reimbursement.* Although psychiatric units of general hospitals and psychiatric units in general hospitals have been exempt from DRG's because of the difficulty of diagnosis and predicting the course of the disease, there are emerging models of DRG's which are likely to be imposed on psychiatry.

3. *Multidisciplinary models of services delivery will become increasingly popular.* One way to reduce costs is to segment the needs of different providers rather than allowing

psychiatrists or other mental health or other mental health providers to deal with any client type. Another alternative may be the reemphasis of a multidisciplinary practice approach which will reduce competition, and enhance cooperation.

4. *The role of the psychiatrist will change.* Psychiatrists will need to more clearly define their services as compared to those other mental health professionals can provide. If not, their share of the market will decrease.

5. *The psychiatrist will be increasingly identified as a provider of medical care.* In order to more clearly differentiate themselves from other mental care providers, in the future psychiatrists will likely move gradually toward subspecialization in areas more closely related to medical practice, such as psychological aspects of physical disorders and biological aspects of mental disorders. They will also likely be less concerned with patients whose problems are primarily psychosocial in origin.

6. *Psychiatrists will have to increase their share of the market for mental health services.* Since third party payers are likely to be reluctant to increase mental health benefits, psychiatrists will need to find new ways to encourage persons who ordinarily consult with general practice physicians or other mental health professionals to use psychiatrists instead.

7. *Use of intensive and long-term services will be severely limited.* Psychiatrists need to be willing to recognize that the overwhelming majority of patients do not require intensive long-term services and that a mechanism, perhaps a modified form of existing peer review, must be developed to justify the provision of long-term services to patients who need them. Progress in such areas will help to ease the existing tensions between psychiatrists and third party payers.

8. *Psychiatrists will become entrepreneurs.* The successful psychiatrist will package inpatient, outpatient, and a variety of other services under his/her control and will try to decrease sole reliance of free-for-service reimbursements.

9. *Psychiatrists will assume gatekeeper roles.* Rather than continuing to seek out the convenience of the private office, psychiatrists will need to increase their consultation with employee assistance programs, health maintenance organizations and other entities designed to reduce the use of more expensive forms of health care.

10. *The locus of psychiatric practice will change.* The locus of practice will shift from the private office to the multidisciplinary clinic or to the general medical unit of hospitals (Biegel, 1986, p. 551).

Certainly, if each of these trends emerge as Beigel predicted, psychiatrists and other mental health providers will be in a great conflict about sites, techniques, and populations.

Such is the stuff of controversy.

COST-EFFECTIVENESS

A final area of controversy which will be discussed in this chapter is the cost effectiveness of mental health services. In some ways, to separate the quest for mental health providers to be eligible to receive third-party payments or to have mental health services included in National Health Insurance or Health Maintenance Organizations from that of the cost-effectiveness of these services is difficult. Such aspirations have been shown in the previous section to cause considerable controversy between psychiatrists and other mental health providers. In a larger sense, attempts to have mental health benefits included in insurance coverage or other third-party payment vehicles creates controversy between Congress or insurance carriers and the collective group of mental health providers with respect to whether or not mental health services reduce the costs of health care generally.

Cost-benefit effects of mental health services are controversial from other vantage points than third-party payment. One such arena is that of accountability of such services to those institutions in which they are employed, to consumers, to whoever pays the costs.

A final cost-benefit controversy relates to which form of mental health services provider or delivery system is less expensive or more productive per dollar. The final section of this chapter will explore each of these areas of controversy associated with cost-benefit effects of mental health services.

Health Care-Mental Health Care: Separate or Integral?

A major area of controversy in the health care system relates to whether or not providing mental health benefits will lead to overutilization of insurance benefits. This question was addressed in the previous section as problems with third-party payment were articulated. Another way of looking at mental health care as a part of general health care coverage is with respect to whether the provision of mental health services reduces costs of general health care or other types of costs which conceivably make the provision of mental health services an economic bargain rather than a drain on already limited funds. To a large degree, this is a cost-effectiveness question.

The central questions of cost-benefit analyses of mental health services are, How much does it cost to have mental health services? How much will it cost not to have such services? What are the economic payoffs or tradeoffs associated with having or not having mental health services of various kinds? Answers to each of these questions are not fully available but there are different forms of data which supply some help in addressing the controversies involved.

Results of Cost-Benefit Analyses

With respect to the question of health care costs, a growing body of literature, primarily in psychology and psychiatry, reports cost benefits in favor of mental health services in relation to physical health care.

A particularly comprehensive set of cost-benefit studies have been undertaken by Cummings (1977) and others to evaluate the economic feasibility of psychotherapy within a comprehensive health system. A basic stimulus to such an approach stems from the generally accepted statistic that 60% of visits to physicians occur from sufferers of emotional distress, not organic illness. Indeed, as Cummings noted:

> Many, if not most, physical illnesses are the result of problems in living (or psychological, emotional distress including psychoneuroses and character disorders). The way we live, eat, drink, smoke, compete, and pollute relate inevitably to strokes, heart attacks, cirrhosis, migraine, suicide, and asthma to list

only a few.... The way we live influences our bodies; conversely, chronic illness and intractable pain create a problem in living. Psychotherapy is a viable form of intervention that can alleviate problems in living and lessen disease, and it belongs in any comprehensive health service until that utopian moment when preventive techniques render it unnecessary. (p. 713)

Cummings has summarized a number of studies examining the experience of providing psychological services as part of the Kaiser-Permanente Health Plan that now serves more than eight million subscribers in several regions: Northern and Southern California; Portland, Oregon; Hawaii; Cleveland, Ohio; and Denver, Colorado. The major studies he reported are summarized as follows.

Follette and Cummings (1967) compared the number and types of medical services sought before and after the intervention of psychotherapy in a large group of randomly selected patients. In doing so, they studied these utilization rates with regard to three groups of patients and a control group. The patient groups were divided into those who received one interview only, brief therapy, and long-term therapy. The findings of the study were as follows:

1. Persons in emotional distress were significantly higher users of both inpatient (hospitalization) and outpatient medical facilities as compared to the health plan average;

2. significant declines occurred in medical utilization in those emotionally distressed individuals who received psychotherapy, as compared to a control group of matched emotionally distressed health plan subscribers who were not afforded psychotherapy;

3. these declines remained constant during the 5 years following the termination of psychotherapy;

4. the most significant declines occurred in the second year after the initial interview, and those patients receiving one session only or brief psychotherapy (two to eight sessions) did not require additional psychotherapy to maintain the lower level of utilization for 5 years; and

5. patients seen 2 years or more in continuous psychotherapy demonstrated no overall decline in total outpatient utilization, inasmuch as psychotherapy visits tended to supplant

medical visits. However, a significant decline did occur in inpatient utilization (hospitalization) in this long-term therapy group from an initial rate several times that of the health plan average, to a level comparable to that of the general, adult, health plan population. (p. 716)

In another study, Cummings and Follette (1968) found that the number of subscribers seeking psychotherapy reached an optimal level and remained constant thereafter. This study was reinforced by a subsequent one (Cummings & Follette, 1976) that indicated that increased demand for psychotherapy will not endanger the health care system because it is not the number of referrals received but the way in which psychotherapy services are delivered that drives up cost or that determines optimal cost-therapeutic effectiveness. Of particular interest here was their finding that one session only, with no repeat psychological visits, can reduce medical utilization by 60% over the following 5 years, as well as the finding of 75% reduction in medical utilization over a 5-year period for patients initially receiving 2 to 8 psychotherapy visits (brief therapy). In an eight-year follow-up study of patients involved in psychotherapy within the health plan (Cummings & Follette, 1976), results reinforced the earlier findings that reduction in medical utilization occurred as a "consequence of resolving the emotional distress that was being reflected in the symptoms and in the doctor's visits" (p. 716)

In reviewing the series of studies of both the therapeutic and cost effectiveness of the psychological services provided, Cummings (1977) reported that only 5.3% of the patients were found to be "interminable," a condition that was effective neither in cost nor in therapeutic benefits. In subsequent work with such patients, Cummings has found that rather than increasing the intensity of psychological services for these persons, the commonly accepted remedy, seeing these persons at spaced intervals of once every two or three months has been found to be both cost- and therapeutically-effective.

Cummings (1977) concluded his review of the studies done within the Kaiser-Permanente Plan by suggesting several global findings. First,

when psychotherapy is properly provided within a comprehensive health system, the costs of providing the benefit are more than offset by the savings in medical utilization.

Second,

> when active, dynamic, brief therapy is provided early and by psychotherapists who are enthusiastic and proactive regarding such intervention, it is the treatment of choice for about 85% of the patients seeking psychotherapy.

Third,

> by providing such brief therapy, it makes economically feasible the provision of long-term psychotherapy to the approximately 10% of the patients who require it for their treatment to be therapeutically effective.

Fourth,

> cost-therapeutically effective programs can be developed for groups with such problems in living as alcoholism, drug abuse, drug addiction, chronic psychosis, problems of the elderly, and severe character disorders. (p. 717)

The impact of psychotherapy on physical health suggested by Cummings (1977) has been further examined by Olbrisch (1977). She reviewed the research literature dealing with the effectiveness of psychotherapeutic intervention upon inappropriate utilizers of medical services, alcohol rehabilitation programs, preparation for surgery, cardiac patients, headache treatment, asthma, skin disorders, gastrointestinal disorders, and other health problems. She found that while the quality of evidence is uneven across these categories, in general the evidence is quite promising, and that in the case of psychotherapeutic preparation for surgery the really solid evidence appears to be for a beneficial effect on physical health. She reported examples in which such beneficial effects are related to cost effectiveness.

In bringing together evidence on cost effectiveness of psychotherapy as related to physical health, Olbrisch indicated that, "In the case of presurgical therapy, much of the evidence of effectiveness lies in cost savings resulting from decreased use of medications and shorter hospitalizations" (p. 774). She noted that the research with overutilizers of medical services suggests potentially enormous cost savings but continued research in the area is of utmost importance. She also noted that private industry "considers a psychotherapy program to be profitable in treating early alcoholism and associated problems while at the same time reducing medical expenses."

Jacobs (1983) has reported on the outcomes of four program evaluation studies undertaken by the Psychology Service at a 500 bed general medical and surgical Veterans Hospital. The findings were as follows:

1. *Effectiveness of an Inpatient Chronic Pain Treatment Program.* Clinical records of a sample of 47 patients who had graduated from a six-week residential pain treatment program were audited. Thirty (30) of the 47 veterans in the sample had histories of heavy narcotic use before entering the pain program. Through use of a graduated "pain cocktail," all former users had been totally withdrawn from narcotics by the time they had completed the program, and all remained free of presciption narcotics for five months after discharge. In the succeeding twenty months the percentage of success slowly dwindled, but stabilized at a 70% rate of non-recidivism to narcotic use. Compared to their pre-treatment pattern, post-treatment effects included a 72% reduction in hospital bed occupancy and a 50% decrease in the frequency of outpatient visits. Three years after treatment, the patients had maintained a 47% reduction from their pre-treatment levels of hospitalization.

2. *Cost Effectiveness of Biofeedback Training.* The effectiveness of a biofeedback training program was examined for a group of 25 patients who had been receiving medical treatment for tension headaches (6), migraine headaches (4), degenerative joint disease with chronic pain (4), stroke with muscle spasticity/paresis (4), intervertebrae disk syndrome with low back pain (3), anxiety disorders with marked psychophysiologic involvement (4). On a pre-to-post basis, the number of in-hosptial days for the group fell from 326 to 120, a 63% reduction.

3. *Vocational Rehabilitation Outcomes for Cases Closed by the Career Center.* Following psychological intervention, "successfully rehabilitated" cases showed an 81% decrease from their former level of utilization of in-hospital beds as well as a major reduction (44%) in their level of subsequent ambulatory care visits. The pre-to-post-utilization levels of inpatient bed use and ambulatory care visits remained essentially unchanged for those veterans who had been closed as "unsuccessfully rehabilitated."

4. *The Job Club.* Also evaluated were the outcomes for forty (40) outpatients who had participated in a four week intensive training program in job finding and job survival skills.

Eighty-seven percent of these veterans became employed or entered formal vocational training upon completion of the program. In a six month follow-up study comparing their before and after utilization of hospital services, the finding was that in-patient days and in-patient sources were virtually eliminated. In addition, post-training visits to outpatient clinics and utilization of related clinic services were reduced by 39% and 57% respectively from pre-training utilization levels shown by this group.

Other studies of mental health benefits beyond psychotherapy per se also show significant cost savings. For example, Goldberg, Krantz, and Locke (1970) found that emphasizing short-term outpatient psychiatric therapy in a major prepaid medical plan led to a reduction of 30% in the overall utilization of the plan after the inclusion of mental health benefits. Reed, Meyers, and Scheidemandel (1972) found similar positive results from the inclusion of psychiatric care in major health plans. With specific respect to the utilization of health plans by those with mental health or psychiatric benefits, some other data are relevant. For example, data from the Blue Cross/Blue Shield Federal Employee Plan which has a generous cost-sharing coverage for psychiatric conditions indicate that the proportion of mental and nervous to total health benefits has stabilized at around 7.5%. In addition, Canadian data about the provincial programs of medical care insurance indicate that the proportion of psychiatric care to total medical payments is between 1.4% and 5.4% in various provinces, depending on the availability of psychiatrists (Reed, 1975).

With regard to alcohol problems particularly, Olbrisch (1977) quoted an unpublished study done at the Kennecott Copper Corporation. This corporation has estimated a return of $5.38 per $1.00 cost per year for its psychotherapy program. This financial impact is estimated from such results as reduced absenteeism, reduced hospital, medical, and surgical costs, and reduced costs of nonoccupational accident and illness.

In a similar study in the Lansing, Michigan, Oldsmobile plant (Alander & Campbell, 1975), the records of 117 workers who participated in an alcohol and drug recovery program were compared with those of 24 known substance abusers who did not participate in such a program. While the latter group worsened in terms of lost work-hours, sickness and accident benefits, leaves of absence, and disciplining actions, the treated employees improved in every category and experienced a large drop in lost wages.

A study of the Employee Counselor Service of New York City Transit Authority found that the program that provided treatment to employees with alcohol-related illnesses had saved one million dollars a year in pay benefits alone. This was early in the program and Joseph M. Warren, Program Director, estimated that by 1978 such pay savings ran to two million dollars annually (Warren, 1978).

Korcok (1978) described a cost-benefit analysis of workplace intervention programs undertaken by the Johns Hopkins School of Public Health. A sample of 12 industrial alcoholism programs available to 134,000 employees saved the corporations involved $500,000 in reduced absenteeism alone during their first year of operation. Fielding (1979) reported on a 1976 cost analysis by Firestone Tire and Rubber Company of their alcoholism program. The benefits of the program over costs were calculated by the company to be $1.7 million for the 723 individual involved or $2,350 per individual. In most of these programs psychotherapy or other direct psychological interventions are included. Sometimes they are described directly as industrial alcoholism programs; in some instances they are parts of Employee Assistance Programs (EAPs) and in more recent classifications, Mental Wellness Programs for employees (Barrie-Borman, Webber, Kiefhaber, & Goldbeck, 1978). Mental wellness programs take a variety of forms. Some have developed from alcohol programs and tend to include such components as the following (Barrie-Borman et al., 1978): alcoholism and alcohol abuse programs; drug abuse programs; psychiatric and psychological services; life crisis counseling, including assistance with financial and legal problems; occupational stress programs; and insured mental health benefits. Many of these programs tend also to include health screening and physical fitness components.

In a collective sense, studies reported here suggest that mental health services included in general health plans do reduce the use of physical care facilities and procedures. Thus, the controversy among third-party payers about the likelihood that including mental health care benefits in insurance plans will lead to overutilization seems not to be the case. In addition, the cost benefit studies available about the provision of mental health services to employees in industrial settings suggest that in such cases the economic benefits of work productivity and reduced absenteeism significantly exceed the costs of providing such services.

Data reported here, however, suggest two other issues which relate to the cost benefit analyses of mental health services. One has to do with the quality of cost-benefit studies and the second with the costs of comparative therapies.

Quality of Cost-Benefit Analyses

Although the cost-benefit studies reported here appear to be well done, concerns are expressed by policy-makers and others about both the lack of such studies and their quality. For example, in a survey of mental wellness programs conducted by the Washington Business Group on Health (1978), many companies report that while their programs had achieved noticeable benefits such as improved employee productivity, reduced absenteeism, improved morale and lower insurance premiums, only a few companies had any confidence in the measurability of costs and benefits and, in general, insufficient data were available. Without doubt cost benefit analyses are sporadic. They need to be conducted systematically throughout the health care system where psychological, social work, or other mental health services are involved. Unless this is done, policy-makers are likely to be continuously dubious about the meaning of such cost-benefit data as now exists.

A second major controversy which emerges from the discussions of the need for and the quality of cost-benefit analyses relates to a major issue of definition and a major need for research. Most of the cost-benefit studies available either lump together all elements of the mental health services program and compare their collective effects to a control group which receives no mental health services or to within group changes. Or, the cost-benefit studies in which psychotherapy is the central treatment modality do not clearly describe what "type" of psychotherapy really took place. In essence, psychotherapy is treated as a singular process rather than one which differs depending upon whether it is dynamic, behavioral, client-centered in orientation, the purposes for which it is implemented, and the populations or settings involved.

Lack of Studies of Comparative Effectiveness of Therapy

The heart of such a controversy is the lack of either comparative research data or cost-benefit data on different therapies. Within this context, Banta and Saxe (1983) discuss the need to link efficacy research about psychotherapy and other mental health services with public policymaking. This involves the assessment of psychotherapy, for example, as a health care technology with includes evaluation by nonpsychological health and economic criteria. Efficacy (or benefit) is seen as the central issue in assessing medical technologies. Obviously, both outcome research and cost-effectiveness tend to converge as major ingredients of policy making related to the support of such technologies.

The problem at issue is that from the U.S. Congress's standpoint, evidence available to it suggests that "over 130 psychotherapies" are available and that there is an "urgent need to determine which of these were effective, which were ineffective, and which were reasonable, given their costs and particular characteristics" (Banta & Saxe, 1983, pp. 919-920).

In conducting its major analysis of psychotherapy for Congress, the Office of Technology Assessment (1980) made several important observations. In significantly telescoped form, the findings included considerable scientific evidence that psychotherapy is effective; it does demonstrate efficacy. In addition, the report found no fundamental problem in applying cost-benefit or cost-effectiveness techniques to psychotherapy. However, because some benefits of psychotherapy are likely to be latent or delayed, the difficulty is in being sure that cost-benefit analyses actually measure psychotherapeutic benefits appropriately and comprehensively. This problem is exacerbated by the difficulty involved in turning some supposed benefits of effective psychotherapy (e.g., happiness, self-confidence) into measurable terms. Perhaps the most important concern in the report was that available outcome data does not in most instances allow Congress or other funding sources to determine which type of psychotherapy in which setting would be "best" or optimal for which patient. Yet, this level of specificity is what insurance carriers and policy makers need if they are going to include mental health services, psychotherapy, or some other psychotherapeutic process in National Health Insurance or other health plans. According to current national mentalities, the reasons for doing so are that health "technology" offers clear benefit, is reproducible and transferable, and is safe. However, there are some persons in Congress and in the mental health professions who do not believe that knowledge exists about comparative mental health techniques to suggest that they meet such criteria or, on the other side of the controversy, that they should have to.

McGuire and Frisman (1983) sharpen the controversy about the interaction between treatment efficacy and cost-effectiveness. They observed, in terms of the current state of efficacy research, that, "The consensus is that psychotherapy—almost any recognized brand of psychotherapy—does work" (p. 935). Such a finding, however, does not really please clinicians, policymakers, nor the research community. The former tend to be disappointed that their pet technique is not singled out as the most effective, the latter are disturbed about selection or design flaws which do not give unequivocal results to one therapy over another (Adelman, 1986). As suggested previously, policymakers would prefer to have clear and unambiguous data about therapies for which they should or should not pay out of insurance or other reimbursement processes. They would, in effect, prefer to have an approved therapies list which is unequivocal based upon "efficacy" outcomes. According to McGuire and Frisman, the latter is really the approach taken by the Food and Drug Administration (FDA), which is to pay only for therapies which are effective but to neglect cost information. Given the current cost containment concerns of the Federal government and of third-party payers, McGuire and Frisman believe that it is necessary to consider both cost and efficacy in treatment decisions and, indeed, in reimbursement policy.

McGuire and Frisman have asked provocative questions about treatment reimbursement. For example, if Therapy A produces some beneficial effect does that mean it is worth paying for? If Therapy A is more effective than Therapy B, does that mean Therapy A is preferred? They contended that the answer is no, not necessarily, until cost information is factored in to the decision. They suggest that if Therapy A is very costly, it may not be preferable to no treatment or its costs may outweigh its advantages over a less costly treatment. Thus, in their view, demonstrated efficacy is an incomplete criterion; cost information needs to be included as reimbursement judgments are made.

McGuire and Frisman go on to contend that more is known about comparative costs of treatments than about the comparative effectiveness of them. Thus, they argued that even where more sophisticated techniques such as meta-analysis are used to compare various types of therapies, clear statements of differences do not emerge. They report the findings of M.L. Smith (1982) which suggest that all therapies work about equally well and the research of Parloff (1982) which stated that, "The present evidence does not permit the identification of any therapy procedures or techniques that are clearly ineffectual or unsafe or any that are clearly more effective than others" (p. 721). Thus, the likelihood of efficacy research being sufficiently definitive about which therapies to pay for and which not to pay for is unclear. However, the utility of such information can be increased by adding cost information into such deliberations.

McGuire and Frisman stated:

> We may not be certain that behavioral therapy works better than psychodynamic therapy, but we do know that 50 visits cost more than 5. We may not know that a 28-day hospital stay for alcoholism is more effective than a 7-day stay without outpatient follow-up, but we do know it is more expensive. We know much more about the relative costs of therapies than about the comparative effectiveness.... In keeping with the limitations of our knowledge, policy aims should be modest. Certainly, however, for some treatments that are very costly, professionally credible and lower cost alternatives to long-term psychotherapy and long inpatient stays for alcohol abuse need to be found. Focus on these two areas alone could have a substantial impact on costs of mental health care. (p. 937-938)

Productiveness of Various Types of Mental Health Services

As one extrapolates from the controversies surrounding the comparative effectiveness of psychotherapies and their costs, a final controversy relates to which mental health provider is most productive or the most cost effective. Part of the issue has to do with inpatient vs. outpatient costs and which provider is more likely to be involved with one kind of mental health care or another. A similar cost relationship can be suggested between different forms of therapy and which provider is likely to use them. While one might argue that a logical cost differential exists among settings, techniques, and provider types, that does not eliminate the controversy which is stimulated by such differentials. Indeed, it serves as the basis for various groups of providers, both core and non-core providers, to argue for their inclusion in the mental health network and particularly for the reimbursement of what they do.

Some selected studies will illustrate the points of controversy. For example, Karon and Vandenbos (1976) have compared the effects, including those relating to cost benefits, of conducting psychotherapy with schizophrenics by psychologists or by psychiatrists. Examining three groups of patients—medicated, psychotherapy conducted by psychiatrists, and psychotherapy conducted by psychologists—they found that total costs of treatment per patient were $17,234, $12,221, and $7,813 respectively. They also conducted a two-year follow-up study in which the finding was that the patients treated by psychologists were hospitalized an average of 7.2 days, as compared with 99.8 for the medicated control group and 93.5 days for patients of psychiatrists. The apparent difference lies with the fact that psychologists tend to effect change in the disordered thought processes of the schizophrenic person whereas the psychiatrist's use of medication alone or adjunctive to psychotherapy brings behavior within acceptable approaches and may reduce original hospitalization time but not reduce total time of hospitalization or use of medication.

Foreyt, Rockwood, Davis, Desvousges, and Hollingsworth (1975) examined the cost-benefit ratio of a token economy program with adult psychiatric patients at the Florida State Hospital, Chattahoochee. Token economy programs are frequently used in guidance and counseling efforts with emotionally disturbed children, juvenile delinquents, and other problems of behavioral control. In their analysis, they studied the hospital costs foregone by getting and keeping patients out of the hospital as well as the extra costs saved if the patient once released did become a consumer of public health benefits or other community services. The researchers calculated hospital costs and other forms of aid in the present and in the future as the bases for their analyses. For example, the cost of a patient hospitalized during 1972 was $4,387. By 1982 the estimate was that these costs would be $6,260. If one is able to obtain the discharge of the patient in 1972 whose life expectancy goes to 1982 or 1992, the calculation is that one will save $46,666 and $92,829 respectively. If the person lives to the year 2012 but is discharged in 1972, the saving is $222,314. Other types of estimates of the cost of aid in the state of Florida in 1972 included average aid to the disabled per year, $968; foster home care, $1,800; per patient cost for community mental health, including staff services and medication, $600; division of vocational rehabilitation, $600 per year. While these costs are high, they are less than hospitalization costs. If one is successful in helping discharged patients remain free of the need for these other community services, a double saving is effected by a successful treatment program.

In considering the cost benefits of the token economy program at Florida State Hospital, the researchers included the hiring of a psychologist for twenty hours a week over a year-and-a-half period ($13,125), clinical psychology graduate students to serve as consultants and behavioral mediators on the wards ($7,500), hospital canteen cards that patients could purchase with tokens earned as behavior is appropriately modified ($8,580). The cost of the total program was $29,205. This staffing arrangement is consistent with other similar programs.

The net economic benefit of the program to the government was calculated to be $2,671,855 if one assumed patients would have been released anyway under typical lengths of hospitalization stay. If one made the assumption that these patients would have spent the rest of their lives in the hospital, the net benefit of the program was calculated to be $10,656,849. Under the first assumption, the cost-benefit ratio was calculated to be 90:1 in dollars saved versus program costs. In the second assumption, the ratio was approximately 360:1. With the ratio of 90:1 a million dollars worth of savings were calculated to occur for each $11,100 of treatment cost.

Sussna (1977) has examined the question of measuring the benefits of a community health center. He begun from the "national view" of the costs and losses resulting from mental illness. His estimates for the year 1976 were as follows:

Losses of Productive Activity:

Reduced by the labor force	$28.60 billion
Loss of homemaking services of women	1.94 billion
Reduction in unpaid activities (volunteer work, recreation, etc.)	.48 billion
	$31.02 billion

Sussna contended that the $31 billion figure cited is a conservative estimate of the production lost and, therefore, the potential social benefits of improved mental health. This is true, he believed, because the values of homemaking services and not-for-pay services are understated. The argument also can be made that many of the important outputs of community mental health centers, like those of other mental health settings, are preventive of future antisocial acts and of reduced productive output but to estimate dollar values with what is represented is extremely difficult to do.

Sussna then estimated that the costs of treatment and prevention in mental health programs for 1977 were as follows:

Inpatient care	$5.00 billion
Outpatient facilities	2.20 billion
Training, research and development	.66 billion
	$7.86 billion

From such perspectives, a substantial dollar difference exists in social benefits over costs in the mental health area. Sussna also has compared the treatment costs per patient in state institutions (in Pennsylvania, for example $12,000 per year) with those in community mental health centers (approximately $400 per year). Obviously, such findings are important for different mental health service providers because community mental health centers are more likely to be staffed by psychologists, professional counselors, clinical social workers, and psychiatric nurse practitioners than by psychiatrists. On the contrary, psychiatrists are likely to be more frequently in state hospitals, general hospital with psychiatric units, or other inpatient facilities.

Berkeley Planning Associates (1975) conducted a study of the costs and effectiveness of vocational rehabilitation service strategies in the state of Washington for individuals most severely handicapped (IMSH). The focus was on services directed at employment, not independent living. The finding was that the average cost for IMSH clients was $598.40 and for non-IMSH clients $471.24. The study suggested that cost effectiveness could be enhanced by better diagnostic and evaluation services that in turn would lead to improved prescription of services. Also the data suggest that rather than rehabilitation counselors focusing only on getting clients employed, attention to providing employment skills that might make them become economically self-sufficient would enhance cost effectiveness of the services available.

Worrall (1978) studied the cost-benefits relationship in a vocational rehabilitation program for a national random sample of 3,743 rehabilitants and 1,063 unsuccessful closures after acceptance. The average case service costs for the rehabilitants was $620.12 and for the nonrehabilitants, $373.76 for FY 1970. Using a conservative model, they found that the rehabilitation program is generally returning more in productivity gains to society than the costs expended. On the average they found a benefit-cost ratio of 5 to 1 although this varied across subpopulations stratified by age, race, marital status, and other demographic characteristics. Of the 180 cost-benefit ratios for different subgroups only 8 were found to be less than 1 (costs exceeding benefits) and 7 of those involved persons over age 54.

Kakalick et al. (1974) studied vocational rehabilitation services—including counseling—for hearing and vision handicapped youth. He investigated program costs and benefits for eight categories of hearing and vision handicapped youth for difference by sex and race. On balance, the returns to society were considered to be substantial. They were found, however, to vary across handicap categories—under the most conservative assumptions the benefit-cost ratio varies from 1.1:1 for the legally blind; 2.7:1 for the partially sighted; 3:1 for the deaf, unable to talk; to 4.4:1 for those with one good eye.

Such findings as those of Berkeley Planning Associates, Worrall, Kakalick et al., give evidence of the important contributions of professional counselors to the needs of different population groups unlikely to be served by either psychiatrists or psychologists. What is more subtle in many of these findings is that many of the psychological processes used in counseling, social work, psychology, and psychiatry demonstrate cost-benefits in different settings and with different populations that are substantial, worthy of note, and important ingredients of the economics of the mental health professions.

CONCLUSION

While this chapter has not exhausted the issues or the controversies which attend the economics of the helping professions, it has suggested the importance and the comprehensiveness of the issues involved. It has demonstrated that economic issues are interactive with the matters of professional identity, status of credentialing, and history that have been described in categories of controversy discussed elsewhere in this book.

The discussion here also has demonstrated that while the economics of mental health services are controversial between and among members of the helping professions, they are very much a matter of controversy between policy-makers, health care economics, insurance carriers, and the helping professions in the aggregate. Debates about third-party payment and the possibility of National Health Insurance have focused attention on some of the central areas in which the mental health professions are most vulnerable, e.g., the availability of definitive outcome data about psychotherapy or other mental health techniques, the comparative costs and effectiveness of different therapies, the economic acumen of practitioners in private practice, clarity of distinction in the competencies or techniques among mental health providers.

Three major foci structured the discussion in this chapter: fee-setting, third-party payment, and cost-effectiveness. Each is comprised of a number of sub-issues and controversies which are more or less distinctive from one focus to another. However, in the larger sense, each of these foci continue to reiterate such major questions as, Who should pay for mental health services? What reimbursement guidelines should apply? Who should be reimbursed for service? How should cost-benefit data inform efficacy research as a basis for economic policy in mental health services? As is illustrated within the chapter, the answers are only partially available.

BIBLIOGRAPHY

BILIOGRAPHY

Abeles, N. (1980). Teaching ethical principles by means of value confrontations. *Psychotherapy: Research and Practice, 17,* 384-391.

Abramson, L.Y., Seligman, M.E.P., & Teasdale, J.D. (1978). Learned helplessness in humans: Critique and reformulation. *Journal of Abnormal Psychology, 87,* 49-74.

Abramson, M. (1984). Collective responsibility in interdisciplinary collaboration: An ethical perspective for social workers. *Social Work in Health Care. 10*(1), 35-43.

Abroms, E.M. (1983). Beyond eclecticism. *American Journal of Psychiatry, 140,* (6), 740-745.

Adams, W. (1968). Clients, counselors and fees—ingredients of a myth? *The Family Coordinator, 17*(4), 280-292.

Adelman, H.S., & Taylor, L. (1984). Ethical concerns and identification of psychoeducational problems. *Journal of Clinical Child Psychology, 13*(1), 16-23

Adelman, H.S. (1986). Intervention theory and evaluating efficacy. *Evaluation Review, 10*(1), 65-83.

Adler, J.S., & Gutheil, T.G. (1977). Fees in beginning private practice. *Psychiatric Annals 7*(2), 35-44.

Alander, R., & Campbell T. (1975). An evaluative study of an alcohol and drug recovery program: A case study of the Oldsmobile experience. *Human Resource Management, 14,* 14-18.

Albee, G.W. (1977). Does including psychotherapy in health insurance represent a subsidy to the rich from the poor? *American Psychologist, 32,* 719-721.

Albee, G.W. (1977). Problems in living are not sicknesses: Psychotherapy should not be covered under national health insurance. *The Clinical Psychologist, 30*(3), pp.3, 5-6.

Albee, G.W. (1982). Preventive psychopathology and promoting human potential. *American Psychologist, 37,* 1043-1050.

Alger, I. (1980). Accountability: Human and political dimension. *American Journal of Orthopsychiatry, 50,* 388-393.

Alley, S., & Blanton, J. (1976). A study of paraprofessionals in mental health. *Community Mental Health Journal, 12*(2), 151-160.

Altmaier, E.M. (1979). Areas of liability arising from the provision of psychological services: Some guidelines for a training agency. *The Counseling Psychologist, 8,* 69-71.

American Association for Counseling and Development. (1983). *AACD and division membership report.* Alexandria, VA: Author.

American Mental Health Counselors Association. (1983) "The last hurrah...." *AMHCA News, 6,* 8.

American Nurses' Association. (1976). *Statement on psychiatric and mental health nursing practice.* Kansas City, MO: Author.

American Nurses' Association. (1973). *Standards: Psychiatric-mental health nursing practice.* Kansas City, MO: Author.

American Nurses' Association. (1982). *ANA Standards of psychiatric and mental health nursing practice.* Kansas City, MO: Author

American Personnel and Guidance Association. (1981). *Ethical standards.* Falls Church, VA: Author.

American Psychiatric Association. (1980). *Diagnostic and statistical manual of mental disorders (Third Edition).* Washington DC: Author.

American Psychiatric Association (1981). *The principles of medical ethics with annotations especially applicable to psychiatry.* Washington, DC: Author.

American Psychological Association (1967). A model for state legislation affecting the practice of psychology: 1967 report of APA Committee on Legislation. *American Psychologist, 22,* 1095-1103.

American Psychological Association (1977). Task force on descriptive behavioral classification. "Progress report." Washington, DC: Author. (Mimeo).

American Psychological Association. (1974, amended 1980). *Criteria for accreditation of doctoral training programs and internships in professional psychology.* Washington, DC: Author.

American Psychological Association. (1981) *Ethical principles of psychologists.* Washington, DC: Author.

American Psychological Association. (August 15, 1985). *Proposed education and credentialing policy goals and revised "Definition of practice" for model licensure guidelines in professional psychology.* Memorandum. The Board of Directors.

Amundson, R. (1985) Psychology and epistemology: The place versus response controversy. *Cognition, 20,* 127-153.

Anastasi, A. (1985) Some emerging trends in psychological measurement: A fifty-year perspective. *Applied Psychological Measurement, 9*(2), 121-138.

Anderson, J.D. (1982). Generic and generalist practice and the BSW curriculum. *Journal of Education for Social Work,18*(3), 37-45.

Anthony, W., & Carkhuff, R. (1977). The functional therapeutic agent. In A. Gurman and A. Razin (Eds.), *Effective psychotherapy,* 103-119. New York: Pergamon.

Arbuckle, D.S. (1965). *Counseling: Philosophy, theory and practice.* Boston: Allyn & Bacon.

Arnold, L.E., Calestro, K., Bates, W. J., & Wasserman, M. (1983). Teaching psychiatric interviewing as a core physician skill. *The Journal of Psychiatric Education, 7*(2), 102-112.

Association, Chapter Submit Briefs supporting Clinical Practice Rights. (1981). *NASW News, 26,* 12.

Atkinson, D.R., Morten, G., & Sue, D. (1979). *Counseling American minorities. A cross-cultural perspective.* Dubuque, IA: Brown.

Bandler, L.S. (1979). The evolution of clinical social work: Continuity and change. In *Change and Renewal in Psychodynamic Social Work: British and American Developments in Practice and Education for Services to Families and Children.* Oxford, England: Proceedings of the Oxford Conference.

Banta, H.D. & Saxe, L. (1983). Reimbursement for psychotherapy, linking efficacy research and public policymaking. *American Psychologist, 38*(8), 918-923.

Barber, B. (1965) Some problems in the sociology of the professions. In K.S. Lynn (Ed.), *Professions in America.* Boston: Houghton Mifflin.

Barrie-Borman, K., Webber, A., Kiefhaber, A., & Goldbeck, W. (1978, December 1-2). *Employee mental wellness programs and issues: An overview.* Background paper for conference on Employee Mental Wellness Programs cosponsored by the Boston University Center for Industry and Health Care and the Washington Business Group on Health Care and the Washington Business Group on Health held in Washington, DC.

Beauchamp, T.L., & Childress, J.F. (1979). *Principles of biomedical ethics.* New York: Oxford.

Beck, C., Rawlings, R., & Williams, S. (1984). *Mental health—psychiatric—nursing.* St. Louis: C.V. Mosby.

Beck, E. (1983). At your beck and call. *AMHCA News, 7*(2), 1-2.

Beis, E. (1983). State involuntary commitment statutes. *Mental Disability Law Reporter, 7*(4), 358-369.

Benedict, R. (1934). *Patterns of culture.* New York: Mentor Books.

Bennett, V.C. (1980). Who is a professional psychologist? (Commentary on professional certification). *The Counseling Psychologist, 9*(1), 28-32.

Bent, R.J. (1976). Professional autonomy and medical supervision. IN H. Dorken (Ed.). *The Professional Psychologist Today.* San Francisco: Jossey-Bass.

Berg, M.R. (1984). Teaching psychological testing to psychiatric residents. *Professional Psychology, 15*(3), 343-352.

Bergin, A.E. (1983). Religiosity and mental health: A critical reevaluation and meta-analysis. *Professional Psychology: Research and Practice, 14*(2), 170-184.

Bergin, A.E. (1985). Proposed values in guiding and evaluating counseling and psychotherapy. *Counseling and Values, 29*(2), 99-115.

Berkeley Planning Associates. (1975) *An evaluation of the costs and effectiveness of vocational rehabilitation service strategies for individuals most severely handicapped.* Preliminary report. Berkeley, CA: Associates, 320 Channing Way.

Berman, J.S. & Norton, N. C. (1985). Does professional training make a therapist more effective? *Psychological Bulletin, 98*(2), 401-407.

Bernal, M.E., & Padilla, A.M. (1982). Status of minority curricula and training in clinical psychology. *American Psychologist, 37,* 780-787.

Berndt, D.J. (1983). Ethical and professional considerations in psychological assessment. *Professional Psychology: Research and Practice, 14*(2), 185-196.

Berzins, J. (1977). Therapist-patient matching. In A. Gurman and A. Razin (Eds.), *Effective psychotherapy,* pp. 222-251. New York: Pergamon.

Biegel, A. (1986). Planning psychiatry's future. *Hospital and Community Psychiatry, 37*(6), 551-554.

Blashfield, R.K, & Draguns, J.G. (1976). Evaluative criteria for psychiatric classification. *Journal of Abnormal Psychology, 85,* 140-150.

Bloch, D.A., & Weiss, H.M. (1981). Training facilities in marital and family therapy. *Family Process, 20*(2), 133-146.

Bloom, M. (1981). *Primary prevention: The possible science.* Englewood Cliffs, NJ: Prentice-Hall.

Blume, G., & Perlman, B. (1981). Perspectives of master's level clinical psychology training coordinators on major issues of subdoctoral education. *Teaching of Psychology, 8*(1), 38-40.

Bornstein, P. J., & Wollershein, J. P. (1978). Scientist-practitioner activities among psychologists of behavioral and nonbehavioral orientations. *Professional Psychology, 9,* 659-664.

Bouhoutsos, J., Holroyd, J., Lerman, H., Forer, B.R., & Greenberg, M. (1983). Sexual intimacy between psychotherapists and patients. *Professional Psychology, 14*(2), 185-196.

British Psychological Society. (1983). Guidelines for a code of conduct for psychologists. *Bulletin of the British Psychological Society, 36,* 242-244.

Brooker, A. E., Bechel, H. P., & Mareth, T. R. (1984). Psychotherapy: Developing a treatment paradigm. *Psychological Reports, 54,* 251-161.

Brooks, D.K., & Weikel, W.J. (1986). History and development: The mental health *counseling movement. Chapter 1 in A.J. Palmo and W.J. Weikel (Eds.), Foundations of Mental Health Counseling.* Springfield, IL: Charles C. Thomas.

Brooks, V.R. (1982). Specializations: Current development and the myth of innovation. *Journal of Education for Social Work, 18*(3), 31-36.

Bugental, J. (1968). Psychotherapy as a source of the therapist's own authenticity and inauthenticity. *Voices: The Art and Science of Psychotherapy, 4*(2), 13-21.

Burns, K. P. (1978). National health insurance: Inclusion of mental health care and clinical psychology. *Professional Psychology, 9*(5), 723-732.

Buss, A. H. (1966) *Psychopathology.* New York: Wiley and Sons.

Cahn, C. H. (1982). The ethics of involuntary treatment: The position of the Canadian Psychiatric Association. *Canadian Journal of Psychiatry, 27*(1), 67-74.

Carter, F. M. (1981). *Psychosocial Nursing.* New York: MacMillan Publishers.

Case, L. P. & Lingerfelt, N.B. (1974). Name-calling: The labeling process in the social work interview. *Social Service Review, 48,* 74-86.

Chodoff, P. (1978). Psychiatry and the fiscal third party. *The American Journal of Psychiatry, 135*(10), 1141-1147.

Chodoff, P. (1984). Involuntary hospitalization of the mentally ill as a moral issue. *American Journal of Psychiatry, 141*(3), 384-389.

Christensen, C. P. (1984). Involuntary hospitalization of the mentally ill as a moral issue. *American Journal of Psychiatry, 141*(3), 384-389.

Clarizio, H.F. (1978). Nonbiased assessment of minority children. *Measurement and Evaluation of Guidance, 11*(2).

Cleveland, S.E. (1980). Counseling psychology: An endangered species? *Professional Psychology, 11*(2), 314-323.

Cleveland, S. E. (1976). Reflections on the rise and fall of psychodiagnosis. *Professional Psychology, 7*(3), 309-318.

Clinical Social Work Council. (1984, March). Definition of clinical social work. *N.A.S.W. News.*

Cohen, L. H. (1979). The research readership and information source reliance of clinical psychologists. *Professional Psychology, 10,* 78-785.

Cohn, J. B. (1983). Harm to third parties in psychotherapy. *American Journal of Forensic Psychology, 1*(2) 15-18.

Cole, N. S. (1981). Bias in Testing. *American Psychologist, 36*(10), 1067-1077.

Colliver, J.A., Havens, R.A., & Wesley, R. M. (1985). Doctoral and Master's level clinical psychologists and MSWs in public mental health setting: A nationwide follow-up. *Professional Psychology: Research and Practice, 16*(5), 634-640.

Commission on Accreditation for Marriage and Family Therapy Education. (1979). *Manual on Accreditation*. Upland, Ca: The Association.

Committee on Definition, Division of Counseling Psychology, American Psychological Association. (1956). Counseling Psychology as a specialty. *American Psychologist, 11*, 282-285.

Corey, G., Corey, M. S., & Callahan, P. (1984). *Issues and ethics in the helping professions (3nd ed.)*. Belmont, CA: Brooks/Cole.

Council on Social Work Education (1984). *Curriculum policy for the Master's degree and baccaleureate degree programs in social work education*. New York: Author.

Corrigan, E. M. (1979). Alcohol knowledge and practice issues. *Health and Social Work, 4*(4), 9-40.

Cronbach, L. J. (1980). Validity on parole: How can we go straight: In W. B. Schrader (Ed.). *New directions for testing and measurement: No. 5 measuring achievement. Progress over a decade*. San Franciso: Jossey-Bass.

Cummings, N.A. & Follette, W. T. (1968). Psychiatric services and medical utilization in a prepaid health plan setting: Part II. *Medical Care, 6,* 31-41.

Cummings, N.A. & Follette, W. T. (1976). Brief psychotherapy and medical utilization: An eight-year follow-up. In h. Dorken and Associates (Eds.), *The professional psychologist today: New developments in law, health, insurance and health practice*. San Francisco: Jossey-Bass.

Cummings, N. A. (1977). The anatomy of psychotherapy under national health insurance. *American Psychologist, 32*(9), 711-718.

Cummings, N.A. (1986). The dismantling of our health system. Strategies for the survival of psychological practice. *American Psychologist, 41*(4), 426-431

Danish S. J., Galambos, N.L. & Laquatra, I. (1983). Life development intervention: Skill training for personal competence. In R.D. Felman, L.A. Jason, J. Moritsuqur, and S. S. Farber (Eds.). *Preventive psychology; Theory, research, and practice,* 49-66. Elmsford, NY: Pergamon.

Danish, S. J., & Smyer, M.A. (1981). Unlimited consequences of requiring a license to help. *American Psychologist, 36*(1), 13-21.

DeLeon, P. H., Uyeda, M. K., & Welch, B. L. (1985). Psychology and HMDS, New partnerships or new adversary? *American Psychologist, 40*(10), 1122-1124.

DeLeon, P. H., Kjervik, D. K., Kraut, A. G., & VandenBos, G. R. (1985). Psychology and nursing: A natural alliance. *American Psychologist 40*(11), 1153-1164.

Delworth, U. (1977). Counseling psychology: A distinct practice specialty. *The Counseling Psychologist, 7*(2), 43-45.

Department of Health and Human Services. (1979). *The Surgeon General's Report on Health Promotion and Disease Prevention.* Washington DC: Author.

DeMuth, N. M., & Kamis, E. (1980). Fees and therapy: Clarification of the relationship of payment source to service utilization. *Journal of Consulting and Clinical Psychology, 48*(6), 793-795.

Denkowski, K. M., & Denkowski, G. C. (1982). Client-counselor confidentiality: An update of rationale, legal status, and implications. *The Personnel and Guidance Journal,* April, 371-375.

Derner, G. F. (1977). Psychology—A health profession or a settled issue, so why the question? *The Clinical Psychologist, 30*(3), 3-4, 5.

Diamond, E. (1976). Minimizing sex bias in testing. *Measurement and Evaluation in Guidance, 9*(1).

Dightman, C. (1970). Fees and mental health services: Attitudes of the professional. *Mental Hygiene, 54*(3), 401-406.

Dohrendwend, B.P., & Dohrendwend, B.S. (1974). Social and cultural influences on psychopathology. *Annual Review of Psychology, 25,* 419-452.

Dohrendwend, B.P., & Dohrendwend, B.S., Gould, M.S., Link, B., Neugebaur, R., & Wunsch-Hitzig, R. (1980). *Mental illness in the United States, Epidemiological estimates.* New York: Praeger Publishers.

Dorken, H. (1980). National health insurance: Implications for mental health practitioners. *Professional Psychology, 11*(4) 664-671.

Dorken, H., & Webb, J.T. (1980). 1976 Third-party reimbursement experiences: An interstate comparison by insurance carrier. *American Psychologist 35*(4), 355-363.

Draguns, J. G. (1985). Psychological disorders across cultures. In P. Pederson (Ed), *Handbook of Cross-Cultural Counseling and Therapy,* 55-62. Westport, Ct: Greenwood Press.

Dujovne, B. (1980). Third-party recognition of psychological services. *Professional Psychology, 11*(4), 574-581.

Dulchin, J., & Segal, A. J. (1982). Third-party confidences: The uses of information in a psychoanalytic institute. *Psychiatry, 45,* 27-37.

Dumas, R. (1983). Social, economic, and political factors and mental illness. *Journal of Psychiatric Nursing and Mental Health Services, 21,* 31-35.

Dunston, P.J. (1983). Culturally sensitive and effective psychologists: A challenge for the 1980's. *Journal of Community Psychology, 11* (October), 376-382.

Edwards, D.W., Greene, L.R., Abramowitz, S.I., & Davidson, C.V. (1979). National health insurance, psychotherapy and the poor. *American Psychologist, 34*(5), 411-419.

Eichelman, B., Wikler, D., & Hartwig, A. (1984) Ethics and psychiatric research: Problems and justification. *American Journal of Psychiatry, 141*(3), 400-405.

Elbert, J.C. (1984). Training in child diagnostic assessment: A survey of clinical psychology graduate programs. *Journal of Clinical Child Psychology, 13*(2), 122-133.

Everstine, L., Everstine, D.S., Heymann, G.M., True, R.H., Frey, D.H., Johnson, H.G., & Seiden R.H. (1980). Privacy and confidentiality in psychotherapy. *American Psychologist, 35*(9), 828-840.

Ewalt, P. (Ed.). (1980) *Toward a definition of clinical social work* Washington DC: Proceedings of the National Association of Social Work Conferences.

Ewing, C.P. (1985). Mental health clinicians and the law: A review of current law governing professional practice. In C. P Ewing (Ed.), *Psychology, psychiatry and the law: A clinical and forensic handbook*. Sarasota, FL: Professional Resource.

Ewing, C.P. (Ed.). (1985). *Psychology, psychiatry and the law: A clinical and forensic handbook*. Sarasota, FL: Professional Resource Exchange.

Ewing, T. N. (1974). Racial similarity and counselor and client satisfaction with counseling. *Journal of Counseling Psychology, 21,* 446-449.

Farina, A., Fisher, J.D., Getter, H., & Fischer, E.H. (1978). Some consequences of changing people's views regarding the nature of mental illness. *Journal of Abnormal Psychology, 87,* 272-279.

Feighner, J.P., & Cohn, J.B. (1985). Double-blind comparative trials of fluoxetine and doxepin in geriatric patients with major depressive disorder. *Psychiatry, 46*(3), 20-25.

Fessler, S.R., & Adams, C.G. (1985). Nurse/social worker role conflict in home health care. *Journal of Gerontological Social Work, 9*(1), 113-123.

Fielding, J.E. (1979). Preventive medicine and the bottom line. *Journal of Occupational Medicine, 21*(2), 79-88.

Fink, P.J. (1978). Politics and funding in primary care—A look to the future. *Psychiatric Opinion, 15*(6), 14-17.

Fischer, L., & Sorenson, G.P. (1985). *School law for counselors, psychologists, and social workers*. New York: Longman.

Fitzgerald, L.F., & Osipow, S.H. (1986). An occupational analysis of Counseling Psychology: How special is the specialty? *American Psychologist 41*(5), 535-544

Flaugher, R.L. (1978). The many definitions of test bias. *American Psychologist 33*(7), 671-679.

Follette, W.T., & Cummings, N.A. (1967). Psychiatric services and medical utilization in a mental health plan setting. *Medical Care, 5,* 25-35.

Ford, J.D. (1979). Research on training counselors and clinicians. *Review of Educational Research, 49*(1), 87-130.

Foreyt, J.P., Rockwood, C.E. Davis, J.E., Desvouges, W.H., & Hollingsworth, R. (1975). Benefit-cost analysis of a token economy program. *Professional Psychology, 6*(1), 73-80.

Forrest, D.V. (1984). Counselor education: Issues for the 1980s. *The School Counselor, 31*(4), 381-384.

Fox, R.E. (1982). The need for a reorientation of clinical psychology. *American Psychologist, 37*(9), 1051-1058.

Frank, G. (1984). The Boulder Model: History, rationale, and critique. *Professional Psychology, 15*(3), 417-435.

Frank, G. (1975). *Psychiatric diagnosis: A review of research.* New York: Pergamon.

Gabbard, G.O. & Smith, W.H. (1982). Psychiatry-psychology conflict: Origins in training. *Journal of Psychiatric Treatment and Evaluation, 4,* 203-208.

Garcia, J. (1981). The logic and limits of mental aptitude testing. *American Psychologist, 36*(10), 1172-1180.

Garfield, S., & Kurtz, R. (1976). Personal therapy for the psychotherapist: Some findings and issues. *Psychotherapy: Theory, Research and Practice, 13,* 188-192.

Garten, J. (1985). Siegel to introduce bill covering marriage and family therapy. *Newsletter. New York Association for Marriage and Family Therapy, 11*(1), 1

George, J.C., & Brooker, A.E. (1984). Conceptualizations of mental health. *Psychological Reports, 55,* 329-330.

Gerson, M.J., & Lewis, K. (1984). Sex role identification and the clinical psychology student. *Professional Psychology, 15*(4).

Gilmore, M.M., & Perry, S.W., III. (1980). The psychiatry internship and the development of professional identity. *American Journal of Psychiatry, 137*(10), 1206-1210.

Gingerich, W.J., Kleczewski, M., & Kirk, S.A. (1982). Name-calling in social work. *Social Service Review, 56,* 366-374.

Glasser, W. (1970). *Mental health or mental illness, psychiatry for practical action.* New York: Harper & Row.

Goldberg, I., Krantz, G., & Locke, B. (1970). Effect of short-term outpatient psychiatric therapy benefits on the utilization of medical services in a prepaid group practice medical program. *Medical Care, 8,* 419-428.

Goldfried, M.R. (1984). Training the clinician as scientist-professional. *Professional Psychology, 15*(4), 477-481.

Goldman, R.D., & Hewitt, B.N. (1976). Predicting the success of Black, Chicano, Oriental and White college students. *Journal of Educational Measurement, 13*(2), 107-117.

Goldschmitt, M., Tipton R.M., & Wiggins, R.C. (1981). Professional identity of counseling psychologists. *Journal of Counseling Psychology, 28,* 158-167.

Goodyear, R.K., & Sinnett, E.R. (1984). Current and emerging ethical issues for counseling psychologists. *The Counseling Psychologist, 12,* 87-98.

Gordon, E.W., & Terrell, M.D. (1981). The changed Social Context of Testing. *American Psychologist, 36*(10), 1167-1171.

Gorenstein, E.E. (1984). Debating mental illness. Implications for science, medicine, and social policy. *American Psychologist, 39*(1), 50-56.

Gottfredson, G.D., & Dyer, S.E. (1978). Health service providers in psychology. *American Psychologist, 33,* 314-338.

Graham, D.L.R., Rawlings, E.I., Halpern, H.S., & Hermes, J. (1984). Therapists' needs for training in counseling lesbians and gay men. *Professional Psychology, 15*(4), 482-496.

Greenwood, E. (1957). Attributes of a Profession. *Social Work, 2,* 45-55.

Grier, W., & Cobbs, P. (1968). *Black rage.* New York: Bantam Books.

Griffith, H. (1982). Strategies for direct third party reimbursement for nurses. *American Journal of Nursing, 82*(3), 408-412.

Grisso, T., & Sales, B.D. (1978). *Law and professional psychology.* Special issues of *Professional Psychology, 9*(5).

Gross, S. (1978). The myth of professional licensing. *American Psychologist, 33,* 1009-1016.

Grossman, J. (1981). Inside the wellness movement. *Health, 13,* 10-15.

Guion, R.M. (1974, May). Open a new window. Validities and values in psychological measurement. *American Psychologist,* 287-296.

Gutheil, T.G. (1980). Restraint versus treatment: Seclusion as discussed in the Boston State case. *American Journal of Psychiatry, 137,* 718-719.

Gutheil, T.G., Shapiro, R., & St. Clair, R. (1980). Legal guardianship in drug refusal: An illusory solution. *American Journal of Psychiatry, 137,* 347-352.

Hahn, M.E., & MacLean, M.S. (1955). *Counseling Psychology.* New York: McGraw Hill.

Halleck, S.L. (1980). *Law in the practice of psychiatry: A handbook for clinicians.* New York: Plenum.

Haney, W. (1981). Validity, vaudeville, and values. A short history of concerns over standardized testing. *American Psychologist, 36*(10), 1021-1034.

Hardcastle, D.A. (1983). Certification, licensure and other forms of regulation. Chapter 37 in A. Rosenblatt and D. Waldfogel, (Eds), *Handbook of clinical social work.* San Francisco, CA: Jossey-Bass.

Hardcastle, D.A. & Katz, A.J. (1979). *Employment and unemployment in social work: A study of NASW members.* Washington, DC: National Association of Social Workers.

Heineman, M.B. (1981). The obsolete scientific imperative in social work research. *Social Service Review,* September, 371-397.

Herbsleb, J.D., Sales, B.D., & Overcast, T.D. (1985). Challenging licensure and certification. *American Psychologist, 40*(11), 1165-1178.

Hertz, M.R. (September 3, 1970). *Projective techniques in crisis.* Address delivered, Society for Projective Techniques and Personality Assessment, Miami, Florida.

Hill, C.E. (1978). Implications of the counseling psychologist's identity for training program. *The Counseling Psychologist, 7*(2), 48-50.

Hinman, S., & Marr, J.N. (1984, May). Training counselors to write behavior-based client objectives. *Rehabilitation Counseling Bulletin,* 291-301.

Hipps, O. (1981). The integrated curriculum: The emperor is naked. *American Journal of Nursing, 81,* 976-980.

Hixson, J., & Epps, E. G. (1975). The failure of selection and the problem of prediction: Racism vs. measurement in higher education. *Journal of Afro-American Issues, 3*(1), 117-128.

Hofling, C. K., & Rosenbaum, M. (1980). The extension of credit to patients in psychoanalysis and psychotherapy. *Bulletin of the Menninger Clinic, 44*(4), 327-344.

Hokenstad, Jr., M.D. (1984). Curriculum directions for the 1980's: Implications of the new curriculum policy statement. *Journal of Education for Social Work, 20*(1), 15-22.

Holroyd, J.C., & Brodsky, A.M. (1977). Psychologists' attitudes and practices regarding erotic and nonerotic psychical contact with patients. *American Psychologists, 32,* 843-849.

Hooper, D., & Roberts, R.J. (1976). Workshop training in psychotherapy. *British Journal of Medical Psychology, 49,* 177-182.

Hopkins, B.R., & Anderson, B.S. (1985). *The counselor and the law.* Alexandria, VA: American Association for Counseling and Development.

Hosford, R.E., Johnson, M.E., & Atkinson, D.R. (1984). Trends and implications for training: Academic criteria, experiential background, and personal interviews as predictors of success in a counselor education program. *Counselor Education and Supervision, 23*(4), 268-275.

Howard, K.I., & Orlinsky, D.E. (1972). Psychotherapeutic processes. In P. Mussen and M.R. Rozenzweig (Eds.), *Annual Review of Psychology 23,* 615-668. Palo Alto, CA: Annual Reviews.

Hudson, W., (1982). Scientific imperatives in social work research and practice. *Social Science Review,* June, 246-257.

Hummel, D. L., Talbutt, L. C., & Alexander, M. D. (1985). *Law and ethics in counseling.* New York: Van Nostrand Reinhold.

Hurst, J. C., & Parker, C. A. (1977). Counseling psychology: Tyranny of a title. *The Counseling Psychologist, 7,* 16-18.

Ingram, R.E., & Zurawski, R.M. (1981). Choosing clinical psychologists: An examination of the utilization of admissions criteria. *Professional Psychology, 12,* 684-689.

Ivey, A.E. (1976). Counseling psychology, the psychoeducator model and the future. *The Counseling Psychologist, 6,* 72-75.

Ivey, A.E. (1982). Credentialism: Protection for the public or the professional? In E.L. Herr and N. Pinson (Eds.), *Foundations for policy in guidance and counseling,* Chapter 10. Falls Church, VA: American Personnel and Guidance Press.

Jacobs, D.F. (1983). *Towards a formula for professional survival in troubled times.* Division 18 (Psychologists in Public Service) Presidential Address delivered at the 91st Annual Convention of the American Psychological Association, Anaheim, California, August 27, 1983.

Jencks, S.F. (1985). Recognition of mental distress and diagnosis of mental disorder in primary care. *Journal of the American Medical Association, 53*(13), 1903-1906.

Johnson, L.C. (1983). *Social work practice: A generalist approach.* Boston: Allyn and Bacon.

Jourard, S. (1964). *The transparent self.* Princeton, NJ: Van Nostrand.

Julius, S.M., & Handal, P.J. (1980). Third-party payment and National Health Insurance: An update on psychology's efforts toward inclusion. *Professional Psychology, 11*(6), 955-964.

Kadis, A., & Winick, C. (1968). Fees in group therapy. *American Journal of Psychotherapy, 22*(1), 60-67.

Kagan, N. (1977). Presidential address, Division 17. *The Counseling Psychologist, 7,* 4-7.

Kakalik, J.S., Brewer, G.O., Doherty, L.A., Fleisehauer, P.D., Genensky, S.M., & Wallen, L.M. (1974). *Improving services to handicapped children with emphases on hearing and vision impairment.* Santa Monica, CA: Rand, R-1240, DHEW.

Kanter, S., & Kanter, J. (1977). Therapeutic setting and management of fees. *Psychiatric Annals, 7*(2), 61-64.

Kardener, S.H. (1974). Sex and the physician-patient relationship. *American Journal of Psychiatry, 131,* 1134-1136.

Karon, B.P., & Vandenbos, G.R. (1976). Cost/benefit analysis: Psychologist versus psychiatrist for schizophrenico. *Professional Psychology, 7*(1), 107-111.

Katz, M.M., Secunda, S., Koslow, S.H., Waas, J.W., Berman, N., Casper, R., Kocsis, J., & Stokes, P. (1984). A multi-vantaged approach to measurement of behavioral and affect states for clinical and psychological research. *Psychological Reports, 55,* 619-671.

Keith-Spiegel, P., & Koocher, G.P. (1985). *Ethics in psychology.* New York: Random House.

Kelly, E.L., Goldberg, L.R., Fiske, D.W., & Kilkowski, J.M. (1978). Twenty-five years later: A follow-up study of the graduate students in clinical psychology assess the VA selection research project. *American Psychologist, 33,* 746-755.

Kiesler, C.A. (1980). Mental health policy as a field of inquiry for psychology. *American Psychologist, 35,* 1066-1080.

Kiesler, C.A. (1985). Prevention and public policy. In J.C. Rosen and L.J. Solomon (Eds.), *Prevention in Health Psychology,* Chapter 16. Hanover, NH: The University Press of New England.

Kilmann, R.H. (1982). A dialectical approach to formulating and testing social science theories: Assumptional analysis. *Human Relations, 36*(1), 1-22.

Kirkpatrick, M. (1983). Sexuality. *The Journal of Psychiatric Education, 7*(1), 32-26.

Kleinman, A. (1980). *Patients and healers in the context of culture. An exploration of the border and between anthropology, medicine, and psychiatry.* Berkeley, CA: University of California Press.

Klerman, G.L., Vaillant, G.E., Spitzer, R.L., & Michels, R. (1984). A debate on *DSM-III. American Journal of Psychiatry, 14*(4), 539-553.

Knapp, S. (1980). A primer on malpractice for psychologists. *Professional Psychology, 11*(4), 511-516.

Knapp, S., & Vandecreek, L. (1982). Tarasoff: Five years later. *Professional Psychology, 13*(4), 511-516.

Koocher, G.P. (1979). Credentialing in psychology. Close encounters with competence. *American Psychologist, 34*(8), 696-702.

Korchin, S.J., & Schuldberg, D. (1981). The future of clinical assessment. *American Psychologist, 36*(10), 1147-1158.

Korchin, S.J. (1976). *Modern clinical psychology: Principles of intervention in the clinic and community.* New York: Basic Books.

Korcok, M. (1978). Dealing with drinkers is just good business. *FOCUS on Alcohol and Drug Issues, 1*(1), February-March.

Krumboltz, J.D., & Menefee, M. (1980). Counseling psycylogy of the future. *The Counseling Psychologist, 8*(4), 46-48.

Kurzman, P.A., & Akabas, S.H. (1981). Industrial social work as an area for practice. *Social Work,* January, 52-60.

Lamb, H.R., & Zusman, J. (1979). Primary prevention in perspective. *American Journal of Psychiatry, 136,* 12-17.

Lancaster, J. (1980). *Community Mental Health Nursing.* St. Louis, MO: C.V. Mosby.

Lanning, W., & Forest, D. (1984). Counselor educators: Comparing NDEA and non-NDEA participants. *Counselor Education in Supervision, 24*(1), 107-113.

Larsen, J.A. (1980). Competency-based and task-centered practicum instruction. *Journal of Education for Social Work, 16*(1), 87-94.

Last, C.G., Barlow, D.H., & O'Brien, G.T. (1983). Comparison of two cognitive strategies in treatment of a patient with generalized anxiety disorders. *Psychological Reports, 53,* 19-26.

Lebensohn, R.M. (1978). Private practice of psychiatry: Future roles. *American Journal of Psychiatry, 135*(11), 1359-1363.

Leighninger, L. (1980, March). The generalist-specialist debate in social work. *Social Science Review,* 1-12.

Levy, C.E. (1981). Improving patient care: Psychologist parity with psychiatrists in hospitals. *Clinical Psychology, 34*(3), 24-25.

Levy, L.H. (1984). The metamorphosis of clinical psychology: Toward a new charter as human services psychology. *American Psychologist, 39,* 486-494.

Lewandowski, D.G., & Saccuzzo, D.P. (1976). The decline of psychological testing. *Professional Psychology,* 177-184.

Lewisohn, P.M., Teri, L., & Hertzinger, M. (1984). Training clinical psychologists for work with older adults: A working model. *Professional Psychology, 15*(2), 187-202.

Liddle, H.A., Vance, S., & Pastushak, R.J. (1979, October). Family therapy training opportunities in psychology and counselor education. *Professional Psychology,* 760-765.

Liddle, H.A. (1982). Family therapy training: Current issues, future trends. *International Journal of Family Therapy, 4*(2), 81-97.

Lieberman, P.B., & Baker, F.M. (1985). The reliability of psychiatric diagnosis in the emergency room. *Hospital and Community Psychiatry, 36*(3), 291-293.

Lindy, J.D., Green, B.L., & Patrick, M. (1980). The internship: Some disquieting findings. *American Journal of Psychiatry, 137*(1), 76-79.

Lipsett, S.M. (1963). *First new nation.* New York: Basic Books.

London, P. (1964). *The modes and morals of psychotherapy.* New York: Rinehart and Winston.

Lorion, R.P. (1974). Patient and therapist variables in the treatment of low-income patients. *Psychological Bulletin, 81,* 344-354.

Losito, W.F. (1980). The argument for including moral philosophy in the education of counselors. *Counseling and Values, 25,* 40-46.

Lowe, J., & Herranen, M. (1978). Conflicts in treatment-understanding roles and relationships. *Social Work in Health Care, 3*(3), 323-330.

Lubin, B., Larsen, R.M., & Mataruzzo, J.P. (1984). Patterns of psychological test usage in the United States: 1935-1982. *American Psychologist, 39,* 451-454.

Mackin, D.K. (1976). Occupational licensing: A warning. *The Personnel and Guidance Journal, 54,* 507, 510-571.

Maher, B. (1982). Mandatory insurance coverage for psychotherapy: A tax on the subscriber and a subsidy to the practitioner. *The Clinical Psychologist, 35*(2), pp. 9-13.

Manuso, J.S.J. (1983). *Occupational clinical psychology.* New York: Praeger.

Manschreck, T.C., & Kleinman, A.M. (1979). Psychiatry's identity crises: A critical rational remedy. *General Hospital Psychiatry, 1*(2), 166-173.

Marks, I.M., Hallam, R.S., Connolly, J., & Philpott, R. (1977). *Nursing in behavioral psychotherapy.* Royal College & Nursing Series. London: Whitefriars Press.

May, R. (1963). Freedom and responsibility re-examined. In E. Lloyd-Jones and E.M. Westervelt (Eds.), *Behavioral Science and Guidance: Proposal and Perspectives,* 95-110. New York: Teachers College Press, Columbia University.

McCaffrey, R.J., & Isaac, W. (1984). Survey of the educational backgrounds and specialty training of instructors of clinical neuropsychology in APA-approved graduate training programs. *Professional Psychology, 15*(1), 26-33.

McCloskey, J., & Grace, H. (1985). *Current issues in nursing* (2nd ed.). Boston: Blackwell Scientific Publications.

McGuire, T.C. (1981). Compulsory insurance for psychotherapy. *The Clinical Psychologist, 34,* 13-14.

McGuire, T.J., & Frisman, L.K. (1983). Reimbursement policy and cost-effective mental health care. *American Psychologist, 38*(8), 935-940.

McGoldrick, M., Pearce, J.K., Giordano, J. (1982). *Family therapy and ethnicity.* New York: The Guilford Press.

McKnight, J. (1977). Professionalized service and disabling help. In I.K. Zola, M. McKnight, J. Caplan, and H. Shaiken (Eds.), *Disabling professions.* London: Marion Boyars.

McLemore, C.W., & Court, J.H. (1977). Religion and psychotherapy—ethics, civil liberties, and clinical savvy: A critique. *Journal of Consulting and Clinical Psychology, 45*(6), 1172-1175.

McNeely, J.D., & Oates, W.E. (1978). Religious symptom pictures of psychiatric patients. In W. Oates (Ed.), *The religious experience of the psychiatric patient,* pp. 65-86. Philadelphia, PA: Westminster.

McNeill, B.W., & Ingram, J.C. (1983). Prevention and counseling psychology: A survey of training practices. *The Counseling Psychologist, 11*(4), 95-96.

Mearig, J.S. (1982). Ethical implications of the children's rights movement for professionals. *American Journal of Orthopsychiatry, 52*(3), 518-529.

Meehl, P.E. (1954). *Clinical versus statistical prediction.* Minneapolis, MN: University of Minnesota Press.

Meyerstein, I. (1981). Family therapy training for paraprofessionals in a community mental health center. *Family Process, 20*(2), 477-493.

Meyerstein, I. (1981). Editorial. Family therapy training: The institutional base. *Family Process, 20*(2), 131.

Mills, M.J., Cummins, B.D., & Gracey, J.S. (1983). Legal issues in mental health administration. *International Journal of Law and Psychiatry, 6,* 39-55.

Mills, M.J., & Gutheil, T.G. (1982). Guardianship and the right to refuse treatment: A critique of the Roe case. *Bulletin of the American Academy of Psychiatry and Law,* 239-246.

Mintz, N. (1971). Patient fees and psychotherapeutic transactions. *Journal of Consulting and Clinical Psychology, 36*(1), 1-8.

Mohammed, Z. & Piercy, F. (1983). The effects of two methods of training and sequencing on structuring and relationship skills of family therapists. *The American Journal of Family Therapy, 11*(4), 64-71.

Monk, A. (1981, January). Social work with the aged: Principles of practice. *Social Work,* 61-68.

Montgomery, R.B. (1977). Current and alternative training models in clinical psychology. *Australian Psychologist, 12*(1), 95-102.

Morris, R. (1979). *Social policy of the American Welfare state: An introduction to policy analysis.* New York: Harper & Row.

Myers, R. (1982). Education and training—the next decade. *The Counseling Psychologist, 10,* 39-44.

NACCMHC. (Undated brochure). *The National Academy of Certified Clinical Mental Health Counselors presents its questions and answers.*

Nadelson, C., Salkt, P., & Notman, M. (1983). Evidence of physical adaptability during the medical training period. *The Journal of Psychiatric Education, 7*(3), 167-182.

Nathan, P.E. (1977). A clinical psychologist views counseling psychology. *The Counseling Psychologist, 7*(2), 36-37.

National Association of Social Workers. (1980). *Code of ethics of the National Association for Social Workers.* Silver Spring, MD: Author.

National Association of Social Workers. (1979). *Code of ethics.* Washington, DC: Author.

Neill, J.R., & Ludwig, A.M. (1980). Psychiatry and psychotherapy: Past and future. *American Journal of Psychotherapy, 34*(1), 39-49.

Nevid, J.S., & Gilden, T.J. (1984). The admission process in clinical training: The role of the personal interview. *Professional Psychology, 15*(1), 18-25.

Newkirk, M. (1983). Economic factors in service delivery. *The Counseling Psychologist, 11*(2), 91-96.

Nichols, K.A. (1985). Psychological care by nurses, paramedical and medical staff: Essential developments for general hospitals. *British Journal of Medical Psychology, 58,* 231-240.

Nichols, W.C. (1979). Education of marriage and family therapists: Some trends and implications. *Journal of Marital and Family Therapy,* January, 19-28.

Office of Technology Assessment. (1980). *The efficacy and cost-effectiveness of psychotherapy. Background paper No. 3: The implication of cost-effectiveness analysis of medical technology.* Washington, DC: U.S. Government Printing Office.

Okon, S.E. (1983). Guidance and counseling services in Nigeria. *The Personnel and Guidance Journal, 61*(8), 457-459.

Olbrisch, M.E. (1977). Psychotherapeutic intervention in physical health, effectiveness and economic efficiency. *American Psychologist, 32*(0), 761-777.

Oldham, J.T. (1978, Fall). Liability of therapists to non-patients. *Journal of Clinical Child Psychology,* 187-188.

Ollendick, T.H. (1984). Training in clinical child psychology: The role of continuing education. *Journal of Clinical Child Psychology, 13,* 90-91.

Osipow, S.H. (1977). Will the real counseling psychologist please stand up? *The Counseling Psychologist, 2,* 93-94.

Osipow, S.H. (1979). Toward counseling psychology in the year 2000. *The Counseling Psycholgist, 8,* 18.

Osipow, S.H., Cohen, W., Jenkins, J., & Dostal, J. (1979). Clinical versus counseling psychology: Is there a real difference? *Professional Psychology, 10,* 149-153.

Padilla, A.M., Ruiz, R.A., & Alvarez, R. (1975). Community mental health services for the Spanish-speaking/surnamed population. *American Psychologist, 30,* 892-905.

Pallone, N.J. (1977). Counseling psychology: Toward an empirical definition. *The Counseling Psychologist, 7*(2), 29-32.

Palmo, A.J. (1981). *Mental health counselor.* Unpublished manuscript prepared for the Board of Directors of the American Mental Health Counselors Association, Washington, DC.

Parloff, M.B. (1982). Psychotherapy research evidence and reimbursement decisions: Bambi meets Godzilla. *American Journal of Psychiatry, 139,* 718-727.

Parsons, T. (1951). *The social system.* Glencoe, IL: Free Press.

Pasternack, S. (1977). The psychotherapy fee: An issue in residency training. *Disease of the Nervous System, 3,* 913-917.

Peabody, D. (1985). *National Characteristics.* Cambridge, England: Cambridge University Press.

Pearlmutter, D.R. (1985). Recent trends and issues in psychiatric-mental health nursing. *Hospital and Community Psychiatry, 36*(1), 56-62.

Pepinsky, H.B., Hill-Frederick, K., & Epperson, D.L. (1978). *The Journal of Counseling Psychology, 25,* 483-498.

Perl, K.G., & Hahn, M.W. (1983). Psychology graduate students' attitudes toward research: A national survey. *Teaching of Psychology, 10*(3), 139-143.

Perlman, B., & Lane, R. (1981). The "clinical" master's degree. *Teaching of Psychology, 8*(2), 72-77.

Perlmutter, F.D. (1982). New directions for mental health promotion. In F.D. Perlmutter (Ed.), *Mental health promotion and primary prevention,* Chapter 1. San Francisco, CA: Jossey-Bass.

Peterson, K.J., & Anderson, S.C. (1984). Evaluation of social work practice in health care settings. *Social Work in Health Care, 10*(1), 1-16.

Pfeiffer, C.M., Jr., & Sedlacek, W.E. (1971). The validity of academic predictors for Black and White students at a predominantly white university. *Journal of Educational Measurement, 8*(4), 253-261.

Phillips, B.N. (1982). Regulation and control in psychology. Implications for certification and licensure. *American Psychologist, 37*(8), 919-926.

Pietrofesa, J.J., Hoffman, A., Splete, H., & Pinto, D. (1978). *Counseling: Theory, research, and practice.* Chicago: Rand McNally.

Piotrowski, C., & Keller, J.W. (1984). Psychodiagnostic testing in APA-approved clinical psychology program. *Professional Psychology, 15*(3), 450-456.

Piotrowski, C., & Keller, J.W. (1984). Attitudes toward clinical assessment by members of the AABT. *Psychological Reports, 55,* 831-838.

Pope, K., Geller, J., & Wildinson, L. (1975). Fee assessment and outpatient psychotherapy. *Journal of Consulting and Clinical Psychology, 43,* 835-841.

Popiel, D.J. (1980). Confidentiality in the context of court referrals to mental health professionals. *American Journal of Orthopsychiatry, 50*(4), 678-685.

Randolph, G. (1975). Experiences in private practice. *Journal of Psychiatric Nursing, 13,* 16-19.

Rappaport, J. (1977). *Community psychology.* New York: Holt, Rinehart, & Winston.

Reavley, W., & Herdman, L.F. (1985). Training nurses in behavioral psychotherapy. *British Journal of Medical Psychology, 58,* 249-256.

Reed, L.S., Meyers, E.S., & Scheidemandel, P.L. (1972). *Health insurance and psychiatric care utilization and cost.* Washington, DC: American Psychiatric Association.

Reed, L.S. (1975). *Coverage and utilization of care for mental conditions under health insurance—various studies, 1973-1974.* Washington, DC: American Psychiatric Association.

Reichert, I. (1982). Human services and the market system. *Health and social work, 7*(3), 173-182.

Reid, W.J. (1981). Mapping the knowledge base of social work. *Social Work, 26,* 124-132.

Reynolds, D.K. (1980). *The quiet therapies: Japanese pathways to personal growth.* Honolulu, HI: The University Press of Hawaii.

Ridley, C.R. (1984). Clinical treatment of the nondisclosing Black client: A therapeutic paradox. *American Psychologist, 39*(11), 1234-1244.

Roberts, K. (1981). The sociology of work entry and occupational choice. In A.G. Watts, D.E. Super, and J.M. Kidd (Eds.), *Career Development in Britain,* Chapter 8. Cambridge, England: Hobson's Press.

Rogers, C.R. (1942). *Counseling and Psychotherapy.* Boston: Houghton Mifflin.

Rogers, C.R. (1951). *Client-centered therapy: Its current practice, implications, and theory.* Boston: Houghton Mifflin.

Romeo v. Youngberg, 644 F.2d 147 (3rd Cir. 1980). Cert. granted 451 U.S. 982. (1982).

Rosen, J.C., & Solomon, L.J. (Eds.). (1985). *Prevention in health psychology.* Hanover, NH: The University Press of New England.

Rosenblatt, A., & Waldfogel, D. (1983). *Handbook of clinical social work.* San Francisco, CA: Jossey-Bass.

Sadoff, R.L., & Showell, R. (1981). *Sex and therapy: A survey of female psychiatrists.* Paper presented at the annual meeting of the American Psychiatric Association, New Orleans, LA.

Saner-Yiu, L., & Saner, R. (1985). Value dimensions in American counseling: A Taiwanese-American comparison. *International Journal of Advancement of Counseling, 8,* 137-146.

Sarason, S.B. (1977). *Work, dying, and social change. Professionals and the one life-one career imperative.* New York: Free Press.

Sarason, S.B. (1981). An asocial psychology and a misdirected clinical psychology. *American Psychologist, 36*(8), 827-836.

Sax, P.R. (1978). An inquiry into fee setting and its determinants. *Clinical Social Work Journal, 6*(4), 305-312.

Schafield, W. (1964). *Psychotherapy: The purchase of friendship.* Englewood Cliffs, NJ: Prentice-Hall.

Schiffer, R.P. (1983). Psychiatric aspects of clinical neurology. *American Journal of Psychiatry, 140*(2), 205-207.

Schindler, F.E., Berren, M.K., & Beigel, A. (1981). A study of the causes of conflict between psychiatrists and psychologists. *Hospital and Community Psychiatry, 32*(4), 263-266.

Schlesinger, S.E. (1984). Substance misuse training in graduate psychology programs. *Journal of Studies on Alcohol, 45*(2), 131-137.

Schmalz, B. (1983). A review of internship training in Ontario. *The Ontario Psychologist, 15*(3), 20-25.

Schneider, L.J., & Gelso, C.J. (1972). Vocational versus personal emphases in counseling psychology training programs. *The Counseling Psychologist, 3*(3), 90-92.

Schofield, W. (1964). *Psychotherapy: The purchase of friendship.* Englewood Cliffs, NJ: Prentice-Hall.

Schonbar, R.A. (1967). The fee as a focus for transference and countertransference. *American Journal of Psychotherapy, 21,* 275-285.

Schuerman, J.R. (1981, December). The obsoletic scientific imperative in social work research: Debate with authors. *Social Service Review,* 144-148.

Sedlacek, W.E. (1977). Test bias and the elimination of racism. *The Journal of College Student Personnel,* 16-20.

Seligman, L. (1984). Before and after licensure. *AMHCA Journal, 6*(1), 2-5.

Senior, J.R. (1976). *Toward the management of competence in medicine. Report of computer-based examination project.* Sponsored by the National Board of Medical Examiners and the American Board of Internal Medicine. Philadelphia, PA, pp. 12-16.

Serban, G. (1981). Sexual activity in therapy: Legal and ethical issues. *American Journal of Psychotherapy, 35*(1), 76-85.

Sevensky, R.L. (1984). Religion, psychology, and mental health. *American Journal of Psychotherapy, 38*(1), 73-86.

Sharfstein, S.S. (1978). Third-party payers: To pay or not to pay. *American Journal of Psychiatry, 135*(10), 1185-1188.

Sharfstein, S.S., Taube, C.A., & Goldberg, I.D. (1977). Problems in analyzing the comparative costs of private versus public psychiatric care. *American Journal of Psychiatry, 135*(10), 1185-1188.

Shanhirzadi, A. (1983). Counseling Iranians. *The Personnel and Guidance Journal, 6*(8), 487-489.

Shectman, F., Hays, J.R., Schuham, A., & Smith, R. (1982). Accountability and confidentiality in psychotherapy with special reference to child treatment. *Clinical Psychology Review, 2,* 201-211.

Shemberg, K., & Keeley, S.M. (1979). Psychodiagnostic training in the academic settings: Past and present. *Journal of Consulting and Clinical Psychology, 34,* 205-211.

Shertzer, B., & Stone, S.C. (1980). *Fundamentals of counseling* (3rd ed.). Boston: Houghton Mifflin.

Shevrin, H., & Schectman, F. (1973). The diagnostic process in psychiatric evaluations. *Bulletin of the Menninger Clinic, 37,* 451-494.

Shimberg, B., & Roederer, D. (1978). *Occupational licensing: Questions a legislator should ask.* Lexington, KY: The Council of State Governments.

Shimberg, B. (1982). Occupational licensing: A public perspective. What is competence? How can it be assessed? In M.R. Stern, *Power and conflict in continuing professional education,* Chapter Two. Belmont, CA: Wadsworth, and Princeton, NJ: Educational Testing Service.

Shultz, S.L., & Russell, A.T. (1984). The emotionally disturbed child psychiatry trainee. *Journal of the American Academy of Child Psychiatry, 23*(2), 226-232.

Siegel, C. (1984). Critical care nurse as independent practitioner. *Focus on Critical Care, 11*(4), 22-26.

Siegel, M. (1979, April). Privacy, ethics, and confidentiality. *Professional Psychology,* 249-258.

Simon, G.C. (1978, May). The psychologist as whistle blower: A case study. *Professional Psychology,* 322-340.

Singer, J.L. (1981). Clinical intervention: New developments in methods and evaluation. In L.T. Benjamin, Jr. (Ed.), *The G. Stanley Hall Lecture Series,* Volume 1. Washington, D.C.: American Psychological Association.

Siporin, M. (1985). Current social work perspectives on clinical practice. *Clinical Social Work Journal, 13*(3), 198-217.

Smith, D. (1982). Trends in counseling and psychotherapy. *American Psychologist, 37*(7), 802-809.

Smith, M.L. (1982). What research says about the effectiveness of psychotherapy. *Hospital & Community Psychiatry, 33,* 457-461.

Smith, R.C. (1978). Psychology and the courts: Some implications of recent judicial decisions for state licensing boards. *Professional Psychology, 9,* 489-497.

Snow, B.M. (1981). Counselor licensure as perceived by counselors and psychologists. *The Personnel and Guidance Journal, 60,* 80-83.

Snygg, D., & Combs, A.W. (1949). *Individual behavior.* New York: Harper and Brothers.

Sporakowski, M.J., & Staniszewski, W.P. (1980). The regulation of marriage and family therapy: An update. *Journal of Marital and Family Therapy, 6,* 335-348.

Stainbrook, E. (1976). Range of curricula in established medical schools. In *Scientific proceedings of the 129th American Psychiatric Association annual meeting,* 227-228. Washington, DC: American Psychiatric Association.

Stern, S. (1984). Professional training and professional competence: A critique of current thinking. *Professional Psychology, 15*(2), 230-243.

Stigall, T.T. (1977). Counseling psychology: Training and credentialing for professional practice. *The Counseling Psychologist, 7*(2), 41-42.

Stone, G.L. (1986). *Counseling psychology: Perspectives and functions.* Monterey, CA: Brooks/Cole.

Stricker, G., Hull, J.W., & Woodring, J. (1984). Respecialization in clinical psychology. *Professional Psychology, 15*(2), 210-217.

Stumphauzer, J.S., & Davis, L.C. (1983). Training Mexican American mental health personnel in behavior therapy. *Journal of Behavior Therapy and Experimental Psychiatry, 14*(3), 215-217.

Sue, D. (1981). *Counseling the culturally different.* New York: Wiley Interscience.

Sue, D.W. (1978). World views and counseling. *The Personnel and Guidance Journal, 56*(8), 458-462.

Sue, O. (1977). Counseling the culturally different. *The Personnel and Guidance Journal, 55,* 422-425.

Sue, S. (1983). Ethnic issues in psychology: A reexamination. *American Psychology, 38,* 583-592.

Sue, S., & McKinney, H. (1975). Asian-Americans in the community mental care system. *American Journal of Orthopsychiatry, 45,* 111-119.

Sugarman, S. (1984, March). Integrating family therapy training into psychiatry residency programs: Policy issues and alternatives. *Family Process, 23,* 23-32.

Super, D.E. (1955). Transition: From vocational guidance to counseling psychology. *Journal of Counseling Psychology, 2,* 3-9.

Sussna, E. (1977). Measuring mental health program benefits: Efficiency or justice? *Professional Psychology, 8*(4), 435-551.

Swagler, R.M., & Harris, D.A. (1977). An economic analysis of licensure and public policy: Evidence from the social work case. *Journal of Consumer Affairs, 11,* 90-101.

Swoboda, J.S., Elwork, A., Sales, B.D., & Levine, D. (1978). Knowledge of a compliance with privileged communication and child-abuse-reporting laws. *Professional Psychology, 9,* 448-457.

Szasz, T. (1961). *The myth of mental illness, foundations of a theory of personal conduct.* New York: Harper & Row.

Tarasoff v. Regents of University of California, 529 P.2d, 553 (Cal. 1974); modified, 551, P.2d 334 (Cal. 1976).

Taube, C.A., Burns, B.J., & Kessler, L.K. (1984). Patients of psychiatrists and psychologists in office-based practice: 1980. *American Psychologist, 39*(12), 1435-1447.

Taube, C.A., & Kessler, L.K. Expenditures for ambulatory mental health care during 1980. *National Medical Care Utilization and Expenditure Survey.* (Data Report No. 5, DHHS Publication No. PHS 84-20000). Washington, DC: U.S. Government Printing Office.

Taylor, C.A., & Mereness, D.A. (1982). *Essentials of psychiatric nursing.* St. Louis: C.V. Mosby.

Thelen, M.H., & Ewing, D.R. (1970). Roles, functions, and training in clinical psychology: A survey of academic clinicians. *American Psychologist, 25,* 550-554.

Thompson, A.J., & Super, D.E. (1964). *The professional preparation of counseling psychologists.* New York: Teachers College Press, Columbia University.

Thoresen, C.E., & Eagleston, J.R. (1985). Counseling for health. *The Counseling Psychologist, 13*(1), 15-87.

Tittle, C.K. (1974). Sex bias in educational measurements: Fact or fiction? *Measurement and Evaluation in Guidance, 6*(4).

Tousley, M. (1982). Certification as a credential: What are the causes? *Perspectives in Psychiatric Care, 20,* 23-26.

Triandis, H.C. (1972). *The analysis of subjective culture.* New York: Wiley.

Triandis, H.C. (1985). Some major dimensions of cultural variation in client populations. In P. Pederson (Ed.), *Handbook of cross-cultural counseling and therapy,* 21-28. Westport, CT: Greenwood.

Tulkin, S.R., & Frank, G.W. (1985). The changing role of psychologists in health maintenance organizations. *American Psychologist, 40*(10), 1125-1136.

U.S. Civil Service Position Classification Standards. (1968). (Psychology Series 180). Washington, DC: Government Printing Office, June 1968.

U.S. Department of Health, Education and Welfare, Public Health Service (July, 1977). *Credentialing health manpower.* DHEW Publication No. (05) 77-50057. Washington, DC: Author.

U.S. Department of Labor. (1984). *Occupational outlook handbook.* Washington, DC: U.S. Government Printing Office.

Uyeda, M.K., & Moldawsky, S. (1986). Prospective payment and psychological services. *American Psychologist, 41*(1), 60-63.

Vaizey, J., & Clarke, C.F.O. (1976). *Education: The state of the debate in America, Britain and Canada.* London, England: Duckworth.

Van Hoose, W.H., & Kottler, J.A. (1978). *Ethical and legal issues in counseling and psychotherapy.* San Francisco: Jossey-Bass.

Van Hoose, W.H., & Paradise, L.V. (1979). *Ethics in counseling and psychotherapy: Perspectives in issues and decision-making.* Cranston, RI: Carroll Press.

VandenBos, G.R., Stapp, J., & Kilberg, R.R. (1981). Health service providers in psychology. *American Psychologist, 36,* 1395-1418.

Vitulano, L.A., & Copeland, B.A. (1980). Trends in continuing education and competency demonstration. *Professional Psychology, 11*(6), 891-897.

Walters, O.S. (1958). Metaphysics, religion and psychotherapy. *Journal of Counseling Psychology, 5,* 253-252.

Waltzer, H. (1980). Malpractice liability in a patient's suicide. *American Journal of Psychotherapy, 34*(1), 89-98.

Warren, J.M. (1978). Changing attitudes of supervisors. *Labor-Management Alcoholism Newsletter, 1,* 9.

Washington Business Group on Health. (1978). *A survey of industry sponsored health promotion, prevention and education programs.* Unpublished interim report prepared for the DHEW National Conference on Health Promotion in Occupational Settings, Washington, DC.

Watkins, C.E., Jr. (1985). Counseling psychology, clinical psychology, and human service psychology: Where the twain shall meet. *American Psychologist, 40*(9), 1054-1056.

Watley, D., & Vance, F.L. (1964). *Clinical versus actuarial prediction of college achievement and leadership ability.* Washington, DC: U.S. Dept of Health, Education, and Welfare.

Weikel, W.J. (1985). The American Mental Health Counselors Association. *Journal of Counseling and Development, 63*(7), 457-460.

Weiskopf, R., & Newman, J.P. (1982). Redesigning internship training programs: A cost-efficient point of view. *Professional Psychology, 13*(4), 571-576.

Weiss, C.S. (1981). The development of professional role commitment among graduate students. *Human Relations, 34*(1), 13-31.

Welch, C.E. (1976). Professional licensure and hospital delineation of clinical privileges: Relationship to quality assurance. In R.H. Egdahl and P.M. Gertman (Eds.), *Quality assurance in health care.* Germantown, MD: Aspen Systems.

Welfel, E., & Lipsitz, N.E. (1984). The ethical behavior of professional psychologists: A critical analysis of the research. *The Counseling Psychologist, 12,* 31-42.

Wellner, A.M. (Ed.). (June, 1977). *Education and credentialing in psychology: IL.* Report of a meeting, June 4-5, 1977. Washington, DC: American Psychological Association.

Wellner, A.M. (Ed.). (May, 1978). *Education and credentialing in psychology: Proposal for a national commission on education and credentialing in psychology.* Washington, DC: American Psychological Association.

Wendt, R.N., & Zake, J. (1984). Family systems theory and school psychology: Implications for training and practice. *Psychology in the Schools, 21,* 204-210.

Wigtil, J.V., & Thompson, A. (1984). Alcohol awareness counselor training: Utilizing a DWI program. *Counseling Education and Supervision, 23*(4), 300-310.

Williams, R.L. (1975). Moderator variables as bias in testing Black children. *Journal of Afro-American Issues, 3*(1), 77-90.

Wilmarth, R. (1983, October/November). A call for unity. *AMHCA News, 7*(2), Vol. 3.

Wilson, S. (1982). Peer review in California: Summary findings in 40 cases. *Professional Psychology, 13*(4), 517-521.

Woodman, N.J., & Lenna, H.R. (1980). *Counseling with gay men and women: A guide for facilitating positive life-styles.* San Francisco: Jossey-Bass.

Woody, R.H. (1969). *Behavioral problem children in the schools: Recognition, diagnosis, and behavioral modification.* New York: Appleton-Century-Crofts.

Woody, R.H. (1980). Introduction: A conceptual framework for clinical assessment. In R.H. Woody (Ed.), *Encyclopedia of clinical Assessment,* Volume 2, pp. xx-xc.

World Health Organization. (1977). *Manual of the international statistical classification of diseases, injuries and causes of death.* 9th Revision, Vol. 1. Geneva, Switzerland: Author.

Worrall, J.D. (1978). A benefit-cost analysis of the vocational rehabilitation program. *The Journal of Human Resources, 13*(2), 285-298.

Wrenn, C.G. (1954). Editorial Comment. *Journal of Counseling Psychology, 1.*

Wrenn, C.G. (1962). The culturally encapsulated counselor. *Harvard Educational Review, 32,* 444-449.

Yiu, L. (1978). Degree of assimilation and its effect on the preference of counseling style and on self-disclosure among Chinese-Americans in Hawaii. Ph.D. dissertation, Indiana University.

INDEX

INDEX

A

Abeles, N. 172, 271
Abramowitz, S.I. 235, 236, 237, 278
Abramson, L.Y. 147, 148, 271
Abramson, M. 42, 271
Abroms, E.M. 13, 14, 194, 271
Academy of Certified Social Workers (ACSW) 35, 41, 131
Accreditation 122
Adams, C.G. 42, 278
Adams, W. 222, 271
Adelman, H.S. 170, 261, 271
Adler, J.S. 31, 225, 226, 271
Akabas, S.H. 114, 284
Alander, R. 257, 271
Albee, G.W. 81, 235, 240, 271
Alexander, M.D. 173, 282
Alger, I. 271
Alley, S. 139, 271
Altmaier, E.M. 161, 271
Alvarez, R. 206, 288
American Association for Counseling and Development (AACD) 54, 55, 59, 132, 271
American Association for Marriage and Family Therapy (AAMFT) 63, 65, 107, 132
American Association of Clinical Psychologists 17
American Association of Family Counselors and Mediators (AAFCM) 65
American Board of Internal Medicine 128
American Certified Social Worker 71
American Medical Association (AMA) 71, 112, 134
American Mental Health Counselors Association (AMHCA) 54, 55, 57, 59, 60, 272
American Nurses' Association 43, 44, 45, 115, 132, 272
American Personnel and Guidance Association 156, 272
American Psychiatric Association 19, 43, 71, 74, 77, 104, 156, 272
American Psychological Association (APA) 5, 19, 25, 26, 27, 28, 30, 33, 54, 58, 59, 74, 112, 131, 132, 134, 135, 136, 137, 143, 144, 156, 272
  accredited training programs 104
  training conference at Vail, Colorado 95
American Psychological Association's Task Force 190
American Rehabilitation Counselors Association (ARCA) 55
American School Counselors Association (ASCA) 55
Amundson, R. 179, 272
Analysis of assumptions
  four classifications 181
  three states 180
Anastasi, A. 203, 209, 272
Anderson, B.S. 173, 281
Anderson, J.D. 114, 272
Anderson, S.C. 39, 288
Anthony, W. 139, 272
Anxiety
  related to fees 225
APA Commission on Legislation 143
Apprenticeship 92
Arbuckle, D.S. 188, 273
Army Alpha and Beta examinations 17
Arnold, L.E. 112, 273
Assessment
  abuses 171
  clinical 183-5
  cross-cultural 196-9
  elements of analysis 171
  language system 187-8
  psychobiological 193-6
  trends 203
  validity 188
Assumptions
  analysis 180
Atkinson, D.R. 104, 110, 273, 282
Authority or regulation of practitioner's behavior 70-2

B

Baker, F.M. 192, 285
Bandler, L.S. 35, 273
Banta, H.D. 259, 260, 273
Barber, B. 68, 273
Barlow, D.H. 193, 273, 284
Barrie-Borman, K. 258, 273
Bates, W. J. 112, 273
Beauchamp, T.L. 170, 273
Bechel, H.P. 196, 274
Beck, C. 44, 273
Beck, E. 55, 273
Behavior
    classification of individual 186
Beigel, A. 24, 290
Beis, E. 160, 273
Benedict, R. 208, 273
Beneficence
    definition 170
Benjamin, L.T., Jr. 292
Bennett, V.C. 135, 273
Bent, R.J. 244, 273
Berg, M.R. 100, 187, 273
Bergin, A.E. 169, 205, 274
Berkeley Planning Associates 265, 274
Berman, J.S. 139, 274
Berman, N. 193, 283
Bernal, M.E. 103, 274
Berndt, D.J. 171, 274
Berren, M.K. 24, 290
Berzins, J. 139, 274
Biegel, A. 249, 251, 274
Biofeedback training 256
Blanton, J. 139, 271
Blashfield, R.K. 189, 274
Bloch, D.A. 63, 64, 65, 66, 274
Bloom, M. 83, 274
Blume, G. 116, 274
Board of Professional Affairs of the American Psychological Association 143
Boards of Psychologist Examiners 56
Bornstein, P.J. 95, 274
Bouhoutos, J. 165, 274
Boulder Conference 94
Boule 157
Boulegenic 157
Bouleuo 157
Brewer, G.O. 266, 283

British Psychological Society 170, 274
Brodsky, A.M. 281
Brooker, A.E. 181, 196, 274, 279
Brooks, D.K. 61, 275
Brooks, V.R. 114, 275
Bugental, J. 222, 275
Bureau of Disability Insurance
    regulations 22
Burns, B.J. 20, 22, 23, 293
Burns, K.P. 243, 275
Buss, A.H. 206, 275

C

Cahn, C.H. 159, 275
Calestro, K. 112, 273
California State Licensure Law of 1968 35
California State Psychological Association 168
Callahan, P. 172, 173, 276
Campbell T. 257, 271
Caplan, J. 286
Carkhuff, R. 31, 100, 139, 272
Carter, F.M. 43, 45, 275
Case
    City of Cleveland v. Cook 56
    Romeo v. Youngberg 290
    State of Ohio vs. Cook 146
    Tarasoff v. Regents of the University of California 165-6
    Weldon v. Virginia State Board of Psychologist Examiners 56
Case, L.P. 181, 275
Casper, R. 193, 283
Certification of Rehabilitation Counselors (CRC) 57
Certification 122, 127-8
Certified Clinical Mental Health Counselor definition 57
CHAMPUS 6, 22, 242
CHAMPVA 22
Chemotherapy 12
Childress, J.F. 170, 273
Chodoff, P. 159, 233, 234, 275
Christensen, C.P. 104, 275
City of Cleveland v. Cook 56
Civil Service Standards 30
Civilian Health and Medical Program of

the Uniformed Services (CHAMPUS) 6, 22, 242
Clarizio, H.F. 199, 275
Clark, Kenneth B. 95
Clarke, C.F.O. 212, 294
Classification system
    four evaluative criteria 189-90
Cleveland, S.E. 29, 30, 31, 198, 275
Clinical assessment 183-5
Clinical psychologists 17-25
    competence 24-5
    effectiveness 21
    in a medical culture 19
    parity 21-3
    skills and expertise 31
Clinical psychology 17-25, 98-100
    distinctions 26-8
    training criteria 18
Clinical social work
    current trends 39-40
    professional controversies 40-3
Clinical Social Work Council 36, 275
Clinical social workers 34-43
    controversies in definition 35-6
    services 41
Clinical training models
    table 97
Cobbs, P. 207, 280
Cohen, L.H. 95, 275
Cohen, W. 33, 288
Cohn, J.B. 194, 275, 278
Cole, N.S. 200, 275
Colliver, J.A. 133, 276
Combs, A.W. 213, 292
Commission on Accreditation for Marriage and Family Therapy Education 63, 276
Committee on Definition, Division of Counseling Psychology, American Psychological Association 276
Committee on the Handicapped (COH) 159
Committee on the Scientific and Professional Aims of Psychology 95
Community Health Centers 12
Community Health Nurse 42
Community interests versus self-interests 69-70
Community mental health 49-51
Community Mental Health Center 22
    regulations 22
Community Mental Health Systems Act of 1963 59
Community sanction 72
Competence 82, 138-42
    assessment of 140-2
    perspectives on 24-5
Confidentiality 166, 167-8
    case of child abuse 166
    definition 166
Connolly, J. 47, 285
Consent
    informed 160-1
    substitute 160
Continuing education
    delivery modes 112-3
Copeland, B.A. 113, 294
Core provider 5-7, 56
    fifth 55
    issues 6-7
Corey, G. 172, 173, 276
Corey, M.S. 172, 173, 276
Corrigan, E.M. 106, 276
Cost studies 263-6
Cost-benefit analyses
    quality of 259
    results of 253-9
Cost-effectiveness 251-66
Costs
    to consumers 148
Council for the Accreditation of Counseling and Related Educational Programs (CACREP) 58
Council on Rehabilitation Education (CORE) 58
Council on Social Work Education (CSWE) 35, 114, 131, 276
Counseling
    cross-cultural 103, 204-15
Counseling psychologists 25-34
    skills and expertise 31
Counseling psychology 98-100
    blurring of the uniqueness 29-34
    distinctions 26-8
    history 28
Counselors
    employment/career 54
    mental health 54
    rehabilitation 54
    school 54
    see professional counselors
Court, J.H. 169, 286

Credentialing 121-52
    educational requirements 130-3
    for consumer protection 146-51
Credentials 70
Criteria
    for psychology program 136-7
    of a profession 68-74
Cronbach, L.J. 200, 276
Cross-culture
    counseling 103
    counseling and therapy 204-15
    implications of counseling and psychotherapy models 205-7
Culture of a profession 72-3
Cummings, N.A. 248, 252, 253, 254, 255, 276, 279
Cummins, B.D. 160, 286
Curriculum Policy Statement (1984) 114

Disaster Relief Act 22
Diversity
    cultural 208-11
    roots of intercultural 211-4
Doherty, L.A. 266, 283
Dohrendwend, B.P. 86, 213, 277
Dohrendwend, B.S. 86, 213, 277
Dorken, H. 230, 244, 277
Dostal, J. 33, 288
Draguns, J.G. 189, 213, 274, 277
Dujovne, B. 242, 277
Dulchin, J. 168, 277
Dumas, R. 115, 277
Dunston, P.J. 103, 277
Duty
    inform 165-7
    warn 165-7
Dyer, S.E. 148, 280

D

Danish S.J. 82, 147, 148, 149, 276
Davidson, C.V. 235, 236, 237, 278
Davis, J.E. 263, 279
Davis, L.C. 112, 293
DeLeon, P.H. 48, 49, 246, 247, 276
Delworth, U. 29, 277
DeMuth, N.M. 235, 277
Denkowski, G.C. 168, 277
Denkowski, K.M. 168, 277
Denton, Senator 55
Department of Health and Human Services 84, 162, 277
Derner, G.F. 239, 240, 277
Desvouges, W.H. 263, 279
Diagnosis
    three requirements 188
Diagnosis Related Groups (DRG) 245-51
Diagnostic and Statistical Manual of Mental Disorders (DSM-III) 77-9, 147, 190-4
    advantages 191-2
    controversial perspectives 191-2
    disadvantages 191-2
    table 191-2
Diamond, E. 199, 277
Dightman, C. 222, 277
Diplomate 73

E

Eagleston, J.R. 85, 93, 294
Eastern psychology 76
Eclecticism
    biopsychosocial 13-4
Economics 217-67
    fee setting 220-8
Education 56-8, 138-9
    differences in 100-2
    of mental health professionals 91-118
Edwards, D.W. 235, 236, 237, 278
Egdahl, R.H. 295
Eichelman, B. 162, 278
Elbert, J.C. 102, 278
Elwork, A. 166, 167, 293
Eminent career award 73
Eminent practitioner 73
Epperson, D.L. 28, 288
Epps, E.G. 202, 281
Ethical issues 155-73
    definition 156
    training 172
Everstine, D.S. 161, 168, 278
Everstine, L. 161, 168, 278
Ewalt, P. 36, 278
Ewing, C.P. 173, 278
Ewing, D.R. 101, 293
Ewing, T.N. 164, 278

F

Family therapists 62-6
  three forces 63
  controversies with other groups 63-6
Family therapy 107-8, 144-5
Farina, A. 147, 278
Federal Employee Compensation Act 22, 230
Federal Employee Health Benefits Acts 230
Federal Employee Health Benefit Program 22
Fee
  beginner anxiety 225
  counseling relationship 223-7
  credit for treatment 226-7
  giving and getting 226
  mandatory coverage 237-8
  medical model 222-5
  medical-nonmedical 228
  practitioner 228
  setting 220-8
  therapeutic issue 222-3
  transference-countertransference 226
  who pays? 237-42
Feighner, J.P. 194, 278
Fellow 73, 74
Fessler, S.R. 42, 278
Fielding, J.E. 258, 278
Fink, P.J. 229, 230, 278
Fischer, E.H. 147, 278
Fischer, L. 173, 278
Fisher, J.D. 147, 278
Fiske, D.W. 95, 283
Fitzgerald, L.F. 29, 278
Flaugher, R.L. 199, 278
Fleisehauer, P.D. 266, 283
Florida State Hospital 263
Follette, W.T. 253, 254, 276, 279
Ford, J.D. 110, 279
Forer, B.R. 165, 274
Forest, D. 98, 284
Foreyt, J.P. 263, 279
Forrest, D.V. 279
Fox, R.E. 32, 279
Frank, G.W. 95, 190, 247, 279, 294
Freedom-of-Choice (FOC) laws 230
Freedom of Choice legislation 56
Freud, S. 9-10, 31
  theories 9-10
Frey, D.H. 161, 168, 278
Frisman, L.K. 260, 261, 262, 286

G

Gabbard, G.O. 15, 16, 17, 279
Galambos, N.L. 82, 276
Garcia, J. 199, 279
Garfield, S. 111, 279
Garten, J. 279
Geller, J. 222, 289
Gelso, C.J. 29, 290
Gemeinschaft 212
Gender 104-5
Genensky, S.M. 266, 283
Generalized Anxiety Disorder (GAD) 193
George, J.C. 181, 279
Georgia statute 145
Gerontology 103
Gerson, M.J. 111, 279
Gertman, P.M. 295
Gestalt psychology 212
Getter, H. 147, 278
Gilden, T.J. 109, 287
Gilmore, M.M. 117, 118, 279
Gingerich, W.J. 181, 279
Giordano, J. 208, 286
Glasser, W. 76, 279
Goldbeck, W. 258, 273
Goldberg, I.D. 236, 257, 279, 291
Goldberg, L.R. 95, 283
Goldfried, M.R. 96, 280
Goldman, R.D. 202, 280
Goldschmitt, M. 29, 280
Goodyear, R.K. 171, 280
Gordon, E.W. 201, 204, 280
Gorenstein, E.E. 80, 81, 280
Gottfredson, G.D. 148, 280
Gould, M.S. 86, 277
Grace, H. 245, 285
Gracey, J.S. 160, 286
Graham, D.L.R. 104, 280
Green, B.L. 118, 285
Greenberg, M. 165, 274
Greene, L.R. 235, 236, 237, 278
Greenwood, E. 68, 280
Grier, W. 207, 280

Griffith, H. 280
Grisso, T. 173, 280
Gross, S. 139, 280
Grossman, J. 84, 280
Guion, R.M. 203, 280
Gutheil, T.G. 159, 160, 225, 226, 271, 280, 286

H

Habilitation
  right to 158-60
Hahn, M.E. 28, 280
Hahn, M.W. 96, 288
Hall, G.S. 32
Hallam, R.S. 47, 285
Halleck, S.L. 161, 281
Halpern, H.S. 104, 280
Handal, P.J. 243, 282
Haney, W. 197, 198, 281
Hardcastle, D.A. 35, 41, 131, 281
Harris, D.A. 147, 293
Hartwig, A. 162, 278
Havens, R.A. 133, 276
Hays, J.R. 291
Health and wellness 84-6
Health Maintenance Organization (HMO) 22, 245-51
  regulations 22
Health Maintenance Organization Act 230
Heineman, M.B. 114, 281
Helper characteristics 108-10
Helping professions
  see mental health professions
Herbsleb, J.D. 150, 281
Herdman, L.F. 48, 289
Hermes, J. 104, 280
Herranen, M. 42, 285
Hertz, M.R. 183, 198, 281
Hertzinger, M. 103, 284
Hewitt, B.N. 202, 280
Heymann, G.M. 161, 168, 278
Hill, C.E. 111, 281
Hill-Frederick, K. 28, 288
Hinman, S. 112, 281
Hipps, O. 115, 281
Hixson, J. 202, 281

Hoffman, A. 205, 289
Hofling, C.K. 227, 281
Hokenstad, M.D., Jr. 114, 281
Hollingsworth, R. 263, 279
Holroyd, J. 165, 274, 281
Hooper, D. 112, 281
Hopkins, B.R. 173, 281
Hosford, R.E. 110, 282
Howard, K.I. 180, 282
Hudson, W. 114, 282
Hull, J.W. 113, 292
Human services psychology 29
Hummel, D.L. 173, 282
Hurst, J.C. 4, 282

I

Iatrogenic 157
Identity 3-51, 75-88
  a reprise 86-8
  functions 4
Immigrants
  techniques 207-10
In-service training 111-3
  delivery modes 112-3
Informed consent 160-1
Ingram, J.C. 94, 109, 282, 286
International Classification of Diseases, Injuries and Causes of Death, Manual of 77, 296
Internship 92, 99
  experience 116-8
Intervention
  psychotherapeutic 11
Isaac, W. 102, 285
Issues 3-51
Ivey, A.E. 27, 32, 100, 138, 149, 150, 282

J

Jacobs, D.F. 255, 282
Jencks, S.F. 195, 282
Jenkins, J. 33, 288
Job club 256-7
Johnson, H.G. 161, 168, 278
Johnson, L.C. 37, 39, 282

Johnson, M.E. 110, 282
Joint Commission on Accreditation of Hospitals 20
Jourard, S. 206, 282
Julius, S.M. 243, 282

K

Kadis, A. 222, 282
Kagan, N. 28, 100, 282
Kakalik, J.S. 266, 283
Kamis, E. 235, 277
Kanter, J. 222, 283
Kanter, S. 222, 283
Kardener, S.H. 283
Karon, B.P. 262, 283
Katz, A.J. 41, 281
Katz, M.M. 193, 283
Keeley, S.M. 291
Keith-Spiegel, P. 173, 283
Keller, J.W. 101, 187, 289
Kelly, E.L. 95, 283
Kessler, L.K. 20, 22, 23, 221, 293
Kiefhaber, A. 258, 273
Kiesler, C.A. 86, 283
Kilberg, R.R. 103, 294
Kilkowski, J.M. 95, 283
Kilmann, R.H. 180, 283
Kirk, S.A. 181, 279
Kirkpatrick, M. 105, 283
Kjervik, D.K. 48, 49, 276
Kleczewski, M. 181, 279
Kleinman, A.M. 10, 12, 13, 213, 283, 285
Klerman, G.L. 190, 283
Knapp, S. 156, 166, 283
Knowledge 141
Knowledge base 68-9
Kocsis, J. 193, 283
Koocher, G.P. 134, 140, 173, 283
Korchin, S.J. 183, 184, 284
Korcok, M. 258, 284
Koslow, S.H. 193, 283
Kottler, J.A. 55, 56, 294
Krantz, G. 257, 279
Kraut, A.G. 48, 49, 276
Krumboltz, J.D. 31, 85, 284
Kurtz, R. 111, 279
Kurzman, P.A. 114, 284

L

Lamb, H.R. 83, 284
Lancaster, J. 48, 49, 284
Lane, R. 115, 288
Lanning, W. 98, 284
Laquatra, I. 82, 276
Larsen, J.A. 117, 284
Larsen, R.M. 101, 285
Last, C.G. 193, 284
Lebensohn, R.M. 12, 284
Legal issues 155-73
    definition 156
    training 172
Leighninger, L. 114, 284
Lenna, H.R. 105, 296
Lerman, H. 165, 274
Levine, D. 166, 167, 293
Levy, C.E. 21, 284
Levy, L.H. 29, 98, 284
Lewandowski, D.G. 198, 284
Lewis, K. 111, 279
Lewisohn, P.M. 103, 284
Licensure 122, 123-7, 139, 142, 147
    occupational 123-4
    prerogative of the state 125
Liddle, H.A. 108, 284, 285
Lieberman, P.B. 192, 285
Lindy, J.D. 118, 285
Lingerfelt, N.B. 181, 275
Link, B. 86, 277
Lipsett, S.M. 212, 285
Lipsitz, N.E. 172, 295
Lloyd-Jones, E. 285
Locke, B. 257, 279
London, P. 205, 285
Lorion, R.P. 236, 285
Losito, W.F. 172, 285
Loss of freedom 159
Lowe, J. 42, 285
Lubin, B. 101, 285
Ludwig, A.M. 10, 11, 17, 287

M

Mackin, D.K. 123, 285
MacLean, M.S. 28, 280
Maher, B. 238, 285

Malpractice 156
Manschreck, T.C. 10, 12, 13, 285
Manuso, J.S.J. 99, 285
Mareth, T.R. 196, 274
Marks, I.M. 47, 285
Marr, J.N. 112, 281
Master of Social Work (MSW) 35
Mataruzzo, J.P. 101, 285
May, R. 205, 285
McCaffrey, R.J. 102, 285
McCloskey, J. 245, 285
McGoldrick, M. 208, 286
McGuire, T.C. 286
McGuire, T.J. 260, 261, 262, 286
McKinney, H. 139, 293
McKnight, J. 147, 286
McKnight, M. 286
McLemore, C.W. 169, 286
McNeely, J.D. 169, 286
McNeill, B.W. 94, 286
Mearig, J.S. 167, 286
Measurement
see assessment
Medicaid Programs 55
Medical model 93-4
Medicare Act 60
Medicare Supplemental Benefits 55
Meehl, P.E. 185, 286
Meichenbaum 31
Menefee, M. 85, 284
Mental health professionals
history 3
who are 5-7
Mental health professions 67-74
Mental health provider 75-88
Mental illness
nature of 76-7
opponents 79-84
Mereness, D.A. 47, 293
Method
actuarial 186
case study 185
clinical 185
statistical 186
studying persons 182-204
Meyer, A. 10
Meyers, E.S. 257, 289
Meyerstein, I. 64-5, 286
Michels, R. 190, 283
Mills, M.J. 159, 160, 286
Minnesota Multiphasic Personality
Inventory (MMPI) 198
Mintz, N. 222, 286
Misconduct
sexual 163-4
Models
cross-cultural implications 205-7
Models of counseling and therapy
transportability 214-5
Mohammed, Z. 107, 286
Moldawsky, S. 248, 249, 294
Monk, A. 114, 286
Montgomery, R.B. 96, 287
Morris, R. 37, 39, 287
Morten, G. 104, 273
Mussen, P. 282
Myers, R. 99, 287

N

Nadelson, C. 111, 287
Nathan, P.E. 28, 33, 287
National Academy of Certified Clinical
Mental Health Counselors
(NACCMHC) 57, 128, 287
National Accreditation Council for
Teacher Education (NCATE) 58
National Ambulatory Medical Care
Survey 195
National Association of Social Workers
(NASW) 1, 36, 112, 131, 132, 156, 287
clinical registry 41
National Board of Certified Counselors
(NBCC) 57, 128
National Career Development
Association (NCDA) 55
National Certified Career Counselors
(NCCC) 57
National Certified Counselor (NCC) 57, 128
National Employment Counselors
Association (NECA) 55
National Federation of Societies of
Clinical Social Work (NFSCSW) 131
National Health Insurance (NHI) 235, 240-2, 251
National Health Insurance Plan 230, 231
National Institute of Mental Health
(NIMH) 5, 17, 18, 43, 44, 240

National Medical Care Utilization and Expenditure Survey 22
National Vocational Guidance Association (NVGA) 55
Neill, J.R. 10, 11, 17, 287
Neo-Freudians 10
Neugebaur, R. 86, 277
Nevid, J.S. 109, 287
New Jersey statute 144-5
Newkirk, M. 223, 287
Newman, J.P. 117, 295
Nichols, K.A. 48, 287
Nichols, W.C. 107, 287
Non-core mental health providers 53-66
Nonmaleficence
   definition 170
Norton, N.C. 139, 274
Notman, M. 111, 287

O

O'Brien, G.T. 193, 273, 284
Oates, W.E. 169, 286
Office of Technology Assessment 260, 287
Okon, S.E. 215, 287
Olbrisch, M.E. 255, 287
Older American Act of 1965 60
Older American Comprehensive Counseling Act of 1983 (HR 2109) 55
Oldham, J.T. 165, 287
Ollendick, T.H. 112, 288
Orientation
   sexual 104-5
Orlinsky, D.E. 180, 282
Osipow, S.H. 28, 29, 33, 278, 288
Overcast, T.D. 150, 281

P

Padilla, A.M. 103, 206, 274, 288
Pallone, N.J. 32, 33, 288
Palmo, A.J. 61, 62, 288
Paradigm
   social science 178-82
Paradise, L.V. 171, 172, 294
Parker, C.A. 4, 282
Parloff, M.B. 261, 288
Parson, T. 212, 288
Pasternack, S. 223, 288
Pastushak, R.J. 108, 284
Patrick, M. 118, 285
Payment
   third-party 228-51
Peabody, D. 210, 288
Pearce, J.K. 208, 286
Pearlmutter, D.R. 115, 288
Pederson, P. 294
Pepinsky, H.B. 28, 288
Pepper, Claude 55
Performance 141
Perl, K.G. 96, 288
Perlman, B. 115, 116, 274, 288
Perlmutter, F.D. 83, 288
Perry, S.W., III 117, 118, 279
Personality measures 101
Persons
   methods of studying 182-204
Peterson, K.J. 39, 288
Pfeiffer, C.M., Jr. 202, 289
Phillips, B.N. 135, 289
Philpott, R. 47, 285
Piercy, F. 107, 286
Pietrofesa, J.J. 205, 289
Pinto, D. 205, 289
Piotrowski, C. 101, 187, 289
Pope, K. 222, 289
Popiel, D.J. 168, 289
Practica 92
Practicum 99
Practitioner fees 228
Practitioner model 94-6
Prediction
   clinical 185-6
   statistical 185-6
Preferred Provider Organization (PPO) 245-51
Primary prevention
   measurement of effectiveness 83-4
Primary prevention 81-4
Privacy 167
Privileged communication 166
   definition 166
   right of the client 167
Procedures
   controversies 177-216
Process

therapeutic 186
Professional associate 131
Professional counselors 53-62
    certification 56-8
    current controversies 60-1
    history 58-60
    identity 59, 61
    training 56-8
Professional member 73
Professions 219-67
Program approval 122
Program credentialing 129-30
Projective techniques 198
Provider of mental health 75-88
Psychiatric nurse 43-51
    community 49-51
    education 115
    nurse-physician relationships 47-9
    role 48
    seeds of controversy 46-7
    standards 45-6
Psychiatric-liaison teams (P-L) 101
Psychiatrists 8-16
    referral sources 243-5
    supervisors 243-5
Psychiatry
    history 9
    identity crisis 12-5
    major tasks facing 194
Psychoanalysis 10
Psychoanalytic therapy 10
Psychodiagnostic 185-90
Psychodynamic 10
Psychological assistant 131
Psychology
    see clinical psychology
    see counseling psychology
Psychology program
    criteria 136-7
Psychometric 185-90
Psychopharmacology 12
Psychotherapeutic 11
Psychotherapy 11

Q

Qualified Mental Health Professional (QMHP) 5

R

Randolph, G. 225, 289
Rank, O. 31
Rappaport, J. 139, 289
Rawlings, E.I. 104, 280
Rawlings, R. 44, 273
Reavley, W. 48, 289
Reed, L.S. 257, 289
Regional Rehabilitation Continuing Education Programs (RRCEP) 112
Registry 122
Registry/registration 128-9
Rehabilitation Act of 1973 22, 230
Reichert, I. 41, 289
Reid, W.J. 39, 40, 289
Relationship
    interprofessional 15-6
    sexual 163-4
Research
    use of clients 162-3
Researcher-practitioner problem 95-6
Rewards symbolic of work achievement 73-4
Reynolds, D.K. 214, 289
Ridley, C.R. 207, 289
Roberts, K. 209, 289
Roberts, R.J. 112, 281
Rockwood, C.E. 263, 279
Roederer, D. 123, 124, 125, 291
Rogers, C.R. 31, 206, 290
Romeo v. Youngberg 290
Rorschach 198
Rosen, J.C. 85, 283, 290
Rosenbaum, M. 227, 281
Rosenblatt, A. 36, 39, 41, 290
Rozenzweig, M.R. 282
Ruiz, R.A. 206, 288
Russell, A.T. 111, 292

S

Saccuzzo, D.P. 198, 284
Sadoff, R.L. 163, 290
Sales, B.D. 150, 166, 167, 173, 280, 281, 293
Salkt, P. 111, 287
Saner, R. 207, 215, 290

Saner-Yiu, L. 207, 215, 290
Sarason, S.B. 17, 18, 290
Sax, P.R. 228, 290
Saxe, L. 259, 260, 273
Schafield, W. 290
Schectman, F. 188, 291
Scheidemandel, P.L. 257, 289
Schiffer, R.P. 194, 290
Schindler, F.E. 24, 290
Schlesinger, S.E. 105, 290
Schmalz, B. 117, 290
Schneider, L.J. 29, 290
Schofield, W. 206, 290
Scholastic Aptitude Test (SAT) 202
Schonbar, R.A. 226, 291
Schuerman, J.R. 114, 291
Schuham, A. 291
Schuldberg, D. 183, 184, 284
Scientist-practitioner model 94-6
Scope of Practice 142-6
Secunda, S. 193, 283
Sedlacek, W.E. 199, 202, 289, 291
Segal, A.J. 168, 277
Seiden R.H. 161, 168, 278
Seligman, L. 56, 291
Seligman, M.E.P. 147, 148, 271
Senior, J.R. 141, 291
Serban, G. 163, 291
Sevensky, R.L. 169, 291
Sexual misconduct 163-4
Sexuality 104-5
Shaiken, H. 286
Shanhirzadi, A. 215, 291
Shapiro, R. 160, 280
Sharfstein, S.S. 231, 232, 236, 291
Shectman, F. 291
Shemberg, K. 291
Shertzer, B. 109, 291
Shevrin, H. 188, 291
Shimberg, B. 123, 124, 125, 127, 141, 142, 291
Showell, R. 163, 290
Shultz, S.L. 111, 292
Siegel, C. 245, 292
Siegel, M. 167, 292
Simon, G.C. 170, 292
Singer, J.L. 32, 292
Sinnett, E.R. 171, 280
Siporin, M. 39, 40, 292
Skills
    cognitive 82
    intrapersonal 82
    life coping 82
    physical 82
Smith, D. 292
Smith, M.L. 32, 261, 292
Smith, R.C. 146, 291, 292
Smith, W.H. 15, 16, 17, 279
Smyer, M.A. 147, 148, 149, 276
Snow, B.M. 133, 292
Snygg, D. 213, 292
Social Security Act 5, 55
Social Security Administration (SSA) 22
    Bureau of Disability Insurance Regulations 22
Social work 35
    concerns 113-4
    curriculum 114
    evolution 37-9
    policy skills 114
    practice skills 114
    professional degree 113
    see clinical social work
    semantics 113-4
Solomon, L.J. 85, 283, 290
Sorenson, G.P. 173, 278
Specialization 102-8
Spitzer, R.L. 190, 283
Splete, H. 205, 289
Sporakowski, M.J., 132, 144, 145, 292
St. Clair, R. 160, 280
Stainbrook, E. 106, 292
Standards for Providers of Psychological Services 25
Staniszewski, W.P. 132, 144, 145, 292
Stapp, J. 103, 294
State Board of Examiners 125
State Board of Psychologist Examiners 41, 134
Statute
    Georgia 145
    mandatory report 167
    New Jersey 144-5
Stern, M.R. 291
Stern, S. 96, 292
Stigall, T.T. 135, 292
Stokes, P. 193, 283
Stone, G.L. 29, 292
Stone, S.C. 109, 291
Strategies
    controversies 177-216
Stricker, G. 113, 292

Stumphauzer, J.S. 112, 293
Sub-doctoral training 115-6
Substance Abuse 105-6
Sue, D.W. 104, 205, 206, 207, 273, 293
Sue, O. 139, 293
Sue, S. 139, 215, 293
Sugarman, S. 107, 293
Sullivan, H.S. 10, 31
Super, D.E. 26, 28, 293, 294
Sussna, E. 264, 293
Swagler, R.M. 147, 293
Swoboda, J.S. 166, 167, 293
Szasz, T. 79, 80, 293

T

Talbutt, L.C. 173, 282
Tarasoff v. Regents of University of California 293
Taube, C.A. 20, 22, 23, 221, 236, 291, 293
Taylor, C.A. 47, 293
Taylor, L. 170, 271
Teasdale, J.D. 147, 148, 271
Techniques
    controversies 177-216
    projective 198
Teri, L. 103, 284
Terminology 156-8
Terrell, M.D. 201, 204, 280
Test bias 196-204
Thelen, M.H. 101, 293
Theme
    credentialing 119-52
    economics 217-67
    education and training 89-118
    ethical and legal standards 153-173
    identity for mental health professions 1-88
    techniques, strategies, and procedures 175-216
Theories
    culture-bound 207-10
Therapy
    arts with psychotherapy 106
    cross-culture 204-15
    effectiveness of 259-62
    family 107-8
    fringe 106-7

    fringe assessment techniques 106
    physical interventions 106
    pop 106
Therapy during training
    personal 110-1
Third-party insurers 168
Third-party payers 54
Third-party payment 6, 148, 228-51
    governmental sources 229
    increase consumption 231-4
    insurance companies 229
    poor benefit 235-7
    recognition of psychological services 242-5
Thompson, A.J. 28, 106, 294, 295
Thoresen, C.E. 85, 93, 294
Tipton R.M. 29, 280
Tittle, C.K. 199, 194
Tools of the mental health professions 177
Tousley, M. 115, 294
Training 56-8
    content 134-8
    differences in 100-2
Training of mental health professionals 91-118
Treatment 81-4
    clinically 159
    institutionalization 159
    involuntary 159
    legally 159
    loss of freedom 159
    psychosocial 14
    religion 169
    right to 158-60
    value conflicts 168-72
Treatment program
    inpatient chronic pain 256
Triandis, H.C. 212, 294
True, R.H. 161, 168, 278
Tulkin, S.R. 247, 294
Turk 31
Types of mental health services
    productiveness of 262-6

U

U.S. Civil Service Position Classification Standards 29, 294

U.S. Department of Health, Education and Welfare, Public Health Service 123, 294
U.S. Department of Labor 61, 294
United States Office of Education 112
University of Pennsylvania 17
Uyeda, M.K. 246, 247, 248, 249, 276, 294

V

Vaillant, G.E. 190, 283
Vaizey, J. 212, 294
Value conflicts 168-72
Van Hoose, W.H. 55, 56, 171, 172, 294
Vance, F.L. 109, 187, 295
Vance, S. 108, 284
Vandecreek, L. 166, 283
VandenBos, G.R. 48, 49, 103, 262, 276, 283, 294
Veterans Administration 17, 22, 29, 30, 31
    Departments of Medicine and Surgery 30
Vietnam Veterans Health Care Bill 22
Vitulano, L.A. 113, 294

W

Waas, J.W. 193, 283
Waldfogel, D. 36, 39, 41, 290
Wallen, L.M. 266, 283
Walters, O.S. 205, 294
Waltzer, H. 166, 295
Warren, J.M. 258, 295
Washington Business Group on Health 259, 295
Wasserman, M. 112, 273
Watkins, C.E., Jr. 98, 295
Watley, D. 109, 187, 295
Webb, J.T. 230, 277
Webber, A. 258, 273
Weikel, W.J. 58, 60, 61, 275, 295
Weiskopf, R. 117, 295

Weiss, C.S. 96, 295
Weiss, H.M. 63, 64, 65, 66, 274
Welch, B.L. 246, 247, 276
Welch, C.E. 112, 295
Weldon v. Virginia State Board of Psychologist Examiners
    case of 56
Welfel, E. 172, 295
Wellner, A.M. 134, 136, 142, 295
Wendt, R.N. 108, 295
Wesley, R.M. 133, 276
Westervelt, E.M. 285
Wiggins, R.C. 29, 280
Wigtil, J.V. 106, 295
Wikler, D. 162, 278
Wildinson, L. 222, 289
Williams, R.L. 199, 295
Williams, S. 44, 273
Wilmarth, R. 56, 295
Wilson, S. 113, 296
Winick, C. 222, 282
Wollershein, J.P. 95, 274
Woodman, N.J. 105, 296
Woodring, J. 113, 292
Woody, R.H. 184, 188, 190, 296
Work Incentive Program 22
World Health Organization 77, 296
    International Classfication of Diseases, Injuries and Causes of Death 77, 296
Worrall, J.D. 265, 296
Wrenn, C.G. 27, 296
Wunsch-Hitzig, R. 86, 277

Y

Yiu, L. 206, 296

Z

Zake, J. 108, 295
Zola, I.K. 286
Zusman, J. 83, 284

ABOUT THE AUTHORS

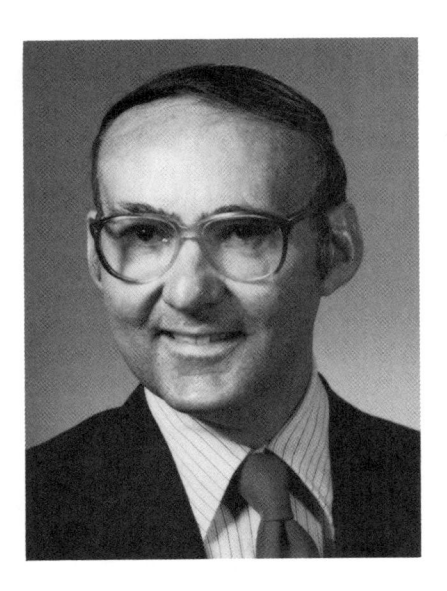

Edwin L. Herr is professor and head, Division of Counseling and Educational Psychology, The Pennsylvania State University. He received his B.S. degree in business education from Shippensburg State College (1955) and his M.A. degree in psychological foundations and his Professional Diploma and Ed.D. in counseling and student personnel administration from Teachers College, Columbia University (1959, 1961, and 1963, respectively).

A former business teacher, school counselor, and director of guidance, Herr previously served as assistant and associate professor of counselor education at the State University of New York at Buffalo and as the founding director of the Bureau of Guidance Services and the Bureau of Pupil Personnel Services, Pennsylvania Department of Education. He has been involved as a visiting professor or researcher in several European universities and in Japan. In 1976, he served as visiting fellow, National Institute for Careers Education and Counseling, Cambridge, England. In 1979 he served as research fellow, Japan Society for the Promotion of Science at Sophia University, Tokyo. In 1978 and 1981 he served respectively as an Asia Foundation Lecturer and as a Yoshida International Education Lecturer. In 1986, he was the recipient of the Eminent Career Award of the National Career Development Association (formerly the National Vocational Guidance Association) for sustained national and international influence on theory, research, and practice in career behavior.

Herr is past president of the American Association for Counseling and Development, past president of the National Vocational Guidance Association, and past president of the Association for Counselor Education and Supervision. He also served as a member of the Executive Committee of the International Round Table for the Advancement of Counselling (1976-84). He is the author of over 200 articles and some twenty books. His most recent books include *Career Guidance and Counseling Through the Life Span: Systematic Approaches* (1984); *Counseling Youth for Employability* (1983); *Foundations for Policy in Guidance and Counseling* (1981); *Guidance and Counseling in the Schools: Perspectives on the Past, Present, and Future* (1979).

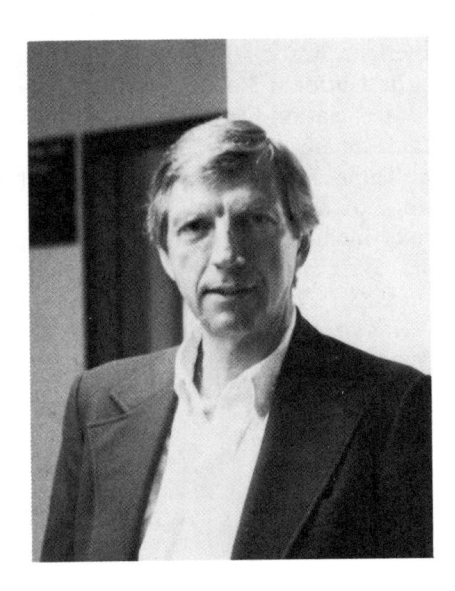

Stanley H. Cramer is Professor and Chair, Department of Counseling and Educational Psychology, State University of New York at Buffalo. He received his B.A. in English (1955) from the University of Massachusetts, an M.A. in English (1957) from State University of New York at Albany, and the Ed.D. in Counseling (1963) from Teachers College, Columbia University. He has been a counselor in several settings, ranging from schools to agencies and, prior to Buffalo, taught part-time at Hofstra, St. John's, and Columbia universities.

He has authored or co-authored 13 books and approximately 45 articles and has served as a consultant to more than 150 schools, colleges, agencies, and organizations. Cramer is a member of the American Psychological Association, a former President of the New York State Association for Counselor Education and Supervision, and has held a variety of other offices in professional associations. He has served in a number of administrative positions in higher education, including Dean of the Faculty of Educational Studies and Associate Vice President for Academic Affairs.

This volume represents his seventh book collaboration with Ed Herr.